Milestones in Neonatal/Perinatal Medicine:

Historical Perspectives from NeoReviews

Edited by Alistair G. S. Philip, MD, FRCPE, FAAP

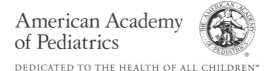

American Academy
of Pediatrics

DEDICATED TO THE HEALTH OF ALL CHILDREN™

American Academy of Pediatrics
141 Northwest Point Boulevard
Elk Grove Village, IL 60007

American Academy of Pediatrics, Elk Grove Village, IL 60007
© 2010 American Academy of Pediatrics. All rights
reserved. Published 2010

ISBN 978-0-578-05484-1

Quantity prices on request. Address all inquiries to:
American Academy of Pediatrics
141 Northwest Point Boulevard
Elk Grove Village, Illinois 60007

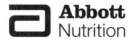

Supported, in part, through an
educational grant from Abbott Nutrition,
a division of Abbott Laboratories.

Dedication

To the countless number of individuals whose contributions to our knowledge and understanding of newborn infants are not specifically recognized with featured commentaries, but who helped to develop the basis for our current management of the preterm or sick infant.

—AGSP, Aug. 20, 2010

CONTENTS

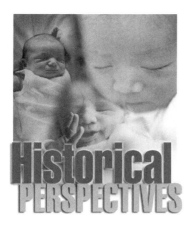

*Milestones in
Neonatal-Perinatal Medicine*

Introduction

As with most disciplines, neonatology developed over many years, however, the rate of progress accelerated rapidly in the late 20th century. In the early part of the 20th century, evaluating and caring for neonates was largely the domain of obstetricians. Pediatricians gradually assumed more and more responsibility for neonates and by mid-century many "premature nurseries" had been established.

Our subspecialty is comparatively young. Indeed, the first use of the terms "neonatology" and "neonatologist" are generally attributed to Dr Alexander Schaffer, who used them in the introduction to the first edition of his book *Diseases of the Newborn* published in 1960. The first examination of the sub-board of neonatal-perinatal medicine of the American Board of Pediatrics was held in 1975 and currently approximately 200 new neonatologists emerge from training programs in the United States each year. In the year 2000, the first volume of the online journal *NeoReviews* was published under the leadership of Drs Bill Hay and David Stevenson, after briefly being incorporated (in print form) into *Pediatrics in Review* for 6 months. This was made possible by the sponsorship of the American Academy of Pediatrics (AAP).

After joining the journal as Associate Editor at the end of 2001, I proposed that we try to highlight some of the seminal articles that had influenced the practice of neonatology in the preceding 40 to 50 years. In a series of "Historical Perspectives" published in *NeoReviews* between 2002 and 2006, we tried to capture the basic essentials of neonatology or as we subtitled the series "The Underpinnings of Neonatal-Perinatal Medicine." These seminal articles can be considered "milestones" on the road to development of our discipline. Although *NeoReviews* is primarily directed toward those working in neonatology, we are closely aligned with our obstetrical colleagues in maternal-fetal medicine. We need to be cognizant of events that may have occurred during pregnancy to understand better why certain problems occur in the neonatal period. For this reason, the section of the AAP that represents neonatologists is called the Perinatal Section and we have a policy committee of the AAP called the Committee on Fetus and Newborn.

Approximately one-quarter to one-third of the original 36 Historical Perspective articles published in *NeoReviews* concern topics that focus primarily on the fetus or events in the delivery room. Many others deal with problems that may have had their origins during the prenatal period. In addition, we have added one "Perinatal Profile" (our historical series continues, with personalities rather than principles), which concerns the introduction of obstetrical ultrasonography. This modality plays such an important role in perinatal medicine that it would be inappropriate to omit it. For this reason, this collection should be of interest to those who practice or are training in maternal-fetal medicine, as well as those in neonatology. By bringing together these varied contributions, we acknowledge the enormous debt we owe to the many physicians who, by their interest, observations, and investigations, blazed the trail in our discipline.

Advances in medicine do not occur in isolation. Our thinking may be influenced by technological advances in other fields. We are influenced in our daily care of patients by many other factors, some of which may be subtle. Experience at one center may not always provide appropriate perspective. In recent years, large randomized controlled trials have attempted to answer important questions in our discipline, which could not be answered by studies from single centers, even over several years. However, there can be little doubt that the contributions highlighted in this series of Historical Perspectives provide the foundation upon which the practice of neonatal-perinatal medicine is based.

The first of these perspectives, which we published in 2002, was devoted to the contribution of Dr Virginia Apgar. It was approximately 50 years since she had first presented her observations at a meeting of anesthesiologists. In republishing these articles in book form, we decided to sequence them in chronological order of the "milestone" articles. For most of these early articles, we believed that it was important to provide the original articles as "data supplements," which can be viewed by going to http://neoreviews.aappublications.org and searching the archives for the pertinent Historical Perspective. In the intervening years, many (but not all) of the original articles have become available in medical libraries through their collections of e-journals.

In some cases, we were fortunate enough to obtain a personal reminiscence from one of the founding fathers (and mothers) of our discipline before they died (eg, William Silverman, Marvin Cornblath, Robert Usher and Paul Polani). For most of the articles, we provided an editorial comment to help put the contribution into present day perspective. For those that did not have an accompanying commentary in the original, I have added a brief commentary for this volume.

This collection is presented in honor of *NeoReviews* reaching its 10-year anniversary. We look forward to providing important review articles in neonatal-perinatal medicine for many years to come. For all but one of these Historical Perspectives, and the one Perinatal Profile, we were able to identify a seminal or "landmark" article that had appeared 30 to 55 years earlier, upon which we could focus. In four cases, the articles were "only" 25 to 30 years old. There may have been earlier reports on some of these topics, and we apologize to those authors whose contributions we may have overlooked. The final article provides an overview of surgery for congenital heart disease and it is not clear when the first procedures were performed on neonates.

All the topics covered have an established place in neonatal-perinatal medicine and their origins are worth understanding. We trust that this collection of "milestones" will provide entertaining and informative reading for our younger readers, while serving as a reminder of "the way it was" for our older readers.

Alistair G. S. Philip, MD, FRCPE, FAAP
Editor-in-Chief, NeoReviews
and
Emeritus Professor of Pediatrics
Stanford University School of Medicine

Chronological Index of Landmark Articles

1948 Exchange Transfusion (Diamond/Pearson)
Diamond LK. Replacement transfusion as a treatment for erythroblastosis fetalis. *Pediatrics.* 1948;2:520–524

1953 Apgar Score (James)
Apgar V. A proposal for a new method of evaluation of the newborn infant. *Curr Res Anesth Analg.* 1953;32:260–267

1954 Chromosomal Abnormalities (Polani)
Polani PE, Hunter WF, Lennox B. Chromosomal sex in Turner's syndrome with coarctation of the aorta. *Lancet.* 1954;ii:120–121

1958 Thermoregulation (William Silverman)
Silverman WA, Fertig JN, Berger AP. The influence of the thermal environment upon survival of newly born premature infants. *Pediatrics.* 1958; 22:876–886

1958 Obstetrical Ultrasound (Donald)
Donald I, MacVicar J, Brown TG. Investigation of abdominal masses by pulsed ultrasound. *Lancet.* 1958;1:1188–1195

1959 Surfactant and RDS (Avery)
Avery ME, Mead J. Surface properties in relation to atelectasis and hyaline membrane disease. *Am J Dis Child.*1959;97:517–523

1961 Group B Streptococci and Perinatal Infection (Philip)
Hood M, Janney A, Dameron G. Beta hemolytic streptococci group B associated with the perinatal period. *Am J Obstet Gynecol.* 1961;82: 809–818

1963 Newborn Metabolic Screen (Guthrie/Levy)
Guthrie R, Susi A. A simple phenylalanine method for detecting phenylketonuria in large populations of newborn infants. *Pediatrics.* 1963;32:338–342

1963 Intravenous Glucose to Reduce RDS Mortality/The Long View (Usher)
Usher R. Reduction of mortality from respiratory distress syndrome of prematurity with early administration of intravenous glucose and sodium bicarbonate. *Pediatrics.* 1963;32:968–975

1964 Transient Symptomatic Hypoglycemia (Cornblath)
Cornblath M, Wybregt SH, Baens GS, Klein RI. Symptomatic neonatal hypoglycemia: studies of carbohydrate metabolism in the newborn infant VIII. *Pediatrics.* 1964;33:388–402

1964 Immediate Feeding in Preterm (Davies)
Smallpeice V, Davies PA. Immediate feeding of premature infants with undiluted breast milk. *Lancet.* 1964;ii:1349–1352

1964 Necrotizing Enterocolitis in the Preterm Infant (Stevenson/Blakely)
Berdon WE, Grossman H, Baker DH, Mizrahi A, Barlow O, Blanc WA. Necrotizing enterocolitis in the premature infant. *Radiology.* 1964;83:879–887

1965 Mechanical Ventilation for RDS (Delivoria-Papadopoulos)
Delivoria-Papadopoulos M, Swyer P. Assisted ventilation in terminal hyaline membrane disease. *Arch Dis Child.* 1964;39:481–484

1967 Birth weight/Gestational Age Classification (Battaglia)
Battaglia FC, Lubchenco LO. A practical classification of newborn infants by weight and gestational age. *J Pediatr.* 1967;71:159–163

1968 Phototherapy for Preterm (Lucey)
Lucey JF, Ferreiro M, Hewitt J. Prevention of hyperbilirubinemia of prematurity by phototherapy. *Pediatrics.* 1968;41:1047–1054

1968 Neurologic Evaluation and Maturity (Amiel-Tison)
Amiel-Tison C. Neurological evaluation of the maturity of newborn infants. *Arch Dis Child.* 1968;43:89–93

1969 Monitoring of Apnea (Daily)
Daily WJR, Klaus M, Meyer HBP. Apnea in premature infants: monitoring, incidence, heart rate changes and an effect of environmental temperature. *Pediatrics.* 1969;43:510–518

1969 Direct Blood Pressure Monitoring (Phibbs)
Kitterman JA, Phibbs RH, Tooley WH. Aortic blood pressure in normal newborn infants during the first 12 hours of life. *Pediatrics.* 1969;44:959–968

1970 Parents in Preterm Nursery (Klaus/Kennell)
Barnett CR, Leiderman PH, Grobstein R, Klaus MH. Neonatal separation: the maternal side of interactional deprivation. *Pediatrics.* 1970;45:197–205

1971 Prenatal Assessment of Lung Maturity (Gluck/Spellacy)
Gluck L, Kulovich MV, Borer RC Jr, Brenner PH, Anderson GG, Spellacy WN. Diagnosis of the respiratory distress syndrome by amniocentesis. *Am J Obstet Gynecol.* 1971;109:440–445

1971 Continuous Positive Airway Pressure (Gregory)
Gregory GA, Kitterman JA, Phibbs RH, Tooley WH, Hamilton WK. Treatment of the idiopathic respiratory distress syndrome with continuous positive airway pressure. *N Engl J Med.* 1971; 284:1333–1340

1972 Antepartum Glucocorticoid Administration and RDS (Liggins)
Liggins GC, Howie RN. A controlled trial of antepartum glucocorticoid treatment for prevention of the respiratory distress syndrome in premature infants. *Pediatrics.* 1972;50:515–525

1972 Total Parenteral Nutrition (Heird/Driscoll)
Driscoll JM Jr, Heird WC, Schullinger JN, Gongaware RD, Winters RW. Total intravenous alimentation in low-birth-weight infants: a preliminary report. *J Pediatr.* 1972;81:145–153

1972 Neonatal Echocardiography (Norman Silverman)
Winsburg F : Echocardiography of the fetal and newborn heart. Invest Radiol 1972;7:152–158.

1973 Methylxanthines for Apnea (Kuzemko)
Kuzemko JA, Paala J. Apneic attacks in the newborn treated with aminophylline. *Arch Dis Child.* 1973;48:404–406

1973 Transcutaneous Blood Gas Measurement (Huch)
Huch R, Huch A, Lübbers DW. Transcutaneous measurement of blood PO_2 ($tcPO_2$): method and applications in perinatal medicine. *J Perinat Med.* 1973;1:183–191

1974 Maternal Serum Alpha-fetoprotein and Fetal Abnormalities (Wald)
Wald NJ, Brock DJH, Bonnar J. Prenatal diagnosis of spina bifida and anencephaly by maternal serum AFP measurement: a controlled study. *Lancet.* 1974;i:765–767

1975 Neonatal Transillumination to Detect Air Leaks (Kuhns/Donn)
Kuhns LR, Bednarek FJ, Wyman ML, et al. Diagnosis of pneumothorax and pneumomediastinum in the neonate by transillumination. *Pediatrics.* 1975;56:355–360

1976 Closure of PDA with Indomethacin (Friedman)
Friedman WF, Hirschklau MJ, Printz MP, Pitlick PT, Kirkpatrick SE. Pharmacological closure of patent ductus arteriosus in the premature infant. *N Engl J Med.* 1976;295:526–529

1978 Fetal Blood Sampling (Rodeck)
Rodeck CH, Campbell S. Sampling pure fetal blood by fetoscopy in second trimester of pregnancy. *Br Med J.* 1978;2:728–730

1978 Prevention of Rhesus Hemolytic Disease (Bowman)
Bowman JM, Chown B, Lewis M, Pollock JM. Rh isoimmunization during pregnancy: antenatal prophylaxis. *Can Med Assoc J.* 1978;118:623–627

1979 Cranial Ultrasound to Detect Intracranial Hemorrhage (Reynolds)

Pape KE, Blackwell RJ, Cusick G, et al. Ultrasound detection of brain damage in preterm infants. *Lancet.* 1979; i :1261–1264

1980 Transcutaneous Bilirubinometry (Yamanouchi/Maisels)

Yamanouchi I, Yamauchi Y, Igarashi I. Transcutaneous bilirubinometry: preliminary studies of noninvasive transcutaneous bilirubin meter in the Okayama National Hospital. *Pediatrics.* 1980;65: 195–202

1982 Magnetic Resonance Imaging (Levene)

Levene MI, Whitelaw A, Dubowitz V, et al. Nuclear magnetic resonance imaging of the brain in children. *Br Med J.* 1982;285:774–776

1985 Extracorporeal Membrane Oxygenation (Bartlett)

Bartlett RH, Roloff DW, Cornell RG, Andrews AF, Dillon PW, Zwischenberger JB. Extracorporeal circulation in neonatal respiratory failure: a prospective randomized study. *Pediatrics.* 1985; 76:479–487

1985 Pulse Oximetry in Neonate (Hay)

Sendak MJ, Harris AP, Rogers MC, et al. Pulse oximetry in newborn infants in the delivery room. *Anesthesiology.* 1985;63:739–740

Difficult to pin-point start date in neonate:

History of Surgery for Congenital Heart Disease (Rudolph)

The Rise and Fall of Exchange Transfusion

Introduction

This month's Historical Perspective deals with a procedure that was once very common, but now is performed infrequently. Despite the fact that pediatric residents today may not have the opportunity to perform an exchange transfusion during their residencies, it is important for younger physicians to appreciate how the procedure was developed and to understand the principles on which it was based.

Although exchange transfusion is performed infrequently these days, the insertion of an umbilical venous catheter is very common. As noted in the accompanying commentaries, the first umbilical venous catheters were inserted for the purpose of exchange transfusion. Consequently, there is a strong connection to modern day neonatology, even though at first glance it may seem that exchange transfusion currently is not relevant.

The original article was written by Dr Louis K. Diamond, [1] who provided his own perspective in a commentary published in 1976 that we reproduce following this introduction. He also provided complete details of how to perform the procedure in a paper published in 1951. [2] In addition, Dr Howard Pearson (who was a fellow in pediatric hematology under Dr Diamond) provides commentary about this important advance from today's perspective. He previously had provided commentary about Dr Diamond's paper in a supplement to *Pediatrics* that drew attention to important papers published in *Pediatrics* in the previous 50 years. [3]

Alistair G. S. Philip, MD, FRCPE, FAAP
Editor-in-Chief, NeoReviews

References

1. Diamond LK. Replacement transfusion as a treatment for erythroblastosis fetalis. *Pediatrics.* 1948;2:520–524
2. Diamond LK, Allen FH Jr, Thomas WO Jr. Erythroblastosis fetalis. VII. Treatment with exchange transfusion. *N Engl J Med.* 1951;244:39–44
3. Pearson HA. Commentary on Dr. Diamond's paper. *Pediatrics.* 1998;102 (suppl):203–205

The following commentary originally appeared in 1976 as one of a series published by Ross Laboratories entitled "Landmarks in Perinatology/ Neonatology" and is reproduced with permission of Abbott Nutrition.

Perspective on Exchange Transfusion

Aphrodite arose full-grown from the sea and the foam. Attractive as that picture is, it seldom occurs so suddenly in the field of science, where advances come relatively slowly in step-like progression. As a result, it is often enlightening to know how a new technique or therapeutic approach came to be. The introduction of exchange transfusion performed through a plastic catheter in the umbilical vein greatly improved the treatment and prognosis of hemolytic disease of the newborn or erythroblastosis fetalis (EF). The historic background of this development is of interest as an introduction to our original publication [please

see data supplement: http://neoreviews.aap publications.org/cgi/data/4/7/e169/DC1/1].

The milieu and the time were particularly favorable. We had a longstanding interest in EF, having published a full review of our cases in 1932, and we continued to accumulate them thereafter. We had established the Blood Grouping Laboratory in 1942 after the Rh blood factor was proved of importance to EF and to transfusion therapy. The Lying-in Hospital encouraged us to organize a special clinic for Rh-negative patients and to see their newborn infants. The combined facilities of this large Obstetric Service and the Children's Hospital newborn ward soon involved us in the care of over 100 affected infants a year. Cooperation with the staff of these hospitals and of others throughout Boston and beyond was ideal. This background made progress rapid and most satisfactory.

Before 1941, transfusions of anemic newborn infants with EF were performed as a lifesaving measure, but with variable results. After the discovery of the Rh factor, more success was achieved through the use of Rh-negative blood. After 1945, four new tests (blocking, slide, albumin, and antiglobulin) proved that the plasma and body fluids of affected infants carried the considerable burden of free maternal anti-Rh antibody, which continued the hemolytic process on newly produced red cells. Thus, it was imperative to remove not only the infant's antibody-coated Rh-positive red cells but the plasma containing free anti-Rh gamma globulin as well. A needle puncture of the longitudinal sinus was too dangerous for this purpose; multiple peripheral veins and arteries were too delicate for routine and lengthy procedures, but there was the umbilical vein, invitingly large and patent. At first, we tried to enter it with large steel needles, but these could not be maintained in situ for long. Rubber catheters became a problem as well as a risk, being too narrow and clot-promoting when blood was withdrawn. Fortuitously, we learned about a plastic, nonwettable, nonirritating polyethylene catheter being used by Dr Franc Ingraham, our pediatric neurosurgeon. He had found that the plastic could be chemically sterilized and reused, was nonirritating to the tissues, and retarded clotting. He had experimented with this as a bypass tube for constant drainage of obstructed ventricles in hydrocephalic patients.

Preliminary in vitro and animal implantation experiments were reassuring, and initial trials of umbilical vein catheterization and blood exchange were successful. Dr Ingraham gave us a generous supply of yards of polyethylene tubing, although we actually required only 18 inches for an umbilical catheterization. This allowed us to distribute trial samples far and wide, as requested. Dr William Thomas, then Chief Resident at the Boston Lying-in Hospital, and I, very soon after the initial trials in October 1946, proceeded to use the technique with assurance. Dr Fred

H. Allen, Jr devised Tuohy adapters and connections for the procedure, and soon thereafter one operator (usually Dr Allen) with a nurse-helper could perform an exchange transfusion expeditiously. After only 6 months, we were able to record successful exchange transfusions in more than 50 infants with EF. At a meeting in London where we reported this (Pediatric Section, Royal Society of Medicine), I distributed a number of the polyethylene catheters and, within a year, papers by Mollison of London, Van Loghem of Amsterdam and others confirmed the successful exchange transfusions of many newborns by this technique. Within 4 years, we had convincing data of its effectiveness in over 350 patients with EF.

The value of exchange transfusion as a therapeutic measure can be appreciated by the statistics; in the 1950s, with about 4 million births per year in the United States, 1/200 infants would have had EF due to maternal Rh sensitization, a conservative estimate of 20,000 infants/year. Before exchange transfusion became routine, mortality was close to 50%, including deaths from kernicterus and its late complications. The new treatment reduced this mortality to 10% or less, so at least 8,000 newborn infants a year were saved in the United States alone. (This does not include the more common form of EF due to ABO incompatibility which, although relatively mild in its hemolytic effect, occasionally does require exchange transfusion. The rarer maternal-fetal blood group incompatibilities which affect Blacks, Orientals, and Caucasians also increase the number of newborns at risk from EF.) Worldwide census figures do not present a reliable estimate of the life-saving potential of exchange transfusion for EF, but the beneficial results could reach millions, since this treatment is also used for infants with hemolytic anemia due to infection, G6PD deficiency, or other red cell defects.

Since 1951, exchange transfusion in the newborn has been used increasingly to combat anemia and to control hyperbilirubinemia with its dread neurologic complication, kernicterus, which causes mental retardation, cerebral palsy, and deafness—all irreparable injuries. In addition, since its introduction for treatment of EF, umbilical vessel catheterization in the newborn has also become an indispensable approach for many other diagnostic, prognostic and therapeutic procedures in the neonatal period. Thus, what began as a simple practical method for treating a single specific disease developed into a widely used mechanism for managing numerous problems in neonatology.

Louis K. Diamond, MD

Linking Exchange Transfusion and Erythroblastosis Fetalis

The history of exchange transfusion is inextricably linked to EF, also designated as hemolytic disease of the newborn. The ascendance and then the virtual disappearance of neonatal exchange transfusions parallel the remarkable changes in the understanding and therapy of this uniquely pediatric disease that have occurred especially over the past 60 years. The earlier history of erythroblastosis is well described in the 1949 monograph of Dr M.M. Pickles. [1]

Before recognition that EF was a hemolytic process, it was assumed that it was caused by hepatic dysfunction, and treatment with purgatives was recommended. After the hemolytic nature of the anemia of EF was accepted, transfusions were advocated to sustain the child's hemoglobin level until spontaneous recovery occurred. In 1932, Drs S.H. Clifford and A.T. Hertig recommended early and repeated transfusions with the blood of either parent until the hemoglobin level was stable. These recommendations were made before the recognition of Rh, and in such transfusions, the father's red blood cells (RBCs) would be obligately Rh positive and the mother's serum would contain Rh antibody. [2] After discovery of the Rh factor, transfusions of Rh-negative RBCs were shown to be far more effective in relieving anemia than Rh-positive RBCs. [3]

Mollison [4] performed RBC survival studies that showed that Rh-negative RBCs had a normal survival, but Rh-positive RBCs were removed rapidly from the circulation of infants who had EF, and it became standard practice to transfuse affected infants only with Rh-negative RBCs. However, the benefit of simple transfusions, even with Rh-negative RBCs, was limited primarily to infants who had anemia after the first postnatal week, and they were largely ineffective in reducing mortality in children who presented early with edema or extreme jaundice. An editorial in *The Lancet* in 1946 stated:

"There is widespread disappointment at the results of (transfusion) therapy although this feeling is rarely expressed in print because few observers publish their failures. Kernicterus is not prevented by the transfusion therapy and the mortality of icterus gravis is still high." [5]

The Rise of Exchange Transfusion

The first use of exchange transfusion (also called exsanguination, venesection, or substitution transfusion) for EF was reported by Dr A.P. Hart from Toronto's Hospital for Sick Children in 1925. [6] He described a severely jaundiced newborn who was the eighth child born to a family in which six previous children had died with jaundice at 3 to 11 days after birth. Although very jaundiced, the infant was only moderately anemic. Believing that there might be "toxins" damaging the liver, Hart persuaded a colleague, Dr J.I. MacDonald, to perform an exsanguination transfusion using a technique developed by Dr Bruce Robertson, a Toronto surgeon. [7] Robertson had developed exsanguination transfusion as treatment for the toxic shock of severe burns and sepsis. The 48-hour-old jaundiced infant was transfused with 350 mL of blood through an ankle vein while 300 mL of blood was aspirated simultaneously from the sagittal sinus through the anterior fontanelle. The infant became less jaundiced and subsequently did well. Hart, in a follow-up of the patient 30 years later, described him as healthy and normal. [8]

Hart's 1925 article went largely unnoticed, and it was not until 1946 that exchange transfusions began to be used as a treatment for EF. Dr H. Wallerstein, in New York, similar to Hart, used the sagittal sinus for removing 50-mL aliquots of blood while infusing Rh-negative blood through a peripheral vein cutdown. [9] Drs A.S. Weiner and I.B. Wexler described another technique that involved transection of the radial artery for removal of blood and simultaneous infusion of blood through a peripheral vein. This required total body heparinization of the infant with its attendant bleeding problems. They exchanged twice the infant's blood volume and showed removal of about 80% of the pre-exchange RBCs. Interestingly, Weiner described testing and evaluation of this procedure on a "mongolian infant" who did not have erythroblastosis! [10]

Both Wallerstein's and Weiner's procedures were technically difficult, had significant complications, and soon were supplanted by a method introduced by Dr L.K. Diamond in 1946. [11] Diamond had demonstrated that the serum of children who had EF and had been transfused with Rh-negative RBCs still contained free maternal anti-Rh antibodies and that all of the remaining RBCs of the infant were coated with antibody. He reasoned that the most effective therapy would be removal of as much of the infant's blood as possible and replacement with Rh-negative blood. This required access to a large and accessible blood vessel. He stated:

"The pediatrician faced with the prospect of finding vascular channels for transfusion cannot help but be attracted to the large and readily accessible vein which presents itself in the umbilical cord." [11]

The umbilical vein had been used previously. In 1923, Dr James Sidbury, a North Carolina pediatrician, administered a blood transfusion through the umbilical vein to treat a newborn who had hemorrhagic disease. [12] Diamond's technique was considerably facilitated by the use of nonreactive polyethylene plastic catheters that had been developed by the neurosurgeons at Boston Children's Hospital. These catheters could be threaded easily into the umbilical vein, through the ductus venosus, and into the inferior vena cava, which was large enough to allow free flow of blood. Using a three-way stopcock, about 20 mL of the infant's blood was alternately withdrawn and replaced with an equal amount of type O Rh-negative donor blood. About 500 mL of blood was exchanged over 1.5 hours, which resulted in replacement of 90% of the infant's antibody-coated RBCs. Diamond described complete recovery of a number of affected infants born to families in which previous children had

died of EF. He noted that before exchange transfusion, the chance of survival of subsequent infants in such families was less than 10%. With the use of exchange transfusion, the survival was increased to 70%. In 1951, Diamond and associates published a virtual *vade mecum,* complete with 10 figures and 5 tables, for performing exchange transfusions. [13] This defined the indications and equipment as well as the technical procedure.

Dr Diamond later remembered that Dr Patrick Mollison first suggested to him that exchange transfusions also might be an effective method of controlling dangerous levels of hyperbilirubinemia and preventing kernicterus and the risk of death and neurologic damage. [14] Diamond's analyses of data from a large number of cases showed that the risk of neurologic damage was low if the level of serum bilirubin did not exceed 20 mg/dL (342 mcmol/L). The management of infants who had EF entailed trying to identify at birth those who were most likely to develop dangerous hyperbilirubinemia and performing early exchange transfusions. Serial serum bilirubin determinations were obtained, and exchange transfusions were performed to maintain the level at less than 20 mg/dL (342 mcmol/L).

Diamond's method of exchange transfusion was relatively simple and safe and was adopted rapidly around the world. If the umbilical cord had been clamped too short to permit easy cannulation, other procedures were suggested. An incision through the skin just superior to the umbilicus could expose the umbilical vein before it penetrated the abdominal wall. The inferior vena cava also could be entered through a cut-down of the saphenous vein in the groin. Umbilical artery catheters could be used for exchange transfusions in small preterm infants. However, these alternate routes for access rarely were necessary.

By the mid-1950s, many pediatricians were performing exchange transfusions in their own hospitals. Traveling exchange transfusion teams were used to serve several hospitals in the Washington, DC, metropolitan area. With the widespread use of exchange transfusion between 1950 and 1960, the mortality associated with EF in the United States

decreased from 70 to 50 per 100,000 live births, although the incidence of maternal sensitization and neonatal incidence of EF were virtually unchanged. [15]

Most infants who had hydrops fetalis were stillborn or died shortly after birth. Because 50% of fetal hydrops deaths occurred after 32 to 34 weeks of gestation, early induction of labor at 35 weeks, followed by exchange transfusions, salvaged some of these severely affected infants. However, in the mid-1950s induction of labor was not considered as an option for infants less than 35 weeks' gestation because of the "dangers of immaturity." The diagnosis of severe EF and the risk of stillbirth usually were based on a history of a previous infant who had EF and high maternal anti-Rh antibody titers (>1/64). However, these criteria often were not specific, definitive, or sensitive.

In 1963, Dr A.W. Liley, using spectrophotometric analysis of amniotic fluid, demonstrated a correlation between the amniotic fluid optical density at 450 μ (the peak spectral absorption of bilirubin) and the severity of anemia at birth and fetal outcome. [16] Very rapidly, amniotic fluid spectroscopy became the standard method for antenatal assessment in sensitized pregnancies. Clinical nomograms of delta OD 450 were constructed to determine the necessity for early induction of labor before fetal death. Improvements in neonatatal management of prematurity made it possible to induce labor for affected infants at 32 to 34 weeks of gestation, but earlier stillbirths remained a problem. Reasoning that early deaths were primarily a consequence of anemia, Liley introduced in 1963 a technique of intrauterine, intraperitoneal transfusions to treat the anemia of severely affected mid-trimester fetuses and prolong their intrauterine lives. [17] This involved transuterine penetration of the fetal peritoneum by a long needle under fluoroscopic guidance and infusion of Rh-negative RBCs into the fetal peritoneum from which they were absorbed into the fetal circulation. Between 1963 and 1968, intrauterine transfusions were used increasingly, and neonatal mortality from EF in the United States decreased from about 60 to 45 deaths per 100,000 live births. [15] The development of ultrasonographic guidance made the procedure more feasible and eliminated radiation exposure. However, intraperitoneal blood transfusions were associated with a significant risk of induction of premature labor and were not effective in hydropic, moribund fetuses.

The development of fetal ultrasonography enabled new approaches to the intrauterine diagnosis and therapy of EF. Percutaneous umbilical blood sampling (PUBS) made it possible to insert a needle reliably and relatively safely through the uterus into the umbilical vein under ultrasonographic guidance. It now was possible to obtain a fetal blood sample as early as 22 to 24 weeks of gestation, allowing measurement of the hemoglobin level and direct assessment of the severity of the hemolytic process. This direct assessment has replaced amniotic fluid spectroscopy almost completely, but spectroscopy still may be used occasionally to indicate the need for PUBS. If indicated, an intravenous transfusion of Rh-negative RBCs then can be administered through the same needle. Since about 1985, it has also been possible to perform intrauterine exchange transfusions in fetuses that have profound anemia (hemoglobin, <8.0 mg/dL [80 g/L]) and those that have hydrops fetalis. The advantages of intrauterine exchange, compared with simple transfusions, are rapid effect and elimination of sensitized Rh-positive fetal RBCs, which decrease the risk of postnatal hyperbilirubinemia. The procedure can be repeated until it is considered safe to induce delivery. Large series of intrauterine exchange transfusions have been reported, with a 60% survival in fetuses that had established hydrops and a 90% survival of profoundly anemic fetuses that did not have hydrops. [18] At birth, almost all of the circulating RBCs of infants who had received intrauterine transfusions were Rh-negative donor RBCs. Because Rh-negative RBCs are not hemolyzed rapidly, postnatal jaundice severe enough to require exchange transfusions usually does not occur, although small simple transfusions sometimes are needed for anemia.

Occasional Rh immunization still is seen in North American and North European women due to prior transfusions, early abortions, sensitization before 21 weeks of pregnancy, or relatively massive fetomaternal transfusions. Elsewhere in the world, Rh erythroblastosis still occurs and is especially frequent in ethnic groups that have a high rate of Rh negativity, including the Basques of Spain (25% to 35%) and the Berbers of Africa and Arabian Bedouins (18% to 30%). In contrast, the rate of Rh negativity is 15% in North European Caucasians, about 5% in African-Americans, and 0 to 2% in Asians. [19]

As a consequence of the large immigration to North America by people from Southeast Asia, an increasing number of infants who have nonimmunologic hydrops fetalis due to homozygous alpha-thalassemia are being reported. Early diagnosis of these infants by ultrasonography has led to intrauterine transfusions and exchange transfusions that have resulted in salvage of some infants. [20]

The Fall of Exchange Transfusion

Other advances that have reduced the need for exchange transfusion include the use of phototherapy (preventive and therapeutic) and in conjunction with exchange transfusions to control hyperbilirubinemia. Phototherapy, when initiated early, often is effective at controlling hyperbilirubinemia in infants who have moderate degrees of hemolysis due to EF or other congenital hemolytic anemias, including ABO hemolytic disease, glucose-6-phosphate dehydrogenase deficiency, and hereditary spherocytosis.

Postpartum administration of Rh immunoglobulin to Rh-negative mothers who have given birth to Rh-positive infants, which was implemented widely after 1968, has resulted in a dramatic decrease in maternal isoimmunization, cases of EF, and the need for exchange transfusions. Kernicterus, phototherapy, and Rh immunoglobulin have been discussed at length by Drs J.M. Bowman, A. Brown, and J.F. Lucey in other issues of *NeoReviews* (see http://neoreviews.aap publications.org/cgi/content/extract/3/11/e223 and http://neoreviews.aappublications.org/cgi/content/extract/4/2/e27).

There is little doubt that prevention of primary isoimmunization of Rh-negative women

with Rh immunoglobulin and the use of phototherapy to control hyperbilirubinemia have had the greatest impact on the virtual elimination of Rh EF and the need for exchange transfusions. Anecdotal testimony suggests the near disappearance of exchange transfusions in most North American medical centers. Dr J.M. Bowman's statistics from his center in Winnipeg, Canada, support this impression. In 1962, 262 exchange transfusions were performed for hemolytic diseases of the newborn at the Winnipeg Health Center, most of which were for Rh EF. In 1994, only one exchange transfusion was performed to treat a newborn who had anti-S hemolytic disease of the newborn. [21]

Exchange Transfusions Today

As the epidemiology of EF has changed dramatically over the past 25 years, most of today's pediatric residents never have observed an exchange transfusion. Very few neonatology fellows have performed one; prenatal exchange transfusions now are being performed by obstetric perinatologists. Most of the generation of American pediatricians who performed many exchange transfusions as part of their routine practices in the 1950s, 1960s, and 1970s no longer are professionally active. Consequently, there is a lack of experienced operators when the infrequent need for exchange transfusion arises and an inevitable increase in the risks of the procedure. Exchange transfusions have a small but significant risk of complications and even mortality resulting from air embolism, portal vein thrombosis, cardiac overload, thrombophlebitis, necrotizing enterocolitis, and the transmission of blood-borne diseases. However, these complications have been infrequent in the hands of experienced exchange transfusionists working in centers that have strong laboratory and pediatric support.

The most common indication for neonatal exchange transfusion today is hemolytic disease of the newborn due to maternal isoimmunization to blood groups other than Rh D. Blood used for routine transfusions is only ABO- and Rh-positive-compatible, and given the large number of RBC antigens, virtually every transfusion is "incompatible" for one or many blood groups! [19]

Exchange transfusions also have been employed for temporary control of severe neonatal hypercalcemia, but peritoneal dialysis and automated hemodialysis appear to be more effective. Partial exchange transfusion using a plasma substitute is effective in reducing the hematocrit in neonatal hyperviscosity syndromes. Exchange transfusions have been used to reduce acutely the hyperammonemia of inherited metabolic diseases of the urea cycle.

Exchange transfusions after the perinatal period also are infrequent. Some indications for exchange transfusions in older patients are to decrease hyperammonemia in Reye syndrome, to replace Hb SS RBCs with normal RBCs in patients who have sickle cell disease and acute chest syndrome, and to reduce the white blood cell count in patients who have leukemia and hyperleukocytosis. These latter conditions often are treated more effectively and easily by erythrocytapheresis and leukopheresis using modern automated apparatus.

Howard A. Pearson, MD
Professor and Chairman of
Pediatrics – Emeritus
Yale University School of Medicine
New Haven, CT

[To read the original article written by Diamond in 1948, please go to: http://neoreviews. aappublications.org/cgi/data/4/7/e169/DC1/1]

References

1. Pickles, MM. *Haemolytic Disease of the Newborn*. London, England: Blackwell Scientific; 1949

2. Clifford SH, Hertig AT. Erythroblastosis of the newborn. *N Engl J Med*. 1932; 207:105–113

3. Levine P. The pathogenesis of erythroblastosis fetalis. *J Pediatr*. 1943;23: 656–675

4. Mollison PL. The survival of transfused erythrocytes in haemolytic disease of the newborn. *Arch Dis Child*. 1943;18:161–172

5. Erythroblastosis foetalis and its treatment [editorial]. *Lancet*. 1946;2:242–243

6. Hart AP. Familial icterus gravis of the newborn and its treatment. *Can Med Assoc J*. 1925;15:1008–1011

7. Robertson BA. Blood transfusions in severe burns in infants and young children: a preliminary report of the treatment of the toxic shock by blood transfusion, with or without preceding exsanguination. *Can Med Assoc J*. 1921;11:744–750

8. Hart AP. Exsanguination transfusion in a newborn infant in 1925. *J Pediatr*. 1948;32:760

9. Wallerstein H. Substitution transfusion: a new treatment for severe erythroblastosis fetalis. *Am J Dis Child*. 1947;73:19–33

10. Weiner AS, Wexler IB. The use of heparin when performing exchange transfusions in newborn infants. *J Lab Clin Med*. 1946;31:1016–1017

11. Diamond LK. Replacement transfusion as a treatment for erythroblastosis fetalis. *Pediatrics*. 1948;2:520–524

12. Sidbury JB. Transfusion through the umbilical vein in hemorrhage of the newborn. *Am J Dis Child*. 1923;25:290–296

13. Diamond LK, Allen FH Jr, Thomas WO Jr. Erythroblastosis fetalis. VII. Treatment with exchange transfusion. *N Engl J Med*. 1951;244:39–49

14. Allen FH Jr, Diamond LK. *Erythroblastosis Fetalis Including Exchange Transfusion Technic*. Boston, Mass: Little, Brown; 1957

15. Birth Defects Branch, Centers for Disease Control. Infant death rates for hemolytic disease of the newborn. Cited in Oski FA, Naiman JL, eds. *Hematologic Problems of the Newborn*. 3rd ed. Philadelphia, Pa: WB Saunders; 1982:323

16. Liley AW. Liquor amni analysis in the management of pregnancy complicated by rhesus sensitization. *Lancet*. 1954;1:1213–1215

17. Liley AW. Intrauterine transfusion of the foetus in haemolytic disease. *BMJ*. 1963;2:1007–1011

18. Poissonnier MH, Brossard Y, Demedeiros N, et al. Two hundred intrauterine exchange transfusions in severe blood group incompatibilities. *Am J Obstet Gynecol*. 1989;161:709–713

19. Diamond LK. Blood transfusion: a history of blood transfusion. The story of our blood groups. In: Wintrobe MM, ed. *Blood, Pure and Eloquent*. New York, NY: McGraw-Hill; 1980:658–715

20. Singer ST, Styles L, Bojanowski J, Quirolo K, Fotte D, Vichinsky EP. Changing outcome of homozygous alpha-thalassemia: cautious optimism. *J Ped HemOnc*. 2000;22:539–542

21. Bowman JM. Immune hemolytic disease. In: Nathan DG, Orkin SH, eds. *Nathan and Oski's Hematology of Infancy and Childhood*. 5th ed. Philadelphia, Pa: WB Saunders; 1993:75

Historical Perspectives: The Rise and Fall of Exchange Transfusion
Alistair G. S. Philip, Louis K. Diamond and Howard A. Pearson
NeoReviews 2003;4;169
DOI: 10.1542/neo.4-7-e169

Remembering Virginia Apgar

Introduction

With this issue of *NeoReviews,* we introduce a feature that should be of interest to all who deal with neonates. "Historical Perspectives: The Underpinnings of Neonatal/ Perinatal Medicine" is a series of reviews that will feature commentary on important contributions from the past. In many cases, we have been able to persuade the author (or one of the authors) of the original contribution to comment on the environment into which the idea was introduced. In other cases, the author(s) is (are) dead, and we have asked a noted authority on the subject or a former colleague to provide the comments.

As our subspecialty has matured, so much has become entrenched in our approach to care that it is difficult to recall (or be reminded) of how different it was not too long ago. Especially for those who have recently embarked on a career in neonatology, it is worth remembering that we all owe a debt of gratitude to the pioneers of our discipline.

Our first commentary comes "from the grave" about a figure who looms large in the assessment of neonates throughout the world: Virginia Apgar. L. Stanley James wrote the piece featured in this issue, which was published originally in a series developed by Dewey Sehring of Ross Laboratories entitled "Landmarks in Perinatology/Neonatology" about 25 years ago. Dr Apgar originally proposed a new method for evaluating the neonate in 1952 and published it in 1953. Thus, this historical perspective might serve as a 50th anniversary celebration. After Dr Apgar died in 1974, Stan James published an appreciation in *Pediatrics.* Subsequently, Dr James, who collaborated on further evaluation of the Apgar score (published in 1958 and 1962), has died. Another suitable candidate to write about Virginia Apgar would have been Joe Butterfield, who was so influential in pushing the United States Postal Service to produce a stamp in her honor (in 1994), but he too has died.

It was my good fortune to meet Virginia Apgar on two occasions. The first was in 1964, when (as a pediatric resident in Honolulu) I was part of a "standing room only" crowd at Kapiolani Maternity Hospital. She talked about neonatal assessment in the delivery room and the importance of having somebody other than the obstetrician perform the assessment and be ready to provide assistance. She subsequently emphasized this point in a 1966 article. I met her again in 1967 when I was a fellow in Neonatology at Boston City Hospital and she had recently become Head of the National Foundation – March of Dimes Division of Congenital Malformations, for whom she was a highly effective spokesperson. One could not help being swept along by her infectious enthusiasm.

Dr Apgar frequently was amused by those who discovered that she was a "real person" and not just an acronym (also courtesy of Dr Butterfield):

A – appearance
P – pulse
G – grimace
A – activity
R – respiratory effort

As Stan James recalled in 1975, she had five careers (anesthesiology, public health, genetics, aviation, and research) as well as many hobbies. Her love of music resulted in her crafting of several stringed instruments, which were purchased by the Perinatal Section of the AAP (again in large measure thanks to Joe Butterfield) and grace the Apgar Memorial String Quartet, whose members played at the dedication of the Apgar stamp. Further details can be found in an article by Skolnick published in 1996, who wrote, "The brilliance of Apgar's simple contribution is that it forced delivery room staff to pay attention to the newborn, so they would recognize when immediate medical attention is needed." Even today, the emphasis on clinical evaluation at birth remains of paramount importance, and the Apgar score continues to be useful to predict short-term outcome, although not long-term neurologic impairment (a purpose for which it never was intended).

Virginia Apgar probably had an even broader influence on neonatology because, as Dr James also recalled, "She was the first person to catheterize the umbilical artery in a newborn infant, and undoubtedly the whole area of newborn intensive care would not be where it is today, were it not for Virginia."

Alistair G. S. Philip, MD, FRCPE, FAAP
Editor-in-Chief, NeoReviews

Suggested Reading

1. Apgar V. A proposal for a new method of evaluation of the newborn infant. *Curr Res Anesth Analg.* 1953;32:260–267
2. Apgar V. The newborn (Apgar) scoring system: reflections and advice. *Pediatr Clin North Am.* 1966;13: 645–650
3. Butterfield LJ, Covey M. Practical epigram of the Apgar score. *JAMA.* 1962;181: 353
4. Butterfield LJ. Virginia Apgar, M.D., Ph.D. (1909–1974). *J Perinatol.* 1994;14:310
5. Butterfield LJ. Virginia Apgar, Physician, 1909–1974. *Perinatal Section News (AAP).* 1994;19:1–2
6. Casey BM, McIntire DD, Leveno KJ. The continuing value of the Apgar score for the assessment of newborn infants. *N Engl J Med.* 2000;344:467–471
7. James LS. Fond memories of Virginia Apgar. *Pediatrics.* 1975;55:1–4
8. Skolnick AA. Apgar quartet plays perinatologist's instruments. *JAMA.* 1996; 276:1939–1940

Historic Perspective of the Apgar Score

The following commentary originally appeared in August 1976 as one of a series published by Ross Laboratories entitled "Landmarks in Perinatology/ Neonatology" and is reproduced with permission from Abbott Nutrition.

In 1949 Dr Virginia Apgar gave up the Chairmanship of the Department of Anesthesiology, Columbia University College of Physicians & Surgeons, to devote her full time to obstetric anesthesia.

Dr Apgar was interested in mortality and morbidity statistics and began to search for a means of characterizing a delivery service in terms of the responsiveness of the infant at birth. She took the course in statistics provided by the School of Public Health and as a result of this developed the idea of quantitating the infant's clinical condition at birth in a numerical fashion. At that time it was customary to consider crying time or breathing time, or even describe the infant's condition as asphyxia livida and pallida. None of these seemed to be satisfactory, so she chose five signs which were classically used by anesthesiologists to monitor the patient's condition throughout surgery. In those years prior to the advent of sophisticated monitoring and the use of paralyzing agents, the anesthesiologist would customarily monitor the heart rate by the temporal pulse, color by appearance of the skin, respiration by chest movement and tone and reflex response by the depth of anesthesia required for the surgery. The experienced anesthesiologist was able to monitor the signs automatically and rapidly. Dr Apgar chose these five signs for evaluating the newborn infant and gave each of them a value of 0, 1 or 2.

In characterizing a delivery service, she hoped:

a. To obtain information on the incidence of vigorous versus depressed infants;

b. To determine the relationship between responsiveness of the infant and outcome, both with regard to morbidity and mortality;

c. To determine the relationship of the responsiveness of different types of anesthesia and analgesia;

d. To determine the relationship between the responsiveness and the type of delivery.

She wished the score to be simple and easy to apply, to enable the physician or nurse to assess the infant's condition rapidly at a glance. She also recognized that time was important and made her observations with a stop watch which she carried around her neck.

The research milieu at the Columbia Presbyterian Medical Center was favorable, with Dr Papper as Chairman of Anesthesiology and Howard Taylor as chairman of Obstetrics and Gynecology. From both of these services she had strong support and no interference.

The research was done during the course of normal clinical care. In preliminary observations she assessed the time of maximal depression of the infants after birth and finally decided on one minute as the time to give the score. She taught the anesthesia residents on the obstetric service to score the infants when she was not herself in the hospital. However, over the years 1950–51 she scored the great majority of infants herself.

She collected and entered the data on anesthesia sheets and then into tables in what she called her black books. In her general activities as obstetrical anesthesiologist she had the assistance of one nurse, but had no grant or special financial support for this work.

As with all of her projects, she approached this with great glee and enthusiasm and mobilized the interest of the obstetric and anesthesia services. She soon found that the obstetricians all wanted to score their babies 10. Some wished to give 12. From this she concluded that it was important that some person other than the one responsible for the delivery should make the score.

She followed every infant with great avidity and believed that her own statistics were more reliable than those of the hospital or the Department of Health. Frequently they were. Infants were observed in either the normal newborn nursery or in the premature nursery, and should complications develop, she followed these infants. For those who died, she usually attended the autopsies herself and was very active in obtaining permission for autopsy, for which she had a near-perfect record. She knew exactly how long it took to process the permission through the various administrative channels till the autopsy could be performed. With a rapid walk, almost amounting to a run, it took exactly one hour to achieve this.

Dr Apgar was always critical about the score and reexamined it in 1958 and 1962 (Apgar V, Holaday DA, James LS, Weisbrot IM, Berrien C. Evaluation of the newborn infant—second report. *JAMA*. 1958; 168:1985; Apgar V, James LS. Further observations on the newborn scoring system. *Am J Dis Child*. 1962;104:419).

She hoped to be able to compare the various delivery services by the distribution of the score and frequently lectured in different parts of the country and the world on the scoring system. In 1957 it was introduced into the NIH Collaborative Project for Cerebral Palsy. This gave the score a very wide application, and the broad mortality statistics from the Collaborative Project with over 30,000 deliveries confirmed what Dr Apgar had found in her 1962 report.

L. Stanley James, MD, FAAP,
Professor of Pediatrics,
Columbia University College of Physicians and Surgeons,
New York, NY

[For the original article by Virginia Apgar, MD, PhD, please see the data supplement: http://neoreviews.aappublications.org/cgi/content/full/3/10/e199/DC1]

Historical Perspectives: Remembering Virginia Apgar

Alistair G. S. Philip and L. Stanley James
NeoReviews 2002;3;199
DOI: 10.1542/neo.3-10-e199

Chromosomal Abnormalities and Clinical Syndromes

Introduction

Fifty years ago, Professor Paul Polani and colleagues described young women who had Turner syndrome and were found to have apparently male "chromosomal sex." (1) At that time, the generally accepted number of chromosomes in humans was 48. Five years earlier, Barr and Bertram described the presence of a prominent mass of chromatin lying close to the nucleolar membrane in neurons of some female cats. (2) This "sex-chromatin" was not found in the males. These "Barr bodies" later were detected in cells grown from skin biopsies. (3)

Then, in 1956, Tjio and Levan reported that the number of diploid chromosomes was 46, (4) which rapidly was confirmed by others. (5) From this ripple, a wave soon developed.

Three years later, the first association of a clinical syndrome with an abnormal number of chromosomes was reported from France (6) and quickly confirmed in Scotland. (7) This was the association of Down syndrome (mongolism) with an extra chromosome number 21 (trisomy 21), although this was called chromosome number 22 at the time. Not long afterward, translocation was noted in a girl who had Down syndrome born to a 21-year-old mother, (8) and translocation was described as a cause of familial mongolism. (9) Other trisomies soon were described. (10)(11)

Based on the realization that the number of sex-chromatin bodies was one less than the number of X chromosomes present, the chromosomes of women who had Turner syndrome and appeared to be chromosomally "male" were investigated. They were found to have 45 chromosomes, with the sex chromosomes being XO. (12)

Many of these exciting chromosomal discoveries were made by Professor Polani and his colleagues. Elsewhere, Professor Polani (now 90 years old) has described in detail the origins and evolution of clinical cytogenetics. (13) In this issue of *Neo Reviews*, we have been fortunate in obtaining his personal reminiscences of these exciting times in the development of pediatrics and genetics. We also provide an extract of a recently published perspective on the importance of chromosomes in the development of human genetics.

Neonatologists rely heavily on their pediatric geneticist colleagues to provide answers to the questions raised when neonates are born with constellations of malformations. The foundation for their evaluations is provided in the accompanying commentaries. Frequently today, answers come from high-resolution chromosomal analysis, but we also may have to go "FISHing for answers" at the molecular level. (14)(15)

Alistair G. S. Philip, MD, FRCPE, FAAP
Editor-in-Chief, NeoReviews

References

1. Polani PE, Hunter WF, Lennox B. Chromosomal sex in Turner's syndrome with coarctation of the aorta. *Lancet*. 1954; ii:120–121
2. Barr ML, Bertram EG. A morphological distinction between neurones of the male and female and the behavior of the nucleolar satellite during accelerated nucleoprotein synthesis. *Nature*. 1949;163:676–677
3. Moore KL, Graham MA, Barr ML. The detection of chromosomal sex in hermaphrodites from a skin biopsy. *Surg Gynecol Obstet*. 1953;96:641–648
4. Tjio JH, Levan A. The chromosomal number of man. *Hereditas*. 1956;42:1–6
5. Ford CE, Hamerton JL. The chromosomes of man. *Nature*. 1956;178: 1020–1023
6. Lejeune J, Gautier M, Turpin R. Etude des chromosomes somatique de neuf enfants mongoliens. *C. R. Acad Sci (Paris)*. 1959;248:1721–1722
7. Jacobs PA, Baikie AG, Court-Brown WM, Strong JA. The somatic chromosomes in mongolism. *Lancet*. 1959;i: 787–790
8. Polani PE, Briggs JH, Ford CE, Clarke CM, Berg JM. A Mongol girl with 46 chromosomes. *Lancet*. 1960;i:721–724
9. Carter CO, Hamerton JL, Polani PE, Gunalp A, Weller SD. Chromosome translocation as a cause of familial mongolism. *Lancet*. 1960;ii:678–680
10. Edwards JH, Harnden DG, Cameron AH, Crosse VM, Wolff OH. A new trisomic syndrome. *Lancet*. 1960;i:787–790
11. Patau K, Smith DW, Therman E, Inhorn SL, Wagner HP. Multiple congenital anomaly caused by an extra autosome. *Lancet*. 1960;i:790–793
12. Ford CE, Jones KW, Polani PE, DeAlmeida JC, Briggs JH. A sex-chromosome anomaly in a case of gonadal dysgenesis (Turner's syndrome). *Lancet*. 1959;i: 711–713
13. Polani PE. Human and clinical cytogenetics: origins, evolution and impact. *Eur J Hum Genet*. 1997;5: 117–128
14. Lin RJ, Cherry AM, Bangs CD, Hoyme HE. FISHing for answers: the use of molecular cytogenetic techniques in neonatology. *NeoReviews*. 2003;4:e94–e98. Available at: http://neoreviews.aappublications.org/cgi/content/full/4/4/e94
15. Reid T. Cytogenetics–in color and digitized. *N Engl J Med*. 2004;350: 1597–1600

Human Cytogenetics

The year was 1959, the year of the "human cytogenetics explosion." For me, it was the year when work over the last 10 years was coming to fruition. Research on congenital cardiac anomalies and my study of human genetics (eg, "moonlighting" at the Galton Laboratory with Penrose) were now falling into place. However, it was my findings and conjectures on Turner syndrome arising out of the congenital heart work and more indirectly on Klinefelter syndrome that were important. They had confirmed cytogenetically my ideas on chromosomal abnormalities, especially sex chromosome complements, and their bearing on sex determination in humans. (It was, in essence, this work and a little more that brought, 14 years later, the Fellowship of the Royal Society, the United Kingdom Academy of Science.) The relatively high frequency of coarctation of the aorta, a male cardiac anomaly, in females who had Turner syndrome suggested to me that these females might be sex-reversed males, and I found that their cell nuclei tested chromatin-negative. (1) The male frequency of red/green color blindness reported in *The Lancet* (2) confirmed the presence of a single X chromosome, but now I thought that patients who had Turner syndrome might be XO (45, X) females, rather than XY sex-reversed males. If this was true, sex determination in humans (and perhaps in mammals generally) could not be as in *Drosophila* (where XOs are male), which was the accepted formula for humans at that time. However, the extrapolation from the XO hypothesis to sex determination in humans seemed too fanciful and unacceptable to a rather clinical journal/readership (much as, conversely, the 1954 Turner "sex chromatin" paper had seemed too clinical for *Nature* but was accepted by *The Lancet*). Incidentally, chromatin-positive males who had Klinefelter syndrome had a female frequency of color blindness, so, by contrast with the putative XO females who had Turner syndrome, they should carry two X chromosomes, as women do.

In 1959, I was research physician (from 1955) for The National Spastics Society (NSS) and, from 1958, director of their Medical Research Section at Keats House of Guy's Hospital Medical School (three, then four strong). I had been assistant director of Pediatrics at Guy's Hospital (Director: Philip R. Evans) from 1950 to 1955 and National Birthday Trust research fellow for the previous 2 years.

During those 10 years, I had had the good fortune to collaborate and work with Maurice Campbell, the cardiologist (and so with Russell Brock, later Lord Brock, the cardiac surgeon in close touch with the Johns Hopkins Blalock/Taussig cardiology group), and especially with Peter Bishop, the sex endocrinologist. I had established a fruitful collaboration with Robert Platt (later Lord Platt, PRCP). Joseph Briggs and Maurice Lessof (later Professor of Medicine at Guy's), Peter Bishop's registrars, and his overseas visitor, Carlos de Almeida (later Head of Cytogenetics, Rio de Janeiro), had been seconded to work with me on sex anomalies. Somewhat later, another of Bishop's overseas visitors, Georgiana Jagiello joined the group and, later still, the new Unit at Guy's (she subsequently became Professor of Human Development and Genetics at the College of Physicians & Surgeons, Columbia University).

In 1955, I sought a direct refutation or confirmation of my unorthodox views on the sex chromosomes in Turner and Klinefelter syndrome and, hence, on human sex determination. I first turned to Gordon Thomas, an expert at Guy's on tissue culture. Although we tried hard and, indeed, saw and counted chromosomes in cultured somatic cells of both patients and controls, we came to no useful conclusion. Having approached Peo Koller unsuccessfully for his excellent expertise with chromosomes, I turned for help to Charles Ford at the MRC Radiobiology Unit, Harwell. I had come to know him in relation to sex chromatin and color blindness work, and we became better acquainted during the 1957 Nuclear Sexing Symposium at King's College Hospital. In fact, I had suggested that Ford be invited to that symposium, given his expertise in general cytogenetics and his recent work on murine chromosomes. I plotted with William Davidson and Robertson Smith, organizers of the Symposium, to involve him in human chromosomes. John Hamerton, later to work with me (and subsequently to become Professor in Winnipeg, Manitoba) and then at Harwell, was at the meeting. The meeting gave the three of us an opportunity to set our future collaboration on chromosomes in human anomalies of sex differentiation.

In the spring of 1958 I received two preprints of the same article that was to appear in *Nature,* one sent by Ford and the other by Laszlo Lajtha, concerning the bone marrow technique for the study of human chromosomes. (3) I immediately sent to Ford bone marrow from patients who had Turner and Klinefelter syndromes (and myself).

At the end of the summer, at the request of the World Health Organization (WHO) Europe, I was seconded by the NSS to work on a large-scale investigation of "pregnancy wastage" that was being planned in the United States. The WHO Europe headquarters was in Copenhagen, where I settled for a while and was given free access to the University Library and an especially welcome chance to discuss sex chromosomes and sex determination with Mogens Westergaard.

I enjoyed browsing, rereading classic human chromosome papers and the more recent ones, especially Ford and Hamerton's meiotic in vivo confirmation (n=23) (4) of Tjio and Levan's finding. (5) It was in this setting that Ursula Mittwoch's paper on a male mongol's meiotic chromosome number (n=24) came to mind. (6) Had she miscounted or was there something wrong with the Down syndrome chromosome number? At the end of 1958 in Copenhagen, I heard from Ford the exciting results of the chromosome work in our two patients: a Turner female who had 45 chromosomes, considered XO, and a Klinefelter male who had 47 chromosomes, seemingly XXY (he also had a normal cell line with 46 chromosomes, probably making him a sex-chromosome mosaic). It was for me, if I may quote Mahlon Hoagland (Judson HE. *The Eighth Day of Creation.* 1979:327), "one of those rare and exciting moments when" observation, surmise, and experimental results snap "into soul-satisfying harmony."

The exciting news from Ford and my Westergaard/Mittwoch scouting needed quick discussion and urgent planning for action. So, in January 1959, Ford and I met at Heathrow (I flew in from Copenhagen and was off to the National Institutes of Health [NIH], Bethesda], the nearest point for us to meet in peace. We published quickly the Turner paper in *The Lancet.* (7) Our XO and XXY (and mosaic) findings obviously suggested, as I had speculated, that sex determination in humans was unlike that in the "paragon" *Drosophila* (in which XO is male and XXY is female); in humans, the Y behaved as a direct, and probably the key, "male determiner" during gonadal differentiation (such as "Westergaard's *Melandrium*" Y chromosome and unlike the fruit fly's Y). In addition, the Klinefelter patient seemed to be a chromosome mosaic, and *Nature* would be the right journal for this information. (8) Independently, Patricia Jacobs and John Strong found an XXY sex-chromosomes complement in a male who had Klinefelter syndrome. (9) The XXY/ mosaic matter also was communicated by Ford to the meeting of the Medical Research Society, of which I was a member, much as, with William Hunter and Bernard Lennox, I had presented in 1954 the sex chromatin story of Turner syndrome.

Sex apart, we urgently began to study the chromosomes of patients who had Down syndrome, believing that trisomy of a small autosome was a possibility. We also decided that, at a later time (depending on our first findings in Down syndrome), we should consider studying Down syndrome patients born to younger women. Such cases were much rarer than those born to older mothers but sibship clustering of being affected had been noted in the young mother group, which suggested that they might represent a distinct subgroup of Down syndrome.

At the NIH, I was attached as a consultant and observer (for WHO Europe) to the National Institute of Neurologic Disease and Blindness, directed by Richard L. Masland (later Professor of Neurology at the College of Physicians & Surgeons of Columbia University). He also was the director of the "Pregnancy Wastage Collaborative Study," on which I was to work. The study stemmed from the obstetric department at Johns Hopkins. The object was to identify, through a prospective in-depth study, factors responsible for abnormal development and subsequent mental, neurologic, and physical abnormality and deviation. To this end, the study was to enlist, from the very beginning of pregnancy, 40,000 women and their offspring. In the 14 collaborating university hospitals, detailed and standardized clinical and biologic investigations would monitor each woman through her pregnancy. The surviving (and non-surviving) offspring were to be studied in comparable detail and assessed at delivery and later using the same standardized clinical and biologic protocols.

In addition to acting as consultant in the planning phase, I was to report whether it seemed desirable and, if so, feasible for parallel work to be undertaken in the Irish Republic, the United Kingdom, and the Scandinavian countries.

No sooner had I arrived at the Bethesda Campus than Ford telephoned to report that Jerome Lejeune had examined the chromosomes of nine children who had Down syndrome. Their chromosome number was 47, documenting that they carried a small extra chromosome. In short, they turned out to be trisomic for the chromosome later defined as number 21. Ursula Mittwoch had counted correctly!

It was likely that Lejeune's patients were children of older women. Accordingly, we proceeded with the study of Down syndrome children born to younger women, as planned, thereby identifying translocation (centric fusion) Down syndrome, "the mongol with 46 chromosomes." (10) The condition, a "hidden" trisomy of the Down syndrome chromosome translocated to another chromosome, could be transmitted genetically through asymptomatic translocation carriers formally with 45 chromosomes. I reported this at the December meeting in New York of the American Neurologic Society at which Lejeune reviewed his work. Later, centric fusion detection allowed us to calculate the mutation rate for that structural chromosome anomaly. (11) At the applied level, this served as the impetus for prenatal detection of the Down anomaly by amniotic cell culture.

My WHO work in the United States, United Kingdom, Dublin, and Denmark required several transatlantic crossings, much traveling in America, and frequent meetings on planning and standardization, an excellent method of acquiring an understanding of the American academic scene and research. Usefully interspersed were seminars and meetings on chromosomes, the effects and pathogenesis of their imbalance on development, and speculation on the relevance of chromosome imbalance and of genic imbalance on oncogenesis and malignancy. Further, there was the opportunity of meeting groups interested in the development of cytogenetics and other human genetics work in the United States.

To me, and in respect of the future direction of my work, the Syracuse, New York, meeting in 1959 was especially rewarding. It gave me the chance to review our work on sex chromosome anomalies and its background (the perennially open and active library at the NIH and its admirable facilities were an immense help), to consider it in a wider context, and to present it to an audience of specialists. The symposium was an opportunity to meet people such as Francis Crick, Barton Childs, James Neel, and William Russell and to hear the latter present parallel work on mice. There were many other geneticists with whom to exchange information and ideas. It was a rich time for

harvesting and for becoming involved in rewarding discussions, some of which might have modified my future and certainly helped in maturing my thoughts on research.

Paul E. Polani, MD, FRCP, FRS
Research Professor Emeritus
London University
Formerly Professor of Pediatric Research at Guy's Hospital Medical School

References

1. Polani PE, Hunter WF, Lennox B. Chromosomal sex in Turner's syndrome with coarctation of the aorta. *Lancet.* 1954; 267:120–121

2. Polani PE, Lessof MH, Bishop PM. Colour-blindness in ovarian agenesis (gonadal dysplasia). *Lancet.* 1956;271:118–120

3. Ford CE, Jacobs PA, Lajtha LG. Human somatic chromosomes. *Nature.* 1958;181: 1565–1568

4. Ford CE, Hamerton JL. The chromosomes of man. *Nature.* 1956;178: 1020–1023

5. Tjio JH, Levan A. The chromosome number of man. *Hereditas.* 1956;42:1–6

6. Mittwoch U. The chromosome complement in a Mongolian imbecile. *Ann Eugen.* 1952;17:37

7. Ford CE, Jones KW, Polani PE, De Almeida JC, Briggs JH. A sex-chromosome anomaly in a case of gonadal dysgenesis (Turner's syndrome). *Lancet.* 1959;276:711–712

8. Ford CE, Polani PE, Briggs JH, Bishop PM. A presumptive human XXY/XX mosaic. *Nature.* 1959;183:1030–1032

9. Jacobs PA, Strong JA. A case of human intersexuality having a possible XXY sex-determining mechanism. *Nature.* 1959;183:302–303

10. Polani PE, Briggs JH, Ford CE, Clarke CM, Berg JM. A Mongol girl with 46 chromosomes. *Lancet.* 1960;278:721–724

11. Polani PE, Hamerton JL, Gianelli F, Carter CO. Cytogenetics of Down's syndrome (mongolism). 3. Frequency of interchange of trisomics and mutation rate of chromosome interchanges. *Cytogenetics.* 1965;104:171–185

Chromosomes and Human Genetics

The following is reproduced with permission from Genetic testing. In: Christie DA, Tansey EM, eds. **Wellcome Witnesses to Twentieth Century Medicine Series. Vol. 17. London, England: Wellcome Trust Centre for the History of Medicine at UCL; 2003:6–8,10–11.**

... I present here a sketchy and condensed view of the importance that chromosomes have had in the modern scientific developments and practical application of human genetics. (1)

So may I start with a few critical dates and names? The starting date is 1956 when Tjio and Levan revealed the chromosome number to be 46 in cultured somatic cells – a finding that broke the technical problem of chromosome handling, as well as the spell of magic 48. (2) Also in 1956, the number 46 was confirmed in vivo by the techniques that Charles Ford and John Hamerton employed on human male meiotic cells at metaphase. (3) Then came 1959 with the discovery of chromosome anomalies, both gono- and autosomal, both numerical and structural. This search was guided by a number of clear clinical indications on where best to harvest, well before chromosome work could be applied effectively to human affairs, using new techniques that have been alluded to. (1)...

We can then skip to the early 1970s, namely to the work of Caspersson and Zech (4) with quinacrine fluorescent banding and to this easier and more complete chromosome identification method than the autoradiography one. Chromosome identification was subsequently made more practical by G-banding and reverse banding.

One can truly say that the scientific uses and practical application of chromosomology revolutionized human genetics and took it out of the doldrums that had been partly due to the influence of eugenics, partly to technical inadequacies, especially, it was felt, of cytological methods.

Medicine too had to come to grips with the practical uses of cytogenetics and genetics in the clinic and so came to realize its fundamental contribution to basic science, level with anatomy and physiology. So the new disciplines of clinical and medical genetics were born.

Although there are many derivatives of the cytogenetic explosion, I discern at least five main lines of descent, and I will look at each of them fairly briefly. The first one was the change of the formal genetics of human sex determination, primary sexual differentiation, already implied in our 1954/56 work on Turner syndrome females, considered quite plausibly to be XO, (5)(6) as well as the studies on Klinefelter syndrome males (7) running in parallel and using in both cases sex chromatin as a cell marker and color vision/color blindness as a genetic marker for the X chromosome. In 1959, as a result of direct X chromosome studies of these two human sex errors, the XO constitution was confirmed in females with Turner syndrome, and the XXY status of males with Klinefelter syndrome was sorted out by the work of Jacobs and Strong and by Ford and ourselves. (8)(9)(10) Thus, the *Drosophila* sex determination pattern, which was a dogma for humans in those days, had to be abandoned in favor of the mammalian Y chromosome as the key sex determiner—the so-called *Melandrium* pattern. At the same time, the reality in humans of chromosome mosaicism was objectively demonstrated.

Later, from 1990, the molecular story of Y-chromosomal control on primary sex determination was being written, to begin with largely by Gubbay, Sinclair, Lovell Badge and Goodfellow, (11) aided by the observations of Jacobs and Ross on the Y chromosome and those of Ferguson-Smith on XX males with Klinefelter syndrome (12)(13) and ourselves on XY females, often with pure gonadal dysgenesis (Swyer syndrome). (14)

The second leitmotif is Mary Lyon's "inactive-X hypothesis" (only one of the two Xs in females is genetically active), proposed in 1961, (15) partly from XO human and murine females, partly from the study of mouse coat color marker genes, and partly from the heterochromy of one X in XX subjects, studied especially by Ohno, (16) and its late DNA synthesis investigated by Taylor and colleagues. (17) Following the pinpointing of the X inactivation (initiation) center, XIC/Xic, and then the discovery of the influence of the inactivation control center, Xce, which affects randomness of X chromosome inactivation, lyonization is a good way towards its molecular resolution, particularly now that the work of Brown and Ballabio on XIST/Xist has identified a control mechanism on the X chromosome which seems to supersede the need to suppress or modulate the activity of individual X-linked genes. (18)... [The other important developments were in cell hybridization for gene mapping and monoclonal antibody production and on chromosomes and genes related to malignancy as well as to single-gene disease such as cystic fibrosis and Duchenne muscular dystrophy.]

...Finally, a few words on the origins of trisomy 21, as a representative of all trisomies, which are about one-third of all recognized pregnancies in women over the age of 40. Only a small proportion of trisomy 21s are inherited in a maternal age-independent manner through centromeric fusion translocation, as we showed in 1959 and 1960. (19)(20) Disregarding the 10% paternal contribution to the origin of trisomy 21, maternal age dependence of nondisjunction of chromosome 21, which lies at the origin of trisomy, seems to result either from the failure of chromosomes 21 to crossover and recombine at meiosis or from a mislocation of chiasma position. The result of either is an error of chromosome partitioning at the first or second meiotic divisions of the mature ovum before or at sperm penetration and fertilization. In either case, namely when no chiasmata form or when chiasmata are mislocated, we know that these recombination errors take place at the meiotic prophase, which, on the female side, is *in fetu* well before she is born, and thus long before she becomes a mother. The fact that meiotic recombination errors *in fetu* are revealed in ova matured and released at advancing maternal age might support the idea that oogenesis follows a production line system. This hypothesis was proposed by Henderson and Edwards in 1968 (21) and, in essence, it says that early entry into meiosis *in fetu* corresponds to exit of the mature ovum soon after puberty, whereas late entry into meiosis *in fetu* yields ova that exit at a late maternal age, a case of first in first out, last in last out; a hypothesis which is supported by our animal experiments. (22)

References

1. Polani P. Human and clinical cytogenetics: origins, evolution and impact. *Eur J Human Genet.* 1997;5:117–128

2. Tjio JH, Levan A. The chromosome number of man. *Hereditas.* 1956;42:1–6

3. Ford CE, Hamerton JL. The chromosomes of man. *Nature.* 1956;178:1020

4. Caspersson T, Zech L, Johansson C, Modest EJ. Identification of human chromosomes by DNA-binding fluorescent agents. *Chromosoma.* 1970;30:215–227

5. Polani PE, Hunter WF, Lennox B. Chromosomal sex in Turner's syndrome with coarctation of the aorta. *Lancet.* 1954;ii:120–121

6. Polani PE, Lessof MH, Bishop PMF. Colour-blindness in ovarian agenesis (gonadal dysplasia). *Lancet.* 1956;ii:118–120

7. Polani PE, Bishop PMF, Lennox B, Ferguson-Smith MA, Stewart JS, Prader A. Colour vision studies and the X chromosome constitution of patients with Klinefelter's syndrome. *Nature.* 1958;182:1092

8. Ford CE, Jones KW, Polani PE, de Almeida JC, Briggs JH. A sex chromosome anomaly in a case of gonadal dysgenesis (Turner's syndrome). *Lancet.* 1959;i:711–713

9. Jacobs PA, Strong JA. A case of human intersexuality showing a possible XXY sex determining mechanism. *Nature.* 1959;183:302–303

10. Ford CE, Polani PE, Briggs JH, Bishop PMF. A presumptive human XXY/XX mosaic. *Nature.* 1959;183:1030–1032

11. Goodfellow PN, Lovell Badge R. SRY and sex determination in mammals. *Annu Rev Genet.* 1993;27:71–92

12. Jacobs PA, Ross A. Structural abnormalities of the Y chromosome in man. *Nature.* 1966;210:353–354

13. Ferguson-Smith MA. X-Y chromosomal interchange in the aetiology of true hermaphroditism and of XX Klinefelter's syndrome. *Lancet.* 1966;ii:475–476

14. Polani PE. Abnormal sex development in man. I. Anomalies of sex-determining mechanisms. In: Austin CR, Edwards RG, eds. *Mechanisms of Sex Differentiation in Animals and Man.* London, United Kingdom: Academic Press; 1981:479–484.

15. Lyon MF. Gene action in the X chromosome of the mouse (*Mus musculus* L). *Nature.* 1961;190:372–373

16. Ohno S, Kaplan WD, Kinosita R. Formation of the sex chromatin by a single X-chromosome in liver cells of *Rattus nor-vegicus. Exper Cell Res.* 1959;18:415–418

17. Morishima A, Grumbach MM, Taylor JH. Asynchronous duplication of human chromosomes and the origin of sex chromatin. *Proc Natl Acad Sci U S A.* 1962;48:756–763

18. Brown CJ, Ballabio A, Rupert JL, et al. A gene from the region of the human X inactivation centre is expressed exclusively from the inactive X chromosome. *Nature.* 1991;349:38–44

19. Polani PE, Briggs JH, Ford CE, Clarke CM, Berg JM. A mongol girl with 46 chromosomes. *Lancet.* 1960;i:721–724.

20. Carter CO, Hamerton JL, Polani PE, Gunalp A, Weller SDV. Chromosome trans-location as a cause of familial mongolism. *Lancet.* 1960;ii:678–680

21. Henderson SA, Edwards RG. Chiasma frequency and maternal age in mammals. *Nature.* 1968;217:22–28

22. Polani PE, Crolla JA. A test of the production line hypothesis of mammalian oogenesis. *Hum Genet.* 1991;88:64–70

Historical Perspectives: Chromosomal Abnormalities and Clinical Syndromes
Alistair G. S. Philip and Paul E. Polani
NeoReviews 2004;5;e315-e320
DOI: 10.1542/neo.5-8-e315

Thermoregulation

Introduction

There can be little doubt that thermoregulation is one of the major concepts underpinning the care of the preterm infant. In the first half of the 20th century in the United States, most preterm infants were maintained with body temperatures lower than term infants. Here we highlight the article that changed that approach, which was written by Bill Silverman and colleagues. (1) In an accompanying piece, Dr. Silverman provides a personal reminiscence of the setting into which this important paper was introduced. This is an extract of a more extensive reflection on lessons learned from randomized controlled trials, which he prepared for the James Lind Library. (2)

Dr. Silverman acknowledges the work of his colleague Richard Day, who many years earlier had demonstrated that preterm infants were homeothermic, but who had his findings dismissed by "the authorities." As Dr. Day noted in 1964, the ability to produce heat in the neonate "rises progressively with cooler and cooler chambers," but shivering was not observed. (3) Further investigation of heat production revealed the importance of brown adipose tissue (or brown fat) and the role it played in "nonshivering thermogenesis." (4) The disadvantage experienced by the "small-for-date" infant in this regard then was emphasized, (5) and the importance of a narrow range of environmental temperatures to minimize energy expenditure gave rise to the concept of a "neutral thermal environment." (6) It should be mentioned that shivering has been seen occasionally in the neonate who has extreme hypothermia, (7) and it has been hypothesized that shivering might occur as "nonshivering thermogenesis" approaches its full potential. (8)

In an accompanying special article in this issue of *NeoReviews*, Dr Sheldon Korones provides a historical review of thermoregulation in the neonate that emphasizes the importance of this topic. In it, he notes that the study by Silverman and colleagues actually was a "rediscovery" of principles formulated in the second half of the 19th century, which continue to underpin neonatal care today.

Alistair G. S. Philip, MD, FRCPE, FAAP
Editor-in-Chief, NeoReviews

References

1. Silverman WA, Fertig JN, Berger AP. The influence of the thermal environment upon survival of newly born premature infants. *Pediatrics*. 1958;22:876–886
2. http://www.jameslindlibrary.org/essays/cautionary/silverman.html
3. Day RL. Thermoregulation of the newly born. In: *Reports of Ross Conferences on Pediatric Research*. Supplement No. 2. Columbus, Ohio: Ross Laboratories; 1964:9
4. Hull D. The structure and function of brown adipose tissue. *Br Med Bull*. 1966; 91:223–234
5. Sinclair JC. Heat production and thermoregulation in the small-for-date infant. *Pediatr Clin North Am*. 1970;17:147–158
6. Hey E. Thermal neutrality. *Br Med Bull*. 1975;31:69–74
7. Brück K. Neonatal thermal regulation. In: Polin RA, Fox WW, eds. *Fetal and Neonatal Physiology*. Philadelphia, Pa: WB Saunders Co; 1992:493
8. Alexander G. Body temperature control in mammalian young. *Br Med Bull*. 1975; 31:62–68

Early Experiences

The following is an excerpt taken with permission from Silverman WA. Personal reflections on lessons learned from randomized trials involving newborn infants, 1951 to 1967. James Lind Library. Available at: www.jameslindlibrary.org.

In 1945, when I began the practice of general pediatrics in New York City, I was appointed to the teaching staff at Columbia University as an instructor at The Babies Hospital. Fortunately for me, as it turned out, Richard Day had just returned to the hospital (he spent the 2nd World War at the US Army's Environmental Research Laboratory working on an improved hand-glove for use in arctic climates). I quickly became one of his most devoted followers. He was the first teacher I ever met who replied to most of my questions with an unapologetic, "I don't know!"

When Dick came across Bradford Hill's book (*Principles of Medical Statistics*) around 1947, he immediately recognized the importance of controlling biases and of statistical arguments in clinical research. He decided to spread the word at our hospital in a series of talks to the staff. But the word "statistics" was off-putting, and attendance was very poor—I was the only one in the audience at his last lecture! Like Dick, I was completely sold on the numerical approach; soon we were making nuisances of ourselves by criticizing the subjective "in my experience" reasoning of our co-workers....

...Following the belated realization that a seemingly benign intervention like oxygen—a time-honored life-saving "drug"—could have such unexpected, unrecognized and devastating consequences, we realized that almost *everything* we were doing to care for premature infants was untested. (At mid-century, before the arrival of ventilators and microchemistry, care of marginally viable newborn infants was essentially "pastoral." Like the approach taken by farmers caring for newborn piglets, conditions considered ideal for survival were provided, and it was assumed that those who were "meant" to survive would do so. But none of these purportedly "ideal conditions" had ever been subjected to formal parallel-treatment trials.)

...at the end of 1954, we undertook the third (in what we thought would be the last) in the series of fixed-sample size trials of atmospheric conditions. This time we sought to compare high humidity (80% to 90% relative humidity) versus moderate humidity (30% to 60% relative humidity). The latter condition had been maintained in American incubators for almost two decades before mist treatment had been introduced.

In the 1954–55 "humidity" trial, we used a fixed-sample size, factorial design (similar to formats used for many years in agricultural field trials), as suggested by John Fertig, professor of biostatistics in the School of Public Health at Columbia University....

...we examined the results of the concomitant "humidity" section of the factorial randomized controlled trial and found another startling result. (1) We did not expect to detect any difference in first-five-day mortality, but found instead that it was *lower* in infants allotted to the "high humidity" arm of the trial! We were puzzled by this outcome because the respiratory retraction scores, incidence of infection and findings at postmortem were virtually the same in both groups. In "dredging" through the records, we found a small but consistent decrease in body temperature among infants reared in "low humidity" (30% to 60% relative humidity).

It seemed very unlikely to us that slightly low body temperature was responsible for an increase in mortality; for more than 20 years, incubator temperatures in America had been intentionally set to maintain relatively low but steady body temperature. This widely accepted practice was based on the findings in a prolonged observational study in Boston in the 1920s (reported in 1933) of the influence of various conditions of the physical environment on the well-being of premature infants. Our unpredicted difference in mortality among babies cared for in the different humidities compared seemed to be a fluke.

Nonetheless, we were now very confident we had a powerful tool to test the "temperature hypothesis" suggested by the associations turned up in the 1953–54 trial.

In March 1956, we began a trial comparing first-five-day mortality among infants housed in incubators maintained at two contrasting levels of ambient temperature (31° to 32°C versus 28° to 29°C) and one level of humidity (80% to 90% relative humidity). (2) A matched-pairs sequential plan (devised by John Fertig and Agnes Berger) was used to allow a running analysis of outcome. In February 1957, a predetermined "decision line" was crossed, indicating that lower mortality was associated with the warmer incubators.

Six years later these results were confirmed independently in trials conducted in Baltimore and in Pittsburgh. Three separate replications confirmed the surprising findings in our 1953–54 trial—small differences in body temperature were associated with measurable differences in mortality—and these findings settled a very old score. Seventeen years before our trial, Dick Day had made some painstaking physiological measurements of thermoregulation in premature infants. His findings—that these babies were truly homeothermic—challenged the widespread practice of caring for newborn infants in slightly cool incubators. But the authorities of the time dismissed his suggestions out of hand, and the everyday custom of maintaining relatively low body temperature in newborn infants continued unchanged for years.

Following these revealing randomized trials, we conducted several more tests of physical environments to tie up some loose ends: a randomized controlled trial comparing two levels of humidity at one body temperature, maintained by a servo-control radiant warmer constructed specifically for this purpose; (3) a trial examining the influence of the thermal environment on acid-base homeostasis in the first hours of life of normal neonates; (4) a randomized controlled trial examining the effect of the thermal environment on growth and on cold resistance of small infants after the first week of life; (5) and, finally, in 1967, a trial of the effects of thermal environment and caloric intake on growth after the first week of life. (6)

Note: These informal comments were written in Greenbrae, California (at the request of my friend Iain Chalmers) in October 2003, on the occasion of my 86th birthday (10/23/03).

William Silverman, MD
Former Professor of Pediatrics Columbia University New York, NY

[To read the original article documenting the influence of the thermal environment on survival of preterm infants written by Dr Silverman and colleagues in 1958, please go to: http://neoreviews.aappublications.org/cgi/data/5/3/e75/DC1/1]

References

1. Silverman WA, Blanc WA. The effect of humidity on the survival of newly born infants. *Pediatrics*. 1957;20:477–486

2. Silverman WA, Fertig JW, Berger AP. The influence of the thermal environment upon the survival of newly born premature infants. *Pediatrics*. 1958;22:876–885

3. Silverman WA, Agate FJ, Fertig JW. A sequential trial of the non-thermal effect of atmospheric humidity on survival of the newborn infant of low birthweight. *Pediatrics*. 1963;31:719–724

4. Gandy GM, Adamsons K, Cunningham N, Silverman WA, James SL. Thermal environment and acid-base homeostasis in human infants during the first few hours of life. *J Clin Invest*. 1964;43:751–758

5. Glass L, Silverman WA, Sinclair JC. Effect of the thermal environment on cold resistance and growth of small infants after the first week of life. *Pediatrics*. 1968;41:1033–1046

6. Glass L, Silverman WA, Sinclair JC. Relationship of thermal environment and caloric intake to growth and resting metabolism in the late neonatal period. *Biol Neonat*. 1969;14:324–340

Historical Perspectives: Thermoregulation
Alistair G. S. Philip and William Silverman
NeoReviews 2004;5;75
DOI: 10.1542/neo.5-3-e75

Perinatal Profiles: Ian Donald and Obstetric Diagnostic Ultrasound

Introduction

One of the things that helps prospective parents to truly understand that they soon will become parents is an ultrasonography scan of the mother's abdomen, which provides a visual image of the fetus – THEIR BABY. This moment of revelation is a comparatively recent development in obstetrics. Less than 50 years ago, the fetus was assessed largely by the palpating hands of the obstetrician.

Alistair G. S. Philip, MD, FRCPE, FAAP
Editor-in-Chief, NeoReviews*

Introduction of Ultrasonography Investigations

In 1958, Professor Ian Donald (Regius Professor of Midwifery at the University of Glasgow) and his colleagues John MacVicar (an obstetrician) and Tom Brown (an engineer) published a paper in *The Lancet* entitled "Investigation of Abdominal Masses by Pulsed Ultrasound." This article described their experience with 100 patients and included 12 illustrations of various gynecologic disorders (eg, ovarian cysts, fibroids) as well as demonstration of obstetric findings such as the fetal skull at 34 weeks' gestation, "hydramnios" (polyhydramnios), and twins in breech presentation. These "B-scope" images were somewhat "grainy" and indistinct compared with today's images, but this was almost certainly the start of a revolution in obstetrics, even if it took many years before most obstetricians were persuaded of the usefulness of such imaging.

It is worth noting that when a future Scottish Professor of Obstetrics visited the United States in 1964 and inquired about interest in ultrasonography diagnosis, he was told to forget it (!) and warned that it was "just a dream of a mad, redheaded Scotsman" that had no future. This characterization of Ian Donald was probably not limited to the United States. Recollections of another

Scottish obstetrician indicate that even by the early 1970s, Glasgow was a "divided city." There were two Professors of Obstetrics and Gynecology in two different institutions in Glasgow, and while Ian Donald was enthusiastically promoting the use of ultrasonography in obstetric diagnosis, his counterpart ("the other professor" in Glasgow) did not accept it.

Early History

Ian Donald was born in 1910 (variously reported to be in Paisley, Scotland, or Cornwall, England), the son and grandson of Scottish doctors. He received most of his early education in Scotland, but obtained a BA from Cape Town University (South Africa) before graduating from St Thomas's Hospital Medical School of the University of London in England in 1937. During the Second World War, he served as a medical officer in the Royal Air Force (RAF), and this allowed him to assimilate knowledge about RADAR (radio detection and ranging) and SONAR (sound navigation and ranging). He realized that echo-sounding SONAR, his preferred term for diagnostic ultrasound for many years, had potential application to clinical obstetrics, but he did not pursue this aggressively until after his appointment as the Regius Professor of Midwifery at Glasgow University in 1954. Earlier (in 1951), he had been appointed as Reader (roughly equivalent to Associate Professor) in Obstetrics and Gynaecology at St Thomas's Hospital in London.

Donald apparently had an intense interest in machines of all kinds from childhood, which persisted during and after his time in the RAF. After World War II, many "bits and pieces" of equipment became available, some of which he acquired. Although his reputation is founded on his work with obstetric ultrasonography, his early research (which involved machines) is of particular interest to neonatologists. While at St Thomas's Hospital, he collaborated with (Professor) Maureen Young of the Physiology Department and published a paper in the *Journal of Physiology* in 1952. This report was followed by two papers published in *The Lancet*; the first, in 1953, included a description of a negative-pressure respirator for neonates and the second, in 1954, concerned a positive-pressure respirator, also for neonates, which was called locally "the puffer." He later bequeathed this positive-pressure ventilator to Dr Herbert Barrie (Consultant Pediatrician at Charing Cross Hospital, London), who recalled that it was a "formidable array of electronics," much of which had been designed by Donald himself and built by his PhD engineers. Barrie later said that it was "basically an electronic finger" that occluded a hole in a tube through which gas was flowing to provide intermittent positive pressure. Professor Osmund Reynolds (University College Hospital, London) has referred to this device as "Ian Donald's puffer ventilator." (Comments from Barrie and Reynolds are both contained in the Wellcome Witnesses report "Origins of Neonatal Intensive Care in the UK.")

Obstetric Ultrasonography

After moving to Glasgow, Donald was based initially at the Royal Maternity Hospital, where the obstetric patients were located, and the Western Infirmary, where the gynecology patients were located and where his ultrasonography equipment was based. In attempting to make gynecologic diagnoses,

*Emeritus Professor of Pediatrics, Division of Neonatal and Developmental Medicine, Stanford University School of Medicine, Palo Alto, Calif.

he relied heavily on collaboration with engineering colleagues, principally Tom Brown, who was "loaned out" by the firm of Kelvin and Hughes Scientific Instrument Company. The initial work was performed using a device that had been designed as a metal flaw detector. As noted in their 1958 article, one of the properties of ultrasound (vibrations whose frequency exceeds 20,000/sec, beyond the range of human hearing) is that it can be propagated as a beam. Reflections of the beam from abdominal interfaces in women being investigated allowed images to be created, which initially were recorded on Polaroid® film.

Although he encountered considerable skepticism over the next few years, it is generally acknowledged (certainly by those with whom he worked in Glasgow) that he had not only vision, but enthusiasm and the courage of his convictions, which kept the entire research enterprise going. With the help of junior colleagues, to whom he gave considerable encouragement, he advanced the capability of ultrasonography in obstetric diagnosis, including diagnosis of placenta previa.

Ian Donald, whose primary responsibilities were as a doctor and a teacher, delivered lectures "with care and enthusiasm." He was the author of "Practical Obstetric Problems," which ran to five editions and was extremely practical (somewhat unusual for the period). Professor Stuart Campbell, who subsequently became one of the foremost practitioners of obstetric diagnostic ultrasonography in the United Kingdom, found Donald to be intimidating when he (Campbell) was a junior doctor. He stated that Donald was "totally brilliant" and noted that although he had a quick temper, this was never directed at patients. For example, if a woman's bladder was overdistended, blame was directed at the junior doctors, not at the patient. Campbell found that the best way to deal with it was " to be quiet and he soon calmed down, because he was an extraordinarily generous man … quite the most ethical and generous senior doctor I have ever [really] met."

It is evident that much of the early research investigation with ultrasonography was possible because Donald was greatly admired by his patients, and the era of written informed consent had not yet arrived. His patients were very willing to cooperate with the studies by Ian Donald and John MacVicar and later with those of James Willocks and Stuart Campbell, who were able to evaluate intrauterine growth using fetal cephalometry (biparietal diameter of the fetal skull) under Donald's tutelage. Various commentators have noted that these studies with ultrasonography would not have been possible today because the unknown effects of the imaging would have made obtaining informed consent difficult. However, it should be mentioned that Donald and his colleagues were very cognizant of the potential for damage from ultrasound and took pains to reassure themselves and others. A large section of their 1958 *Lancet* article was devoted to the "Possibility of Harmful Effects of Diagnostic Ultrasound," with heat production and cavitation being major concerns. They reported on several experiments that had been performed either in vivo or in vitro by themselves or others. In particular, kittens "exposed to more than 30 times the dose of ultrasound necessary in its diagnostic use produced no detectable neuro-pathological change."

For approximately a decade, Donald split his time between two hospitals. In the early days, diagnostic ultrasonography studies on pregnant patients necessitated transporting the patients by private car to the ultrasound equipment, which was very bulky. In 1964, the new Queen Mother's Hospital opened at Yorkhill in Glasgow, allowing Donald to see obstetric and gynecologic patients in the same hospital. Ultrasonography equipment also was evolving; the B-scope images that were presented in 1958 were followed by scan conversion (which converted to "peak memory" and allowed a photograph to be taken after looking at the image) and later by real-time scanners. Stuart Campbell saw the ADR linear array scanner in 1974 and called it "one of the most staggering innovations in ultrasound I had experienced in my life."

Conclusion

Throughout his academic career, Ian Donald was recognized as one of the leaders in obstetrics and gynecology, who attracted attention from scholars around the world. He received many honors during his lifetime. His legacy is not confined to Scotland or the continued advances in obstetric ultrasonography. In 1981, the Ian Donald Inter-University School of Medical Ultrasound was founded in Dubrovnik, Croatia, by Professor Asim Kurjak. In addition, the International Society of Ultrasound in Obstetrics and Gynecology (ISUOG) awards the Ian Donald Gold Medal annually.

He died in 1987, approximately 2 weeks after traveling to London to receive an Honorary Fellowship from the Royal College of Physicians, London. However, he apparently had been in ill health for almost half of his life, having had major cardiac surgery (for mitral valve stenosis) three times. During one of these hospitalizations, he self-diagnosed a retroperitoneal hematoma, which he was able to demonstrate to his doubting cardiac colleagues using ultrasonography! After the second operation, he published a "moving, yet wryly humorous essay" (in the words of John Fleming, one of his colleagues in Glasgow), which was published anonymously in the *Lancet* in 1969 (November 22 issue, pp 1129–1131), and apparently was very comforting to "many terrified patients about to undergo a similar ordeal." After his third operation, he took careful notes and wrote an additional article that was published in the *Scottish Medical Journal* in 1976, entitled "At the Receiving End." This article was intended to show others undergoing repeat cardiac surgery "that they need fear no worse than what they have survived previously; in fact, noticeably less." Donald added, "Patients must not be lied to and must be given every opportunity to face and stand up to the truth, as I was."

Today, we take for granted the remarkably clear images of the fetus that can be obtained with modern equipment. Such imaging allows for early detection of a wide variety of congenital abnormalities and for transfer of mother and baby to specialized centers for medical and surgical care. While this advance might have occurred eventually, the vision and unwavering dedication to the cause by Ian Donald undoubtedly contributed in large measure to where we are today.

Suggested Reading

Selected Articles by Ian Donald

Donald I, Young IM. An automatic respiratory amplifier. *J Physiol.* 1952,116:4P

Donald I, Lord J. Augmented respiration: studies in atelectasis neonatorum. *Lancet.* 1953;1:9–17

Donald I. Augmented respiration: an emergency positive-pressure patient-cycled respirator. *Lancet.* 1954;1:895–899

Donald I, MacVicar J, Brown TG. Investigation of abdominal masses by pulsed ultrasound. *Lancet.* 1958;1:1188–1195

Willocks J, Donald I, Campbell S, Dunsmore IR. Intrauterine growth assessed by ultrasonic fetal cephalometry. *J Obstet Gynaecol Br Commonw.* 1967;74:639–647

Donald I, Abdulla U. Placentography by sonar. *J Obstet Gynaecol Brit Commonw.* 1968;75:993–1006

Donald I. Sonar as a method of studying prenatal development. *J Pediatr.* 1969;75:326–333

Donald I. On launching a new diagnostic science. *Am J Obstet Gynecol.* 1969;103:609–628

Donald I. At the receiving end: a doctor's personal recollections of second time cardiac valve replacement. *Scott Med J.* 1976;21:49–57

Development of Ultrasonography in Obstetrics

Christie DA, Tansey EM, eds. *Looking at the Unborn: Historical Aspects of Obstetrical Ultrasonography.* Wellcome Witness Seminar. March 10, 1998. Available at: http://www.ucl.ac.uk/histmed/ [Look under Publications and then go to Wellcome Witnesses to Twentieth Century Medicine, Volume 5]

Additional detailed information about the development of obstetric ultrasonography is available at http://www.ob-ultrasound.net/history1.html

Donald's Contribution to Neonatology

For commentary about his role in development of assisted ventilation, see: http://www.ucl.ac.uk/histmed/ [Look under Publications and then go to Wellcome Witnesses to Twentieth Century Medicine, Volume 9: Origins of Neonatal Intensive Care in the UK]

Historical Perspectives: Perinatal Profiles: Ian Donald and Obstetric Diagnostic Ultrasound

Alistair G. S. Philip

NeoReviews 2007;8;e195-e198

DOI: 10.1542/neo.8-5-e195

Surfactant Deficiency to Surfactant Use

The Discovery of Surfactant

Although there was a significant lag time between the discovery of surfactant and its clinical application, the seminal paper was written by Mary Ellen Avery and Jere Mead in 1959. (1) Treatment of respiratory distress syndrome (hyaline membrane disease) took a giant step forward when surfactant was approved by the United States Food and Drug Administration for use in neonates more than a decade ago.

In addition to the original paper by Avery and Mead, we also have permission to reproduce two pieces by Dr. Avery, which tell the story of the discovery of the role of surfactant and its modern application. The first was published in the Ross series, "Landmarks in Perinatology/ Neonatology" in February 1977, and the second comes from a presentation that Dr. Avery recently made in Japan, which will be published in the *Journal of the Japan Society for Premature and Newborn Medicine*.

Finally, more details of how this discovery "really happened" are available in another recent review. (2)

Alistair G. S. Philip, MD, FRCPE, FAAP
Editor-in-Chief, NeoReviews

References

1. Avery ME, Mead J. Surface properties in relation to atelectasis and hyaline membrane disease. *Am J Dis Child.* 1959;97:517–523
2. Avery ME. Surfactant deficiency in hyaline membrane disease: the story of discovery. *Am J Respir Crit Care Med.* 2000;161:1074–1075

Historic Perspective on Surfactant Deficiency

The following commentary originally appeared in 1977 as one of a series published by Ross Laboratories entitled "Landmarks in Perinatology/ Neonatology" and is reproduced with permission of Abbott Nutrition.

The demonstration of deficient surface-tension-lowering substances in lung extracts of infants who died with hyaline membrane disease was a step in a series of observations that had previously set the stage. Peter Gruenwald, the pathologist, had wondered about the abnormal patterns of aeration in lungs of premature infants and doubted as early as 1947 that hyaline membranes were not responsible for resorption atelectasis. Richard Pattle, the student of foams and anti-foam agents at the Chemical Defense Establishment in England, had discovered the surface-tension-lowering properties of the alveolar lining layer and wondered if a deficiency of it could be responsible for poor aeration of premature lungs.

After Pattle's original note in *Nature* in 1955 on stability of bubbles from lungs, and before his definitive paper in the *Proceedings of the Royal Society of Medicine* in 1958, we had decided to measure surface tension in lungs of infants who died of many causes. Only those with atelectasis and hyaline membranes showed the expected behavior related to a lack of surface-tension-lowering materials (later called by John Clements the pulmonary surfactants). Excited by these findings, we suggested that an immaturity of the lung with respect to the capability to synthesize surfactants could result in atelectasis and that postnatal induction of this capacity would be consistent with the 3 to 4 day course of the disease. The next series of questions and 20 years of work were obvious: what was the surface-tension-lowering material, where and how synthesized, what were the regulators of synthesis, storage and secretion, what were optimal conditions for function, what could be done to accelerate synthesis, or conserve limited stores? Now, nearly 20 years later, we have many answers, and more than enough questions for the next 20 years.

The setting for the 1957 to 1959 observations was the physiology department of the Harvard School of Public Health and the nurseries of the Boston Hospital for Women. It was while pondering the origin of foam in pulmonary edema, and its nature, that I was led to Pattle's article. Pulmonary edema meanwhile had been a topic of long-standing interest at the Harvard School of Public Health since the days of Cecil Drinker, and the effects of foam on the mechanical properties of the lungs were of concern to my preceptor, the physiologist, Jere Mead.

It was Jere Mead's work with Edward Radford on surface forces in lungs that stimulated John Clements to measure surface tension of lung extracts. Jere Mead suggested I visit Clements (then at Edgewood, Maryland) to adapt his methods to the solution of my problem, which was to examine the surface tension properties of fetal and neonatal lungs. During Christmas vacation in 1957 I made that visit; later Jere Mead assembled a surface balance, and by March we knew we had made an exciting observation. The communication of that excitement was difficult, however, and took several years, since few pediatricians or pathologists were comfortable with the idea of the dependence of surface tension on surface area, which is the central issue with respect to alveolar stability. That finding was first made by John Clements in 1957, who commented that the alveolar lining layer served as an antiatelectasis factor.

It is perhaps pertinent to note that the studies done in 1957 to 1959 were as a special fellow of the National Institute of Neurological Diseases and Blindness, but without any separate grant support. The facilities and supplies were provided by the Department of Physiology, Harvard School of Public Health, but since all the equipment was assembled from laboratory leftovers, the cost was minimal. I made the first trough from a wooden slide box lined with paraffin; only after the original observations did we splurge on a Teflon trough, made by a plastics manufacturer in Cambridge.

The essential attribute in the environment was the encouragement to pursue new ideas and a receptivity even to their initial halting presentation. The subsequent pursuit of ideas was made possible by continuing grant support from the National Institutes of Health and the American Thoracic Society, and my own personal support as a faculty member at Johns Hopkins was greatly helped by the John and Mary Markle Foundation.

Mary Ellen Avery, MD
Boston, Massachusetts

Suggested Reading

Clements JA. Surface tension of lung extracts. *Proc Soc Exp Biol Med.* 1957;95:170

Gruenwald P. Surface tension as a factor in the resistance of neonatal lungs to aeration. *Am J Obstet Gynecol.* 1947;53:996

Mead J, Whittenberger JL, Radford EP. Surface tension as a factor in pulmonary volume-pressure hysteresis. *J Appl Physiol.* 1957; 10:101

Pattle RE. Properties, function and origin of the alveolar lining layer. *Nature.* 1955;175:1125

Pattle RE. Properties, function and origin of the alveolar layer. *Proc Roy Soc (London).* Series B. 1958;148:217

The Story of Neonatology: Personal Perspectives

The following commentary was presented by Dr. Avery to the 46th Annual Meeting of the Japan Society of Premature and Newborn Medicine and is reprinted with permission from the Journal of the Japan Society for Premature and Newborn Medicine. *2002;14: 13–16.*

Modern neonatology arose from the advances in many disciplines, especially pulmonary physiology, microbiology, and nutrition. Technological advances, including micro-chemical determinations, and ventilators, were pivotal in the survival of ever more premature infants.

My interest in these infants began as a medical student about 1950, when virtually no survivors under 1 kg birth weight were reported, with the exception of some small-for-gestational-age infants. As new knowledge of developmental biology and especially physiology became available, the challenge to apply it to the care of the low-birth weight infants was exciting. A major stimulus in my training came from the book *Physiology of the Newborn Infant* by Clement A. Smith. He summarized the existing studies, principally on lambs, that had elucidated changes in fetal development and adaptations at birth. The first edition was published in 1945, and the third and last edition was in 1959, when I was one of his research fellows at Boston Lying-In Hospital and Harvard Medical School. The last half of the 20th century was witness to a crescendo of research on many aspects of human reproduction that collectively resulted in a fall in infant mortality from about 16 per 1,000 live births to less than 5 per 1,000 live births, with fewer than 4 infant deaths per 1,000 live births in Japan and Sweden. Maternal mortality is very rare. The major challenge is to prevent preterm births and make neonatal care available to all.

One of the major advances in the last half of the 20th century has been awareness that the lung has an alveolar lining layer composed of surfactants that stabilize the airspaces at end-expiration by achieving a low surface tension at the alveolar-air interface. On inflation, the surface tension increases and contributes to the elastic recoil of the expanded lung. The ability of the surface layer to change with surface area depends on the presence of phospholipids and hydrophilic and hydrophobic proteins.

Many individuals have contributed to our knowledge of surface tension phenomena in lungs, especially the pathologists Gruenwald and, in England, Pattle, who worked in the Chemical Defense establishment, and Clements at the Army Chemical Center, Edgewood, Maryland, unlikely sites for studies that eventually have saved thousands of babies' lives. They realized that infants born prematurely, and especially infants of diabetic mothers, had normal lungs at birth, but with the need to breathe after birth, gradually developed respiratory distress. The first publication that related deficiency of surfactants in some preterm infants was in 1959, but wide acceptance of the idea took about 20 years, with many neonatologists focused on the "hyaline membrane" now known to be secondary to ventilation in a surfactant-deficient lung. The 1- to 3-day course of the respiratory distress syndrome represents acceleration of the time of appearance of surfactants by endogenous glucocorticoids in preterm infants. If they survive a few days, most will recover completely. If they require mechanical ventilation, some will develop a more chronic lung disorder, bronchopulmonary dysplasia.

The composition of the alveolar-air interface is now known to be saturated phospholipids (especially disaturated phosphatidyl choline) and lipoproteins, all of which are synthesized, stored as osmiophilic bodies, and secreted by an exocrine process by the alveolar type II cell.

The molecular biologists have determined that the structure of the proteins that are known as "collectins" resemble the better known mannose-binding proteins. They have been named in order of their discovery, surfactant-associated proteins A, B, C, D, abbreviated SP-A, SP-B, etc. SP-A and SP-D are hydrophilic, and the others are hydrophobic. The relative contribution of each to alveolar stability is disputed. It is clear now that B and C are essential since "knock-out" mice die with arrested development of alveoli. A surprise was the finding that SP-A is absent in lungs of infants who died from hyaline membrane disease. However, mice who have had the gene for SP-A "knocked-out" do not have tubular myelin *or* die of respiratory distress syndrome, but rather die of sepsis. SP-B-deficient mice have a disorder similar to that in humans, known as hereditary alveolar proteinosis, that is often lethal in infancy, although affected infants can live for some months. The group in St. Louis has followed a number of such infants and has reported no success with surfactant replacement. In some, lung transplantation has been effective.

SP-C is the most hydrophobic of the proteins, and its cysteines have been found to be dipalmitoylated lipopeptides. It is the only surfactant protein known to be synthesized by the Clara cell as well as the type II alveolar cell. Some interactions between SP-B and SP-C have been found essential for optimal biophysical function of lipid bilayers.

SP-D, the most recent surfactant-associated protein to be discovered, has been extensively studied and found to be a potent opsonin. It facilitates the ingestion by macrophages of viruses, bacteria and parasites. The chemical structure of SP-D is the mirror image of SP-A. It resembles a member of the group that includes the better known mannose-binding protein.

Most recently, Stahlman and colleagues have used a highly specific antibody to detect SP-D (from Whitsett in Cincinnati) to search for SP-D in samples of tissues from infants who died. The surprise finding was the evidence of SP-D throughout the respiratory tract and many secretory epithelial cells. They include lacrimal and salivary glands, upper gastrointestinal tract, uterine cervix and skin. It is tempting to marvel at the beauty of a design that put the innate immune system protein wherever exposure to the environment could lead to deposition of microorganisms. Incidentally, have you noticed how often animals lick their wounds? The story of these proteins continues to evolve.

There is another side to my personal perspectives and that is the route from discovery, to confirmation, to acceptance of efficacy, and eventually the license of a drug for widespread use among premature infants born with insufficient pulmonary surfactants. During my second trip to Japan as head of the American Delegation to honor the international year of the child in 1979, I went to Akita at the invitation of Tetsuro Fujiwara at the end of a marvelous visit to many cities. He had devoted many years to the quest for a suitable way to provide premature infants at risk of hyaline membrane disease with a surfactant. Others had established lack of efficacy by aerosol, but had also demonstrated the possibility of instillation of natural materials from lavage of mature rabbits' lungs into the trachea of preterm rabbits (by Enhorning and Robertson in Sweden). The Fujiwara group in Morioka had used minced cows' lung as the source of surfactant to treat newborn lambs that were preterm and deficient in surfactants. The results were dramatic, and of special interest were radiographs of an infant in whom the intratracheal tube was in a bronchus, so that only one lung received the surfactant. The post-treatment film showed good aeration in the treated lung only. Fujiwara commented that this was the first evidence of the primacy of surfactant deficiency as the cause of hyaline membrane disease. Before then, the association of deficiency of surfactant with the respiratory distress syndrome could have been a secondary effect to pulmonary ischemia or even heart failure (the prevailing views in 1979).

Fujiwara established a relationship with a Japanese pharmaceutical company that produced the product from minced cows' lungs that could be given to infants. Safety and efficacy were reported in *Lancet* in a small study in 1980. It was labeled TA surfactant for Tokyo Tanabe-Akita surfactant. This material was given to me by Dr. Fujiwara for our group to analyze and eventually evaluate in a prospective, randomized trial that was published in 1987. Meanwhile, Abbott Laboratories arranged with the Japanese Company to license it to them for further study and modification that resulted in their trade name *Survanta*. Multiple clinical trials confirmed prompt increase in aeration after instillation into the lung via an endotracheal tube. The Food and Drug Administration of the United States licensed Survanta in 1989 for use in low birth weight infants.

Surfactant replacement in premature infants has become routine, with continuing redefinition of eligibility with respect to "prevention" or "treatment." There is some debate about which preparation is most effective, although small differences were documented when phospholipids alone were evaluated in comparison with the more effective "natural" preparations that contained the surfactant proteins.

Much interest is focused on a fully synthetic preparation now being studied in Germany and the United States. Although no adverse events have been documented from the preparations from animal lungs, a lingering concern is the remote possibility of prion disorders with a prolonged incubation period. The German Product (*Venticute*) developed by Byk Gluden Pharmaceuticals Konstanz contains recombinant SP-C. A preliminary report from Spragg et al shows promise in treatment of adult respiratory distress syndrome. Another synthetic surfactant that consists of phospholipids and a synthetic peptide KL4 (4 lysine groups) was developed at Scripps Research Institute in La Jolla, California, by Revack and others. It is under investigation at this time (2001).

In conclusion, much is known and much more needs to be known about pulmonary metabolism. I am encouraged by invitations such as this to show some aspects of the process of discovery of the role of surface forces in lung aeration and an ever-increasing interest in surfactant replacement in disease. The impressive results in preterm infants with surfactant deficiency depend on replacement of a deficit in surfactant at their birth; but after birth, most infants over 1,000 grams birth weight acquire the capacity to synthesize their own surfactants within a few days. Meanwhile, as little as one dose is often sufficient. More than two doses add very little to the outcome.

Mary Ellen Avery, MD
Boston, Massachusetts

Historical Perspectives: Surfactant Deficiency to Surfactant Use

Alistair G. S. Philip, Mary Ellen Avery and Mary Ellen Avery

NeoReviews 2002;3;239
DOI: 10.1542/neo.3-12-e239

Group B *Streptococcus* in Neonatal Sepsis: Emergence as an Important Pathogen

The Preantibiotic Era

In the preantibiotic era, the group A beta-hemolytic *Streptococcus* was much more likely to be associated with serious bacterial infection of women and infants than was group B beta-hemolytic *Streptococcus* (GBS). Soon after the introduction of penicillin and other antibiotics, the most likely organisms to be cultured from neonates who had sepsis were gram-negative bacilli, most notably *Escherichia coli*. When penicillin-resistant staphylococci emerged, *Staphylococcus aureus* became prominent.

By 1958, a review of neonatal sepsis (septicemia) indicated that GBS could be a devastating organism. (1) Between 1933 and 1943, two cases of neonatal sepsis due to GBS (also called *S agalactiae*) were reported, and four more were seen between 1943 and 1947. Of the six infants, four had meningitis and two had pneumonia; all died. (1) Over the next few years, the importance of GBS in perinatal infection began to emerge.

Alistair G. S. Philip, MD, FRCPE, FAAP
Editor-in-Chief, NeoReviews

Emergence of GBS

First documented as an important organism in the perinatal period (for both women and infants) by Hood and associates in 1961, (2) early-onset meningitis caused by GBS was reported in 1962, (3) and the role of GBS in neonatal infection was emphasized by Eickhoff and colleagues in 1964. (4) During the next decade, the ascendancy of GBS continued, to the extent that by 1973, McCracken (5) considered it to be "the new challenge" and a year later, with a colleague, described a wide spectrum of disease resulting from GBS infection. (6)

The emergence of GBS infection was not limited to the United States; it appeared to be widespread throughout Europe. In the early 1970s, there were reports in the language of the country of infection from Bulgaria, France, Germany, Hungary, and the United Kingdom. (7) At about this time, the idea of "early-"and "late-"onset infections was proposed (8) and was well established by the end of the decade. (9) The possibility of nosocomial transmission had been reported, (10) and the importance of the various serotypes was documented at about this time. (11) Reports from Scandinavia and the rest of the world soon followed, indicating that this organism would be a player on the infection stage for many years to come.

Preterm Infants and Chest Radiographs

Those caring for newborns during that era had a great sense of foreboding that preterm infants might fall victim to overwhelming infection with GBS because of the high case-fatality rate for all infected infants, especially those born preterm. This was emphasized further by the difficulty encountered in trying to distinguish preterm infants who had respiratory distress syndrome (RDS) from those who had early-onset group B streptococcal pneumonia. It was noted that the diseases could be indistinguishable radiographically, (12) which probably was attributable to the finding of hyaline membranes (the hallmark of RDS) in infants who died from GBS pneumonia. Hyaline membranes of GBS pneumonia included cocci within them. Indeed, similar findings of hyaline membranes were observed with other types of bacterial infection, with organisms (most notably gram-negative rods) comprising the bulk of the hyaline membranes. (13)

Early Diagnosis

Because of the difficulty in distinguishing RDS from GBS and other types of pneumonia, it became routine to initiate antibiotics early in the postnatal course of all preterm infants. This "indiscriminate" use of antibiotics (with the implicit sense that resistant organisms would emerge) bothered me, and in the mid-1970s I began to look for ways to distinguish the infected from the noninfected infant. (14) With many other investigators, I examined a wide variety of acute-phase proteins and other markers over the next 2 decades, but a definitive test has remained elusive. Although the combination of leukocyte counts and C-reactive protein concentrations has proved useful when evaluated serially, (15)(16) the perfect test has yet to be found. Among the many agents evaluated more recently, interleukin-6, procalcitonin, and serum amyloid A have shown the most promise, but they have not been adopted universally. There is hope that polymerase chain reaction (17) or fluorescent in situ hybridization techniques (18) will provide definitive answers in the future.

Early Prophylaxis

Some infants who had GBS sepsis had a fulminant course and died despite early and apparently appropriate antibiotic therapy (according to in vitro sensitivities). However, it was difficult to distinguish such infants based on maternal factors, birthweight, or gestational age, although mortality (case-fatality) clearly was higher in the very preterm or very low-birthweight infants. Because of this, the focus became prevention.

It had been documented earlier that antepartum prophylaxis was ineffective in eliminating GBS colonization at delivery, but by the late 1970s and early 1980s, both intrapartum and postpartum prophylaxis had demonstrated efficacy in the prevention of early-onset GBS infection. (19)(20) Although these studies were encouraging, there was concern (which I shared) that widespread use of prophylactic ampicillin or penicillin would contribute to the emergence of resistant organisms or suppress gram-positive organisms at the expense of allowing gram-negative organisms to predominate. In addition, the attack rate in neonates was only 1 in 50 to 1 in 100 of those who were colonized, suggesting that not all maternal carriers required treatment. (21) This enigma was resolved partially with the discovery that serotype-specific antibody transferred from mother to baby was (is) protective, (22)(23) but most pregnant women lacked immunity to GBS, regardless of colonization status. It should be mentioned that in early epidemiologic studies of pregnant women, only about 5% were colonized with GBS, but this number currently is closer to 25%.

Further concern about postpartum prophylaxis came from a large randomized, controlled trial in Chicago of infants whose birthweights were less than 2 kg, which showed no difference between those receiving prophylactic penicillin and controls. (24) Early-onset GBS sepsis was found in 10 of 589 infants (17%) in the early treatment group compared with 14 of 598 (23%) in the control group. Fatality rates among affected infants were similar (6 of 10 [60%] died in the early treatment group versus 8 of 14 controls [57%]).

At about the same time, another group in Chicago demonstrated that selective intrapartum chemoprophylaxis with ampicillin could interrupt mother-to-infant transmission in high-risk situations. Although not emphasized in their abstracts, this group used a combination of intra-partum and neonatal chemoprophylaxis. In 1986, they published a randomized, controlled trial of this combined approach documenting no GBS infection in 85 infants of treated mothers compared with five GBS infections in 79 controls, a difference that was statistically significant. (25) Other groups subsequently confirmed these findings.

Clinical Manifestations

The clinical manifestations of group B streptococcal infection are diverse. In addition to the usual presentations of sepsis, pneumonia, and meningitis reported earlier, Howard and McCracken (6) described infants who had septic arthritis, osteomyelitis, facial cellulitis, ethmoiditis (in a 9-week-old preterm twin), conjunctivitis, and empyema associated with pneumonia. They also reported that four infants had "asymptomatic" bacteremia. To this wide-ranging list of clinical presentations, an unusual association of group B streptococcal infection with right-sided diaphragmatic hernia was added later. This was described initially in 1975, and 26 cases had been reported by 1989. (26) Whether this is an "acquired" lesion or a "congenital" lesion that is revealed remains uncertain, but the age at recognition ranged from 3 to 45 days. Cellulitis-adenitis was added to the list of presentations in 1982, (27) and isolated cervical lymphadenitis was recorded recently. (28)

Prophylactic Strategies

A little more than a decade ago, both the American College of Obstetricians and Gynecologists (ACOG) and the American Academy of Pediatrics (AAP) issued statements that concentrated on preventive approaches to maternal and infant infection. In addition, the spectrum of group B streptococcal disease was broadened to include nonpregnant adults, especially those who had underlying disease such as diabetes mellitus and cancer. (29) The primary prevention strategy employed was intrapartum chemoprophylaxis, although efforts to find appropriate immunoprophylaxis continued. It was known that serotypes Ia, Ib, II, and III accounted for more than 90% of neonatal disease, with type III most usually associated with "late-onset" disease (especially meningitis), but serotypes IV, V, and VI had been described. (29) More recently, serotypes VII and VIII have been added, and serotype V was found to be associated commonly with GBS colonization. (30)

Although the ACOG and AAP statements in the early 1990s had a modest impact on the incidence of GBS infection in the neonate, a marked decrease in incidence has been seen since the publication in 1996 of consensus guidelines for GBS prevention developed by the AAP, ACOG, and the Centers for Disease Control and Prevention (CDC). (31) These guidelines suggested either a risk factor-based strategy or a screening-based strategy (using antenatal culture status). More recently, the CDC documented the superiority of the screening-based strategy. (32)(33) A combined maternal and neonatal chemoprophylaxis strategy also has proved helpful. (34)

Although such chemoprophylaxis strategies have had a significant impact, decreasing the incidence of early-onset GBS infection, attempts to produce a multivalent vaccine to provide widespread immunoprophylactic protection against the most virulent strains of GBS continue. (35) Such a vaccine could minimize the prophylactic use of antibiotics and diminish the potential for development of antibiotic-resistant organisms.

Conclusion

GBS emerged as an important pathogen in neonatal infection as early as the 1940s, but it was well established (and feared) by the early 1970s. Recent efforts focusing on chemoprophylaxis have resulted in a marked reduction in neonatal GBS infection, but it still is important to develop a multivalent vaccine against the most common GBS serotypes.

Alistair G. S. Philip, MD, FRCPE, FAAP
Professor of Pediatrics Stanford University
School of Medicine
Palo Alto, Calif.

References

1. Nyhan WL, Fousek MD. Septicemia of the newborn. *Pediatrics*. 1958;27:268–278

2. Hood M, Janney A, Dameron G. Beta hemolytic streptococci group B associated with the perinatal period. *Am J Obstet Gynecol*. 1961;82:809–818

3. Keitel HG, Hananian J, Ting R, Prince LN, Randall E. Meningitis in the newborn infant. *J Pediatr*. 1962;61:39–43

4. Eickhoff TC, Klein JO, Daly AK, Ingall D, Finland M. Neonatal sepsis and other infections due to group B beta hemolytic streptococci. *N Engl J Med*. 1964;271:1221–1228

5. McCracken GH Jr. Group B streptococci: the new challenge in neonatal infections. *J Pediatr*. 1973;82:703–706

6. Howard J, McCracken GH Jr. The spectrum of group B streptococcal infections in infancy. *Am J Dis Child*. 1974;128:815–818

7. Harper IA. The importance of group B streptococci as human pathogens in the British Isles. *J Clin Pathol*. 1971;24:438–441

8. Quirante J, Ceballos R, Cassidy G. Group B beta-hemolytic streptococcal infection in the newborn. I: Early onset infection. *Am J Dis Child*. 1974;128:659–665

9. Baker CJ. Group B streptococcal infection in neonates. *Pediatr Rev*. 1979;1:5–15

10. Steere AC, Aber RC, Warford LR, et al. Possible nosocomial transmission of group B streptococci in a newborn nursery. *J Pediatr*. 1975;87:784–787

11. Baker CJ, Barrett FF. Group B streptococcal infections in infants: the importance of the various serotypes. *JAMA*. 1974;230:1158–1160

12. Ablow RC, Driscoll SG, Effman EL, et al. A comparison of early-onset group B streptococcal neonatal infection and the respiratory distress syndrome of the newborn. *N Engl J Med*. 1976;294:65–70

13. Jeffrey H, Mitchison R, Wigglesworth JS, Davies PA. Early neonatal bacteremia: comparison of group B streptococcal, other gram-positive and gram-negative infections. *Arch Dis Child*. 1977;52:683–686

14. Philip AGS, Hewitt JR. Early diagnosis of neonatal sepsis. *Pediatrics*. 1980;65:1036–1041

15. Philip AGS. Response of C-reactive protein in neonatal group B streptococcal infection. *Pediatr Infect Dis J*. 1985;4:145–148

16. Philip AGS. Neonatal sepsis and C-reactive protein [letter]. *Pediatrics*. 1994;93:693

17. Ke D, Bergeron MG. Molecular methods for rapid detection of group B streptococci. *Expert Rev Mol Diagn*. 2001;1:175–181

18. Artz LA, Kempf VA, Autenrieth IB. Rapid screening for *Streptococcus agalactiae* in vaginal specimens of pregnant women by fluorescent in situ hybridization. *J Clin Microbiol*. 2003;41:2170–2173

19. Yow MD, Mason EO, Leeds LJ, Thompson PK, Clark DJ, Gardner SE. Ampicillin prevents intrapartum transmission of group B streptococcus. *JAMA*. 1979;241:1245–1247

20. Siegel JD, McCracken GH Jr, Threlkeld N, Milvenan B, Rosenfeld CR. Single-dose penicillin prophylaxis against neonatal group B streptococcal infections: a controlled trial in 18,738 newborn infants. *N Engl J Med*. 1980;303:769–775

21. Feigin RD. The perinatal group B streptococcal problem: more questions than answers [editorial]. *N Engl J Med*. 1976;294:106–107

22. Baker CJ, Kasper DL. Correlation of maternal antibody deficiency with susceptibility to neonatal group B streptococcal infection. *N Engl J Med*. 1976;294:753–756

23. Vogel LC, Boyer KM, Gadzala CA, Gotoff SP. Prevalence of type-specific group B streptococcal antibody in pregnant women. *J Pediatr*. 1980;96:1047–1051

24. Pyati SP, Pildes RS, Jacobs NM, et al. Penicillin in infants weighing two kilograms or less with early-onset group B streptococcal disease. *N Engl J Med*. 1983;308:1383–1389

25. Boyer KM, Gotoff SP. Prevention of early-onset neonatal group B streptococcal disease with selective intrapartum chemoprophylaxis. *N Engl J Med*. 1986;314:1665–1669

26. Rescorla FJ, Yoder MC, West KW, Grosfeld JL. Delayed presentation of a right-sided diaphragmatic hernia and group B streptococcal sepsis. *Arch Surg*. 1989;124:1083–1086

27. Baker CJ. Group B streptococcal cellulitis-adenitis in infants. *Am J Dis Child*. 1982;136:631–633

28. Fluegge K, Greiner P, Berner R. Late-onset group B streptococcal disease manifest by isolated cervical lymphadenitis. *Arch Dis Child*. 2003;88:1019–1020

29. Wessels MR, Kasper DL. The changing spectrum of group B streptococcal disease. *N Engl J Med*. 1993;328:1843–1844

30. Hickman ME, Ranch MA, Ferrieri P, Baker CJ. Changing epidemiology of group B streptococcal colonization. *Pediatrics*. 1999;104:203–209

31. Benitz WE. Perinatal treatment to prevent early-onset group B streptococcal sepsis. *Semin Neonatol*. 2002;7:301–314

32. Schrag SJ, Zell ER, Lynfield R, et al, Active Bacterial Core Surveillance Team. A population-based comparison of strategies to prevent early-onset group B streptococcal disease in neonates. *N Engl J Med*. 2002;347:233–239,

33. Centers for Disease Control and Prevention. Prevention of perinatal group B streptococcal disease. *Morbid Mortal Wkly Rep MMWR*. 2002;111:541–547

34. Velaphi S, Siegel JD, Wendel GD Jr, Cushion N, Eid WM, Sanchez PJ. Early-onset group B streptococcal infection after a combined maternal and neonatal group B streptococcal chemoprophylaxis strategy. *Pediatrics*. 2003;111:541–547

35. Paoletti LC, Madoff LC. Vaccines to prevent neonatal GBS infection. *Semin Neonatol*. 2002;7:315–323

Historical perspectives: Group B *Streptococcus* in Neonatal Sepsis: Emergence as an Important Pathogen

Alistair G. S. Philip

NeoReviews 2004;5;e467-e470
DOI: 10.1542/neo.5-11-e467

Newborn Metabolic Screening

The topic of metabolic screening of the newborn is perhaps not as exciting to the average neonatologist as some of the other topics in this book. Apart from anything else, most metabolic screening occurs in the well-baby nursery. However, the impact of metabolic screening on the lives of countless apparently well babies with metabolic disorders is a major accomplishment in neonatology. The ability to prevent neurobehavioral disorders with devastating consequences, by modifying the diet of these children, is truly remarkable. Although the primary role in counseling may be assumed by the geneticist, neonatologists should be familiar with these disorders.

Dr Harvey Levy describes the enormous contribution of Dr Robert Guthrie and the introduction of screening for phenylketonuria (PKU) and several other disorders. Somewhat later, the ability to screen for congenital hypothyroidism (which is considerably more common than PKU) provided additional impetus for the continuation of newborn metabolic screening (1). Recent expansion of metabolic screening from the five to six disorders that were evaluated for several decades to the 30 to 40 disorders that can be detected today by means of tandem mass spectrometry (2) is another leap forward. However, it also brings with it several ethical controversies that must be considered (3).

Alistair G. S. Philip, MD, FRCPE, FAAP
Editor-in-Chief, NeoReviews

References

1. Dussault JH, Coulombe F, Laberge C et al. Preliminary report on a mass screening program for neonatal hypothyroidism. *J Pediatr.* 1975;86:670–674.
2. Cowan TM. Neonatal screening by tandem mass spectrometry. *NeoReviews.* 2005;6:e539–e547.
3. Ross LF. Ethical and policy issues in newborn screening. *NeoReviews.* 2009;10:e71–e81.

Introduction

It began with Bob Guthrie's second child. John was mentally retarded. Because of this, Guthrie was stimulated toward research that could prevent mental retardation and other developmental disabilities.

In 1957, Guthrie was conducting cancer research at the Roswell Park Cancer Institute in Buffalo, NY. Because of John, Bob and his wife Margaret were very active in the Buffalo chapter of the New York State Association for Retarded Children. As Vice-President of the chapter, he was responsible for the program at the monthly meeting. He had heard that Dr Robert Warner, director of the newly established Children's Rehabilitation Center at Buffalo Children's Hospital, was doing work in developmental disabilities, so he invited Dr Warner to speak about his work at one of the meetings. At the meeting, Dr Warner discussed his work in treating children with mental retardation, some of whom had metabolic disorders. Over coffee after the meeting, Guthrie mentioned his interest in the prevention of mental retardation.

As a result of the meeting and especially the discussion after the meeting, the two kept in touch. About a year later, Dr Warner introduced Guthrie to phenylketonuria (PKU). Dr Warner explained that PKU was an inborn error of phenylalanine metabolism that caused mental retardation, but that when these retarded children received a special phenylalanine-restricted diet, not only did their blood phenylalanine levels decrease, but their behavior improved substantially. One problem in administering the diet, Dr Warner explained, was the difficulty with tests required to measure the blood phenylalanine levels for close monitoring of the patients. This persuaded Guthrie to try to produce a simpler method for measuring blood phenylalanine.

Guthrie thought such a test might be possible by modifying the *Bacillus subtilis* or *Escherichia coli* bacteria assays he was using to screen for different antimetabolites in blood from patients who were being treated for cancer. In those assays, he put a filter paper disc of serum from a patient on a bacterial plate containing agar not supplemented with thiamine or its pyrimidine moiety. If there was inhibition of bacterial growth around the disc and this inhibition was abolished when a second disc of serum from the patient was put on a plate containing supplemented agar, the serum contained the antimetabolite. In other words, the thiamine or its pyrimidine moiety effectively competed with the antimetabolite in the serum, and growth occurred.(1) Using this principle of competitive inhibition, he could develop a very simple test for serum phenylalanine by adding the well-known phenylalanine antagonist beta-2-thienylalanine to the agar. Instead of the antimetabolite that inhibited bacterial growth being in the serum and the competitor added to the agar, the antimetabolite was added in the phenylalanine assay, and the phenylalanine in the serum competed with the antimetabolite to allow growth. The greater the amount of phenylalanine in the serum, the more effective was the competition with the set amount of antimetabolite in the agar, and, hence, the greater the bacterial growth. He used this assay to monitor the serum phenylalanine levels in the individuals with PKU treated by Dr Warner.

From Cancer Research to the PKU Test

In 1958, Guthrie transferred from Roswell Park to Buffalo Children's Hospital, where he began to apply his bacterial assay system to the identification of PKU in retarded children. Initially, he tested urine from these children because it was easier to obtain than blood. However, during this time, a pivotal event occurred. His wife's 15-month-old niece who was developmentally delayed and autistic was diagnosed with PKU on the basis of the urine ferric chloride reaction, the standard diagnostic test used at that time. This greatly stimulated his interest in PKU. (2) He sought more information and learned that if dietary treatment began in the newborn period, the mental retardation from PKU could be prevented. (3) He also learned that the blood phenylalanine level in children who have PKU is increased within the first days after birth. (4) He then realized that perhaps his phenylalanine assay could be used to test every newborn, allowing those found to have PKU to be given the diet immediately and averting the mental retardation. At that point, he had used only serum for his test, and he knew that newborns could not be tested routinely if a venipuncture was required. The answer was to have the assay respond to blood dropped from a heel stick onto a filter paper. So, he used filter paper discs of whole blood for his assay, which worked as well as serum. He now had proof of principle.

The next step was to prove that his blood test could indeed detect PKU. He arranged for blood specimens to be collected in filter paper from residents of a school for the mentally retarded in upstate New York. All of the residents known from urine testing to have PKU were identified by his blood test as well as four additional residents with PKU who had not been detected by urine screening.

Newborn Screening for PKU

Convinced that his test could be used for routine screening of newborns for PKU, he exhibited his phenylalanine assay and its potential application to newborn screening at the 1961 annual meeting of the American Public Health Association. Dr Arthur Lesser, who was then the Director of the Maternal and Child Health Division of the United States Children's Bureau, saw the exhibit and immediately advocated a national trial of the test. In 1962, funds from the Children's Bureau were provided for this purpose. At the same time, the phenylalanine assay was set up at the Erie County Department of Health, which included Buffalo, and offered to newborn nurseries in the area hospitals. After 800 infants were screened, the first baby with PKU was identified.

At that point, Guthrie knew the test could detect PKU in newborns. Now the task was to get all newborns tested, which required a public health approach. For this, he needed to package the test for easy use in public health laboratories. The laboratories needed simply to open the package, mix the elements of the assay according to the directions, and perform the test with existing personnel rather than hire trained bacteriologists. The funds

from the Children's Bureau allowed for the rental of sufficient space to establish a small "factory" for preparing enough kits to screen 1 million infants. Each kit contained a plastic tray, glucose-salt medium powder, a bottle of agar powder to be combined with the medium powder, a vial of the beta-2-thienylalanine inhibitor, a vial of powdered *B subtilis* spores, a strip of filter paper containing spots of dried blood with known quantities of phenylalanine to be used as standards, and instructions for performing and interpreting the test. Training sessions were held in Buffalo for technicians from public health laboratories throughout the United States. At the completion of the 4-day session, the technicians were given the kits and filter paper cards for collection of blood specimens.

It is worth noting that one of the "technicians" who took the course was Dr Robert MacCready, Director of the Diagnostic Laboratory of the Massachusetts Department of Health. Dr MacCready was a physician who, like Guthrie, had a personal interest in the prevention of mental retardation because he had a child who had Down syndrome. Dr MacCready brought a test kit back to the Massachusetts laboratory, set it up in one of the rooms of the Diagnostic Laboratory, and asked pathologists in hospitals throughout the state to obtain blood specimens from newborns just before the babies were discharged from the nursery. By the fall of 1962, almost all newborns in Massachusetts were being screened for PKU, establishing the first universal newborn screening program in the world.

Publication of the PKU Test

The time had come to publish the test in a peer-reviewed journal so it would become widely known and accepted by the medical and scientific communities. Dr Guthrie thought that the journal should be one widely read by pediatricians. Late in 1962, after the testing of more than 100,000 newborns, he submitted the manuscript to a prominent pediatric journal. To his amazement and great disappointment, the manuscript was rejected. Instead, the journal published an article criticizing the test based on the screening of only 95 neonates. (5) An accompanying editorial

stated that routine newborn screening for PKU was premature and that attention instead should be devoted to case finding among high-risk populations and families that had a history of PKU. (6) Guthrie then submitted the manuscript to *Pediatrics,* where it was accepted, but not until he agreed to an additional delay of 6 months so a committee report on PKU screening could be included in the same issue. This seminal paper appeared in 1963. (7) Subsequently, Dr MacCready published letters to the editor in several prominent journals supporting the reliability of the test and its value in identifying PKU in the newborn based on the Massachusetts experience. Notable in one of these letters was the surprising information that among the first 53,000 newborns screened, nine cases of PKU were detected. (8) (This turned out to be "beginner's luck" because the frequency of PKU in Massachusetts now is known to be no greater than 1:12,000.) The "Guthrie test" for PKU was substantiated, eventually leading to establishment of the value of newborn screening and to the current much more comprehensive metabolic screening throughout the world. (9)

Newborn Screening Becomes a Reality

Although this marked the beginning of routine newborn screening, it took more than a publication or two to make universal newborn screening a reality. Guthrie and others knew that with the reluctance of many physicians to relinquish any authority over diagnosing disease and the lack of any organization among the many newborn nurseries spread throughout a state, having every newborn properly tested as a routine procedure would be extremely difficult. Already opposition to PKU screening was being voiced. (10) However, Guthrie was nothing if not determined. So, he spoke to lay groups throughout the country, especially local groups of the National Association for Retarded Children, about the value of his test in preventing mental retardation, and over the next few years, these groups persuaded their state legislators to pass laws requiring PKU screening of all newborns. The first such law was enacted in Massachusetts in 1963. By 1965, 32 states had passed a similar law. (11) Newborn screening was on its way.

Beyond PKU Screening

Guthrie did not stop with PKU. He knew of other metabolic disorders that seemed to fit into the same category as PKU in that the presence of a biochemical marker detectable in the blood of newborns caused mental retardation or other disabilities postnatally and was amenable to preventive dietary treatment. These disorders included maple syrup urine disease, homocystinuria, and galactosemia. He also learned that by substituting beta-2-thienylalanine as the chemical inhibitor with an analog of the amino acid he wanted to measure, his bacterial assay would respond to other amino acids (eg, leucine to detect maple syrup urine disease and methionine to detect homocystinuria). In addition, he and Dr Kenneth Paigen developed a different bacterial assay that responded to galactose for the detection of galactosemia. (12) These tests were added to newborn screening in several states and proved to be successful.

Thus began the multiple newborn screening we know today.

The Guthrie Specimen

Of the two components of Guthrie's system for newborn screening—the filter paper blood specimen and the bacterial assay for phenylalanine—the more lasting and the one with the most far reaching effect has been the specimen. Of course, newborn screening would not have begun without the simple assay for phenylalanine or without identifying a disorder that had the impact of PKU. However, the bacterial assay has been largely supplanted by newer technology. (9) The heel stick filter paper dried blood specimen (the "Guthrie specimen") is different. It is the key to newborn screening. It is collected easily and safely and transported efficiently to a central laboratory, the analytes are stable without special conditions of storage at least as long as required for screening, and there is sufficient blood for the continuing addition of screening tests. The Guthrie specimen now is used even well beyond newborn screening (eg, for secondary testing in newborn screening

programs and extensively for molecular testing and research). (13)

Newborn screening has revolutionized the field of metabolic disorders and has led to advances in endocrinology and hematology. With the current advances in genetics, there is little reason to doubt that many more genetic and quasi-genetic disorders will be screened in the future in the Guthrie specimen collected from the newborn or beyond the newborn period. As the future unfolds, we should remember that it all began with the dedication and simple genius of Bob Guthrie.

Harvey L. Levy, MD
Senior Associate in Medicine/Genetics
Children's Hospital Boston
Department of Pediatrics
Harvard Medical School
Boston, Mass.

[To read the original article on PKU testing written by Guthrie and Susi and published in *Pediatrics* in 1963, please go to: http://neoreviews.aappublications.org/cgi/full/6/2/e57/DC1 or http://pediatrics.aappublications.org/cgi/content/full/102/1/51/236]

References

1. Guthrie R, Loebeck ME, Hillman MJ. Sensitivity to analogs of thiamine pyrimidine associated with resistance to amethopterin or purine antagonists. *Proc Soc Exp Biol Med*. 1957;94:792–794

2. Koch JH. *Robert Guthrie – The PKU Story*. Pasadena, Calif: Hope Publishing House; 1977

3. Horner FA, Streamer CW, Clader DE, et al. Effect of phenylalanine-restricted diet in phenylketonuria II. *Am J Dis Child*. 1957;93:615–617

4. Horner FA, Streamer CW. Phenylketonuria treated from earliest infancy. *Am J Dis Child*. 1959;97:345–347

5. Scheel C, Berry HK. Comparison of serum phenylalanine levels with growth in Guthrie's inhibition assay in newborn infants. *J Pediatr*. 1962;61:610–616

6. Wright SW. Mass screening for phenylketonuria. *J Pediatr*. 1962;61:651–652

7. Guthrie R, Susi A. A simple phenylalanine method for detecting phenylketonuria in large populations of newborn infants. *Pediatrics*. 1963;32:338–342

8. MacCready RA. Phenylketonuria screening programs. *N Engl J Med*. 1963;269:52–53

9. Fearing MK, Levy HL. Expanded newborn screening using tandem mass spectrometry. *Adv Pediatr*. 2003;50:81–111

10. Kretchmer N, Day RW, Knudson A, et al. Phenylketonuria, and the Guthrie inhibition assay screening procedure. *Pediatrics*. 1963;32:344–346

11. Andrews LB. *State Laws and Regulations Governing Newborn Screening*. Chicago, Ill: American Bar Association; 1985

12. Guthrie R. Screening for "inborn errors of metabolism" in the newborn infant – a multiple test program. *Birth Defects Orig Art Ser*. 1968;4:92–98

13. Levy HL, Albers S. Genetic screening of newborns. *Annu Rev Genomics Hum Genet*. 2000;1:139–177

Historical Perspectives: Newborn Metabolic Screening
Harvey L. Levy
NeoReviews 2005;6;e57-e60
DOI: 10.1542/neo.6-2-e57

Transient Symptomatic Neonatal Hypoglycemia

Introduction

The accompanying article by Dr. Marvin Cornblath provides an excellent example of an all-too-common problem in medicine: The magnitude of concern about a medical disorder often is inversely related to the amount of accurate data defining it. In this case, Dr. Cornblath describes how concern for neonatal hypoglycemia has grown exponentially over the past 50 years. He also points out that those characteristics of low glucose concentration that might cause irreversible neuronal injury remain relatively undocumented and poorly defined. This problem likely will continue, because, despite Dr. Cornblath's repeated admonitions to conduct prospective studies, no one will conduct a prospective study in human infants to determine under what conditions low glucose concentrations cause "brain damage." We are left, then, with experimental observations that cells in culture stop working and eventually die when deprived of glucose (and alternative energy substrates) and that animals subjected to prolonged, severe glucose deficiency in time develop irreversible neuronal injury. We also know that iatrogenic hypoglycemia can lead to seizures and neurologic impairment. How should we proceed?

Charles Stanley argued in a 1999 *New England Journal of Medicine* editorial that normal infant glucose concentrations should be used as standards. (1) He took this stance primarily because he did not want anyone to miss rare but more severe forms of hypoglycemia, such as genetically defective potassium channels that cause persistent hyperinsulinemic hypoglycemia, (2) which are difficult to diagnose and treat and commonly are associated with neurodevelopmental impairment. Earlier, Alan Lucas (3) had argued in a 1988 *British Medical Journal* article that repeated low glucose concentrations (<47 mg/dL [2.6 mmol/L]) in preterm infants were associated with delayed neurodevelopment. Also, Srinivasin and associates (4) showed in the *Journal of Pediatrics* in 1986 that "normal" preterm infants, like "normal" term infants, achieved and maintained plasma glucose concentrations above approximately the same value estimated by Lucas by 12 hours after birth. In addition, Marconi and colleagues (5) showed in a 1996 article in *Obstetrics & Gynecology* that human fetuses who were born "normal" and "healthy" at term had umbilical venous glucose concentrations above 50 mg/dL (2.8 mmol/L) from mid-gestation (about 16 to 20 weeks) through term. Together, these disparate clinical data should reasonably define the lower limit of the statistically "normal" glucose concentration range in healthy infants as somewhere above approximately 45 mg/dL (2.5 mmol/L). They do not, however, define the glucose concentration below which brain damage necessarily occurs.

Beyond these clinical observations, we really do not know how low a glucose concentration must decline, for how long, and with what set and degree of contributing factors. There are many contributing factors, most of which have not been studied systematically with respect to their interaction with hypoglycemia on neurologic impairment and long-term abnormal developmental outcome. These include, but are not limited to, effect of prematurity, growth restriction, maternal diabetes, low concentrations of alternative energy substrates (eg, ketoacids and lactate), previous or concurrent hypoxia, hypotension, acidosis, anemia, polycythemia, hyperviscosity, reduced cerebral blood/plasma flow rate, and sepsis. Based on many reports, it is clear that transient (minutes to a few hours) low glucose concentrations (25 to 45 mg/dL [1.4 to 2.5 mmol/L]) in otherwise healthy infants are not associated directly with abnormal neurodevelopmental outcome. In fact, such "transient hypoglycemia" appears to be physiologic and even might be important in stimulating postnatal glycogenolysis and gluconeogenesis. At the least, therefore, we should be less strict about interpreting low glucose concentrations as universally bad (or a sign of malpractice) and pay more attention to recognizing and managing infants who are at risk for or actually have low glucose concentrations. Healthy infants should regulate their blood glucose concentrations into the normal range. Physicians should be alert to when this might not happen, and when it does not happen, try to determine the mechanism. Obviously, they also should try to correct the problem. This would satisfy the concerns raised by Dr. Cornblath and the many other interested parties, particularly the infants who are at the center of this controversial disorder.

William W. Hay, Jr, MD, FAAP
Co-Editor, NeoReviews

References

1. Stanley CA, Baker L. The causes of neonatal hypoglycemia [editorial]. *N Engl J Med.* 1999;340:1200–1201
2. Stanley CA. Hyperinsulinism in infants and children. *Pediatr Clin North Am.* 1997;44:363–374
3. Lucas A, Morley R, Cole TJ. Adverse neurodevelopmental outcome of moderate neonatal hypoglycemia. *BMJ.* 1998;297:1304–1308
4. Srinivasin G, Pildes RS, Cattamanchi G, et al. Plasma glucose values in normal neonates: a new look. *J Pediatr.* 1986;109:114–117
5. Marconi AM, Paolini C, Buscaglia M, et al. The impact of gestational age and fetal growth on the maternal-fetal glucose concentration difference. *Obstet Gynecol.* 1996;87:937–942

A Personal View of a Bittersweet Journey

Although blood sugar values have been measured in newborns since 1911, there was relatively little interest in this substrate during the first half of the 20th century. By 1930, it was known that blood sugar levels were lower in term newborns and even lower in preterm infants (<2.5 kg) than in older infants and children. In 1937, in the first extensive clinical study, Hartmann and Jaudon reported nine neonates among 285 infants and children who had varying degrees of severity of hypoglycemia defined as:

- Mild: 40 to 50 mg/dL (2.2 to 2.8 mmol/L) "true sugar" values
- Moderate: 20 to 40 mg/dL (1.1 to 2.2 mmol/L) "true sugar" values
- Extreme: <20 mg/dL (1.1 mmol/ L) "true sugar" values

These "true sugar" values were equivalent to glucose concentrations reported today.

However, Hartmann and Jaudon's important report had little to no impact on identifying or reporting additional neonates who had hypoglycemia. In the next 22 years between 1937 and 1959, only 10 additional infants who had hypoglycemia were reported. Nevertheless, the definitions and concepts of Hartmann and Jaudon, while still relevant, often are ignored today. They emphasized that all deviations from biologic norms represent a continuum of severity. They also pointed out the need for specific, accurate analytic methods that require only small amounts of capillary blood, remove nonglucose-reducing substances, and prevent glycolysis.

During the years after World War II (1947 to 1960), marked advances in biochemical and physiological measures of neonatal adaptation occurred, with the availability of micro-analyses in clinical biochemistry and physiology. These included specific micro determinations for assaying glucose that allowed surveys of relatively large numbers of preterm and term neonates both here and abroad for defining expected glucose values. Bedside techniques were developed for repetitive blood gases and pH determinations as well as oxygen and energy requirements.

As a result of these surveys, the consensus grew that even extremely low (0 to 10 mg/dL [0 to 0.56 mmol/L]) glucose concentrations were of no significance because they occurred both with and without clinical manifestations. Then, within a 10-month period during 1957, six newborns presented with symptomatic hypoglycemia during the first days after birth. In 1959, these infants plus two others from earlier in the decade were reported in an article as "Symptomatic Neonatal Hypoglycemia Associated With Toxemia of Pregnancy." By 1964, 50 additional patients who had similar presentations as well as 24 infants investigated personally had been reported. Although predominantly male, most of the infants were small for gestational age and were born to mothers who had toxemia (preeclampsia/eclampsia) of pregnancy (50%). All infants had clinical signs of hypoglycemia that included changes in levels of consciousness, episodes of tremors, irritability, lethargy, apnea, cyanotic spells, feeding poorly after feeding well, hypothermia,

seizures, hypotonia, limpness, and coma. All had laboratory blood and/or cerebrospinal fluid (CSF) glucose determinations of less than 10 to 25 mg/dL (0.56 to 1.4 mmol/L). Symptoms and laboratory values recovered promptly after therapy with feedings or infusions of glucose with or without steroids and did not recur.

The widespread and perhaps justified skepticism in the 1950s about the significance of low blood sugars in neonates required several strict criteria for diagnosis, including duplicate blood or CSF glucose analyses and satisfaction of Whipple's Triad:

- The presence of characteristic clinical signs
- Coincident low blood and/or CSF glucose concentrations measured accurately with sensitive and precise methods
- Resolution of clinical signs within minutes to hours once normoglycemia was re-established

Only when all the requirements were met was it possible to consider the diagnosis of clinically significant hypoglycemia.

If the signs did not clear with treatment, the hypoglycemia had to be considered secondary to an underlying condition that required different management. Such secondary hypoglycemia occurred with CNS pathology (infection, malformations, intraventricular hemorrhage), sepsis (gram-negative), congenital heart disease (left-sided anomalies), hypoxia, ischemia, endocrine deficiencies, or multiple congenital anomalies (trisomy 18 and 21). Similar manifestations without hypoglycemia may occur in newborns who have perinatal asphyxia, respiratory distress syndrome, other metabolic disorders, as well as intrauterine stresses and abnormalities throughout pregnancy, labor, and delivery. It is interesting to speculate what changes occurred in the 1950s and 1960s that resulted in the sudden appearance of this "syndrome" in so many newborns worldwide.

Initially, symptomatic neonatal hypoglycemia was accepted in most nurseries worldwide. Because hypoglycemia could be treated, it was considered possible to reduce the frequency of mental retardation and other consequences (eg, developmental delays). This coincided with one of the major objectives

of the newly created (1963) National Institute of Child Health, Human Development and Aging. Although severe, persistent, or recurrent hypoglycemia was reported to cause mental retardation and abnormalities of neurologic development, this causal relationship with transient symptomatic neonatal hypoglycemia was and remains tenuous at best. Both can occur together, but causation still remains uncertain and has never been tested in a prospective controlled clinical trial.

Nevertheless, the possibility of instituting early intervention prompted a search for methods to anticipate symptomatic and identify "asymptomatic" hypoglycemia. Indeed, the clinical reports of transient symptomatic hypoglycemia and studies of glucose metabolism in neonates revealed that low glucose concentrations were present hours before clinical signs occurred. In addition, the availability of the micro glucose methods made screening of "normal" term and preterm newborns practical. This allowed definition of statistical expressions for "hypoglycemia," "normoglycemia," and "hyperglycemia" and permitted intervention prior to the appearance of clinical signs. Because the "normal" concentrations depend on feeding practices and clinical support interventions, "abnormal" values derived from screening are arbitrary and of questionable value without follow-up data to indicate any untoward long-term effects. Yet, this concept and the resulting "cut-off value" defining abnormalities in glucose concentrations continue to be popular.

Concurrent with the flurry of publications, interest in neonatal carbohydrate metabolism and hypoglycemia increased exponentially with the availability of micro techniques to measure circulating concentrations of hormones and substrates. It became possible to develop protocols to examine both the potential mechanisms that caused and the damage, if any, that resulted from the low blood glucose levels. Thus, a significant fall in plasma glucose concentration provoked a measurable counterregulatory hormonal response in both adults and children. The increases in serum epinephrine, growth hormone, cortisol, and glucagon, together with free fatty acids, glycerol, and ketone bodies, could be defined. In addition, several studies over the next decade demonstrated the ability of the fetal and neonatal brain to use alternate fuels, such as ketone bodies and lactate, for oxidative metabolism, often in preference to glucose.

In the following years (1970 to 1988), while a number of new causes for and associations with hypoglycemia were being discovered, a group of investigators announced new definitions for hypoglycemia in newborns. Similar to definitions applied in adults, hypoglycemia was defined as glucose concentrations less than 40 mg/dL (2.2 mmol/L). By fiat, the defining levels increased from less than 20 to 25 mg/dL (1.1 to 1.4 mmol/L) in low-birthweight infants and less than 30 mg/dL (1.7 mmol/L) for term infants to less than 40 mg/dL (2.2 mmol/L) for all infants. There was no rationale or evidence for this change. On the positive side, new hypoglycemic syndromes that were reported included deficiencies in fructose diphosphatase, carnitine, and glucagon and multiple acyl-CoA dehydrogenase deficiency syndromes. New approaches were developed for congenital hypopituitarism, which was found to occur with congenital optic nerve hypoplasia, and the genetics of familial hyperinsulinemic hypoglycemia of infancy, which contributed to a better understanding of nesidioblastosis.

At this same time, more newborns were being screened with an ongoing series of "improved" bedside strip tests that continued to be inaccurate, especially in low glucose ranges (<45 mg/dL [2.5 mmol/L]), and inappropriate for diagnosing significant hypoglycemia during the first hours and days after birth even until today. These arbitrary definitions of hypoglycemia increased the frequency of hypoglycemia in otherwise healthy newborns.

In 1988, two publications changed the definition of transient neonatal hypoglycemia again. In a large, well-controlled feeding study of 661 infants whose birthweights were less than 1,850 g, 6,808 blood glucose levels were accumulated as part of the database. After multiple regression coefficients and correlation analyses, the authors concluded that five or more first morning glucose analyses of less than 47 mg/dL (2.5 mmol/L) any time during the first 2 months after birth were significantly correlated with poor Bayley Scores and an increased incidence of neuromotor function delays at 18 months of age. Interestingly, all of these poor outcome correlations disappeared by 8 years of age, although this result was not published until 1999 in a response letter to the editor. In another study, transient changes in brainstem auditory evoked responses occurred in five neonates who had hypoglycemia. In one, a minimal wave change was seen at glucose levels of 47 mg/dL (2.5 mmol/L), with obvious changes at levels of 13 to 29 mg/dL (0.72 to 1.6 mmol/L) in all. As a result, the level for defining neonatal hypoglycemia became less than 47 mg/dL (2.5 mmol/L). Neither study provided compelling evidence for this change, which resulted in an increased incidence of "hypoglycemia" and further confusion. A 1-day international meeting to define a rational normal blood glucose value in the neonate was unable to clarify the situation or arrive at a consensus.

At about the same time, other neuroglucopenic responses to induced hypoglycemia were found. Three hours of glucose values less than 30 mg/dL (1.67 mmol/L) in neonates weighing less than 1,800 g increased cerebral blood flow and epinephrine and norepinephrine responses. However, to demonstrate a causal relationship of these physiologic responses with significant hypoglycemia alone, a reversal of these responses following adequate glucose administration will need to be documented. Further research is needed to correlate acute changes in function with long-term effects on the brain.

Low neonatal glucose levels may be quite different in duration in those infants who may develop long-term damage. Defining the harmful parameters and the associated long-term sequelae will require new, carefully conducted and controlled prospective clinical trials in populations of infants who have different clinical and metabolic circumstances. The relaxation of specific criteria for diagnosis, including clinical symptoms and their response to therapy, continues to make management and diagnosis of neonatal hypoglycemia difficult.

Concurrent experimental work in adult rats and neonatal monkeys indicated that the former required an isoelectric electroencephalogram (EEG) and glucose level of less than 18 mg/dL (1.0 mmol/L) for 30 minutes to produce neuronal necrosis, and the latter tolerated 6 to 10 hours of glucose levels of less than 16 mg/dL (0.89 mmol/L) after birth without any significant sequelae. These further findings put in doubt the value of the new definitions of hypoglycemia.

Then, in 1999, again by fiat from Philadelphia, it was proclaimed that all glucose values less than 60 mg/dL (3.3 mmol/L) were hypoglycemic at any age in the neonate. To date, no basis for this recommendation has been published. Yet, newborns whose glucose concentrations are less than 60 mg/dL (3.3 mmolL) are being given intravenous glucose in the neonatal intensive care unit at great expense, pain to the neonate, and emotional trauma to parents and families without any known basis for doing so. Again, laboratory studies did not support these recommendations, when it was reported that neonatal pigs had to be maintained at blood glucose values of less than 10 mg/dL (0.56 mmol/L) with an isoelectric EEG before there was significant release of glutamate, a neurotoxic amino acid believed to be important in brain damage due to hypoglycemia.

Since the 1970s, a powerful factor influencing the definitions and lack of critical prospective, long-term, controlled studies of neonatal hypoglycemia has been the ever-increasing number of medical litigations involving "low" sugars and every type of neurologic or intellectual handicap known. Any glucose values a few milligrams less than the "cutoff" value between normo- and hypoglycemia for any period of time became the crucial fact that resulted in huge tax-free medical malpractice awards to plaintiffs and their lawyers. Thus, the arbitrary increases in glucose values defining "hypoglycemia" in the neonate have minimal medical effects, but far-reaching societal effects that are extremely costly.

I know of no way to stop these recent recommendations or their further escalations for defining blood glucose levels in newborns as hypoglycemia. Therefore, I suggest discarding the term "neonatal hypoglycemia" entirely except for those conditions with known cause and/or rational explanation. These would include any condition that involves severe, recurrent, or persistent low blood glucose (eg, glycogen storage disease, hyperinsulinemia, hypopituitarism, acyl-CoA dehydrogenase deficiency, etc). Obviously, this information would not be known initially. Therefore, those "adaptive fluctuations" in glucose levels occurring during the first days after birth that can be supported should not be designated as "hypoglycemia," with its connotation of disease, but rather should be defined by a new, different, nondisease term. "Operational thresholds" were suggested in May 2000 to indicate a range of values when interventions to raise the concentration of glucose might be considered. Other possible terms include "glucose operational scales" or "transient physiologic oligoglycemia." Follow-up would be critical to determine if extremely low levels of glucose occur, persist, or recur and are associated with other problems. Criteria for the application of these new designations would be similar to those recommended for "operational thresholds" (see the section on Operational Thesholds in the 2001 *Pediatrics* article available at http://www.pediatrics.org/cgi/content/full/105/5/1141). In addition, a return to clinical criteria, including reliable glucose determinations and notes reporting whether a response to glucose treatment occurred, would be an important addition to the evaluation and care plan.

Marvin Cornblath, MD
Lecturer in Pediatrics
Johns Hopkins University School of Medicine
Clinical Professor of Pediatrics
University of Maryland School of Medicine
Baltimore, MD

[For the original article by Dr. Cornblath and colleagues reporting the 24 infants who had symptomatic neonatal hypoglycemia, please go to: http://neoreviews.aap publications.org/cgi/data/4/1/e1/DC1 or http://pediatrics.aappublications/cgi/content/abstract/33/3/368]

Suggested Reading

Cornblath M, Hawdon JM, Williams AF, et al. Controversies regarding definition of neonatal hypoglycemia: suggested operational thresholds. *Pediatrics.* 2001;105:1141–1145

Cornblath M, Odell GB, Levin, EY. Symptomatic neonatal hypoglycemia associated with toxemia of pregnancy. *J Pediatr.* 1959;55:545–562

Cornblath M, Schwartz R, Aynsley-Green A, Lloyd JK. Hypoglycemia in infancy: the need for a rational definition: A Ciba Foundation discussion meeting. *Pediatrics.*1990;85:834–837

CornblathM, Wybregt SH, Baens GS, Klein RI. Symptomatic neonatal hypoglycemia: studies of carbohydrate metabolism in the newborn infant VIII. *Pediatrics.* 1964;33:388–402

Stanley CA, Baker L. The causes of neonatal hypoglycemia [editorial]. *N Engl J Med.* 1999;340:1200–1201

Historical Perspectives: Transient Symptomatic Neonatal Hypoglycemia
William W. Hay, Jr and Marvin Cornblath

NeoReviews 2003;4;1
DOI: 10.1542/neo.4-1-e1

Immediate Feeding of Preterm Infants

Introduction

In 1985, Thomas E. Cone, Jr, published his book *History of the Care and Feeding of the Premature Infant*. (1) In it, he provides a detailed historical perspective of the management of infants in the preceding century. One of the areas that set pediatricians apart in the first half of the 20th century was the attention they gave to feeding and nutrition. However, feeding the preterm infant was long considered a difficult task, with many differing opinions. In a recent Historical Perspectives, we highlighted how some of the difficulties were circumvented by the introduction of total parenteral nutrition, with a commentary by Heird and Driscoll. (2)

This month's perspective is provided by Dr. Pamela Davies, who collaborated with Dr. Victoria Smallpeice to introduce very early enteral feeding with human milk in preterm infants in 1964. (3) With the benefit of 40 years of hindsight, it may be difficult to appreciate how "against the grain" this approach was. Dr. Davies has been retired for more than 10 years now, but recalled their original contribution in an article published in 1991, (4) a significant portion of which (at her suggestion) we produce (with permission).

Although parenteral nutrition remains the preferred method for early feeding of the extremely low-birthweight infant (<1,000 g), an increasing tendency in recent years has been to introduce small amounts of enteral feeding to these tiny babies early in the postnatal period. Such "minimal enteral" or "trophic" feedings seem to provide benefits such as improved milk tolerance, better postnatal growth, and reduced rates of sepsis. (5) The research by Smallpeice and Davies dealt with babies whose birthweights were 1,000 to 2,000 g. In the upper half of this weight category, it is now "standard practice" to provide early feeding with human milk. We are pleased to highlight their significant contribution.

Alistair G. S. Philip, MD, FRCPE, FAAP
Editor-in-Chief, NeoReviews

References

1. Cone TE Jr. *History of the Care and Feeding of the Premature Infant.* Boston, Mass: Little, Brown & Co; 1985
2. Heird WC, Driscoll JM Jr. Total parenteral nutrition. *NeoReviews.* 2003;4:e137–e139. Available at: http://neoreviews. aappublications.org/cgi/content/full/4/6/e137
3. Smallpeice V, Davies PA. Immediate feeding of premature infants with undiluted breast milk. *Lancet.* 1964;ii:1349–1352
4. Davies PA. Low birth weight infants: immediate feeding recalled. *Arch Dis Child.* 1991;66:551–553
5. McClure RJ. Trophic feeding of the pre-term infant. *Acta Paediatr Suppl.* 2001;90:19–21

Low Birthweight Infants: Immediate Feeding Recalled

The following excerpts are taken from the article printed in Archives of Disease in Childhood. *1991;66:551–553 with permission.*

… At the beginning of the century it was felt that feeding should begin as soon as possible after birth to prevent death from inanition. But for Julius Hess, an American physician renowned then for his pioneering care of low birthweight infants in Chicago, and an advocate of an early start, this meant giving nothing the first 12 hours of life and one to three feeds of human milk, obtained from a wet nurse if necessary, in the second 12 hours, "if the infant's condition warrants." (1) The fear of aspiration of milk into the lungs was great. With feeble or absent sucking and swallowing reflexes in the most immature infants, and the tools for the job confined to spoon, pipette, or fountain pen filler, this is not surprising. However, some 27 years later Hess was to counsel that the period of starvation for babies weighing less than 1200 g should be 24–48 hours, subcutaneous injections of physiological saline being given in the interim. (2) Mary Crosse, who started the first "premature baby unit" in the United Kingdom, also changed her mind. In the first edition of *The Premature Baby*, published in 1945, she advised a 12 hour initial fast with dilute milk delayed to the third or fourth day. In the third, fourth, and fifth editions (the latter published in 1961) she advised that the first 24–96 hours should be without fluids of any kind. (3)

This was despite the fact that feeding techniques were advancing, for oesophageal gavage feeding with rubber tubes had been practiced in the 1940s and plastic indwelling nasogastric tubes became available in the early 1950s. And although two voices opposed the prolonged starvation period, (4)(5) "scientific" rather than practical reasons for the delay were appearing. Clement Smith, noted for his work on the physiology of the newborn infant in Boston, Massachusetts, proposed in 1949 that as many low birthweight infants were oedematous and excreted large amounts of urinary sodium and potassium in the first days of life, oedema would be increased and prolonged if solutions containing sodium were given. (6) Smith was an influential voice in the United States and United Kingdom. He had persuaded Gaisford and Schofield in Liverpool to impose further extremes of starvation, even up to 111 hours, (7) and at a meeting in Finland disagreed with Yllpo, who believed starved babies became acidotic and should be given 5% glucose solution in the first 24 hours.

Hints of a change in attitude, however, were evident from 1960 onwards. In America Bauman reported a controlled trial in which preterm infants were given either 5% dextrose in 0.45% saline by nasogastric drip starting six hours after birth or nothing until the age of 36 hours, when both groups started milk feeds. Neither beneficial nor detrimental effects were recorded. (8) …. In the United Kingdom Laurance and Hutchinson-Smith also reported less jaundice among pre-term infants fed early rather than late with undiluted breast milk. (9) Clement Smith, in his Borden Award address in 1962 considered he had been wrong in 1949 to put oedema forward as a reason for delaying feeding; most preterm infants were not oedematous at birth, though various stresses such as cold might make them so. He believed feeding techniques were improving fast so that aspiration was less common. He still nevertheless felt that the low birthweight infant could manage without added energy initially as he considered the babies had enough stored glycogen and fat, and tissue protein available for catabolism, to prevent them dying of inanition. (10)

Victoria Smallpeice, clinical director of the pediatric department in the United Oxford Hospitals, had felt increasingly uneasy about such a practice for some time. She argued that the nourishment afforded the fetus via the placenta was continuous and that it made little sense to stop supplying it abruptly at birth and over the period of highest mortality.... She heard the professor of surgery at the Institute of Child Health, London – Andrew Wilkinson – speak at an international congress of pediatrics in Lisbon in 1962 on the metabolic costs of starvation in newborn infants undergoing surgery and the reparative effect of early feeds of undiluted breast milk on this chemical chaos. This fitted in with McCance's concept of continued growth being all important in the maintenance of normal homeostasis. (11) These ideas excited her, and she returned home from the Lisbon meeting resolved to start feeding low birthweight infants very soon after birth with expressed undiluted human milk. Her colleague Hugh Ellis generously allowed all infants weighing 1000–2000 g born in or admitted to the Nuffield Maternity Home at the Radcliffe Infirmary to be under her care for a trial period. This started in November 1962 and continued until the end of March 1964, by which time 111 infants had been included. Eight of the original 119 of the stipulated weight range had to be excluded: two because of oesophageal atresia, one whose admission was delayed until the fourth day, and five during the early part of the trial who died within four hours after birth without being fed.

The babies were fed via an indwelling nasogastric polyvinyl tube and were given 60 ml/kg of undiluted human milk in the first 24 hours of life, 90 ml/kg on the second day, 120 ml/kg on the third, and 150 ml/kg on the fourth. That this break with traditional care was introduced with apparent ease was largely due to the enthusiasm and skill of the young nursing staff. The trial was uncontrolled, but comparison was made with the first 45 infants of the same birthweight cared for at the Churchill Hospital, Oxford, over the same time period, by the same medical staff, but fed later. The early fed infants had lower mean serum bilirubin concentrations and passed their first meconium and regained birthweight at earlier mean times (all p<0.05). Twenty seven of the 111 (24%) early fed infants died, as did 12 of 45 (27%) of the later fed.

The paediatric section of the Royal Society of Medicine held its summer meeting in Oxford in 1964, and these results were reported there. (12)

I think it is fair to say they were listened to with some interest, but doubt and skepticism were also evident. The results were later recorded in more detail in the *Lancet,* (13) and a few months later an editorial there adopted a rather lofty tone of disapproval, implying that any possible advantages were outweighed by the risks, and that if "nature" had created the healthy mature human infant to observe "temperance and moderation" over his first drink, then presumably she also knew best where the preterm infant was concerned. (14) The nature argument did not cut much ice with Smallpeice and Davies, who knew that many full term infants would suck avidly at the breast within a short time of birth given the chance, and who felt she was a poor model for the preterm infant, mortality in that situation being nearly 100%. But was the *Lancet* editorial right about the risk? Perinatal mortality for infants weighing 1000–2000 g at the Radcliffe Infirmary was lower in the single full year of the trial (1963) than in any year since records were first available there (1952), but this was not a controlled trial. Towards the end of 1965 Wharton and Bower published the results of such a trial undertaken at the Sorrento Maternity Hospital, Birmingham, the unit from which Mary Crosse had lately retired. (15) A total of 239 infants were involved, alternate admissions being fed within two to eight hours (usually within two to four hours of birth) using volumes similar to those used at Oxford, the remainder being fed at 12 to 16 hours with much smaller amounts. The mortality in the early fed group was 17%, and in the later fed group 6% (p<0.01). When deaths considered inevitable or "due to factors other than immediate feeding" were excluded, a substantial difference (13.8% compared with 5.8%) remained but did not reach significance. Wharton and Bower reported that in some very preterm infants in the early fed group "apnoeic attacks with cyanosis and circulatory failure were regularly occurring after each feed"; six of 20 infants who died in this group were considered to have aspirated feeds. Bilirubin concentrations were significantly lower and birthweight was regained significantly earlier in the immediately fed group (p<0.01 for both). Symptomatic hypoglycaemia occurred in four of the later fed group, one of whom died, but in none of the early fed group. The authors reported they intended to continue early feeding with undiluted breast milk, but reduce the volumes by a third. In Oxford, no change was made....

Were there harmful effects of immediate feeding? The increased mortality of the alternate case trial at Birmingham has already been referred to; careful review of the Wharton and Bower paper led us to believe the verdict was not proved. But in any event both trials have been largely overtaken by the increasing survival of very immature babies, and a single regimen of feeding suitable for all low birthweight infants can no longer be prescribed. The larger number of infants with birthweights less than 1000 g now surviving was the spur for further research into their nutritional requirements. (16) The skill and care with which young doctors and nurses developed parenteral feeding were in no small measure responsible for lowering mortality. Few would deny that it can occasionally have serious, even lethal, complications, but used for short periods in the transitional stage after birth when respiratory illness is most likely it has proved invaluable. I resisted it for too long....

Drillien recorded particularly poor results at follow up of low birth-weight children in

Edinburgh in two years (1953 and 1954) when fluid had been withheld completely for the first three to four days of life there, milk not being introduced until the fifth to ninth days, a truly Spartan regimen. (17) While no one today would venture feeding breast milk within an hour or two of birth to a 500 g infant, I think it is likely that those of low birthweight will ever again be starved as they largely were when Victoria Smallpeice – with vision and not a little courage – inaugurated her trial of early feeding with human milk in 1962. Her belief that their nutrition should be interrupted as briefly as possible so that growth could be resumed soon after birth is likely to endure....

Pamela A. Davies, MD, FRCP, HON. FRCPCH, DCH

[To read the original article on immediate feeding of preterm infants with undiluted human milk written by Smallpeice and Davies in 1964, which was reprinted with permission from Elsevier (*The Lancet.* 1964;ii: 1349–1352), please go to: http://neo reviews.aappublications.org/cgi/content/full/5/2/e29/DC1]

References

1. Hess JH. *Premature and Congenitally Diseased Infants.* Philadelphia, Pa: Lea and Febiger; 1922:179

2. Hess JH, Lundeen EC. *The Premature Infant. Medical and Nursing Care.* Philadelphia, Pa: JB Lippincott Co; 1949:115

3. Crosse VM. *The Premature Baby.* London, United Kingdom: J & A Churchill; 1945:42–72. (3rd ed 1952, 4th ed 1957, 5th ed 1961)

4. Yllpö A. Premature children. Should they fast or be fed in the first days of life? *Ann Paediatr Fenn.* 1954–55;1:99–104

5. Gleiss J. Zum Frühgeborenenproblem der Gegenwart. IX. Mitteilung. Uber futterungs-und umweltbedingte Atemstörungen bei Frühgeborenen. *Zentral Kinderheil.* 1955;76:261–268

6. Smith CA, Yudkin S, Young W, Minkowski A, Cushman M. Adjustment of electrolytes and water following premature birth (with special reference to edema). *Pediatrics.* 1949;3:34–48

7. Gaisford W, Schofield S. Prolongation of the initial starvation period in premature infants. *BMJ.* 1950;i:1404–1405

8. Bauman WA. Early feeding of dextrose and saline solution to premature infants. *Pediatrics.* 1960;26:756–761

9. Laurance BM, Hutchinson-Smith B. The premature baby's diet. *Lancet.* 1962;1:589–590

10. Smith CA. Prenatal and neonatal nutrition. Borden Award address. *Pediatrics.* 1962;30:145–156

11. McCance RA. The maintenance of stability in the newly born. 1. Chemical exchange. *Arch Dis Child.* 1959;34:361–370

12. Smallpeice V, Davies PA. The immediate feeding of babies weighing 1,000–2,000 g with breast milk. *Proc R Soc Med.* 1964;57:1173–1175

13. Smallpeice V, Davies PA. Immediate feeding of premature infants with undiluted breast-milk. *Lancet.* 1964;ii:1349–1352

14. Anonymous. The first drink [editorial]. *Lancet.* 1965;1:791–792

15. Wharton BA, Bower BD. Immediate or later feeding for premature babies? A controlled trial. *Lancet.* 1965;ii:969–972

16. Shaw JCL. Growth and nutrition of the very preterm infant. *Br Med Bull.* 1988;44:984–1009

17. Drillien CM. *The Growth and Development of the Prematurely Born Infant.* Edinburgh, Scotland: E & S Livingstone; 1964:302–308

Historical Perspectives: Immediate Feeding of Preterm Infants
Alistair G. S. Philip and Pamela A. Davies
NeoReviews 2004;5;29
DOI: 10.1542/neo.5-2-e29

Neonatology: The Long View

Introduction

This month's contribution to our series of Historical Perspectives is a slight departure from our standard format. Instead of focusing on a seminal paper or important topic in the development of neonatology, Robert Usher, MD, provides a personal view of the evolution of neonatology during the past half century or so. Dr Usher is one of the true pioneers in North American neonatology who has made an enormous contribution to neonatal/perinatal medicine, not only in Quebec, but also in many other parts of the world (recognized by his receipt of the Apgar Award in the year 2000). His contributions are diverse, but, as noted in the following section, started with his evaluation of the metabolic component of the respiratory distress syndrome (RDS).

As a pediatric resident, I learned about the "Usher regime" for managing neonates who had RDS using continuous intravenous glucose and bicarbonate supplementation. A visiting professor agreed that Dr Usher's results were impressive, but expressed the opinion that it might be the selfless devotion of Dr Usher to his patients rather than the regime itself that produced these good results. Almost certainly, it was a combination of the two.

As a fellow in neonatology, my research centered on the role of placental transfusion and its effect on circulating blood volume and hematocrit. This was an area previously studied by Dr Usher both with Professor John Lind at the Karolinska Institute in Stockholm [1][2] and on his return to Montreal. [3] The role of placental transfusion in preventing RDS was being postulated at that time, and Dr Usher and colleagues later provided support for this hypothesis. [4]

I made another connection with Dr Usher's work when I later became intrigued with observations he made with Kenneth Scott on bone development in term infants born with intrauterine growth restriction (IUGR), which they called fetal malnutrition syndrome. [5] I was able to add some observations about fontanelle size (and membranous bone growth) to their observations on delayed epiphyseal ossification at the knee. [6]

Subsequently, Dr Usher's work on developing a regionalized system of care for the province of Quebec and his evaluation of neonatal mortality in the region had an important influence on my own participation in a regional perinatal program and consideration of factors influencing neonatal outcome. [7]

Bob Usher always has held strong opinions and had a very direct and enthusiastic teaching style (at least in formal lectures). In the following section, he provides one man's opinion of important factors that changed the way we practice neonatology and what still needs to be done to overcome persistent problems. It is interesting to note how many of the contributions that he considers important have generated previous Historical Perspectives. Others may disagree with his comments, but I hope that this stimulates some discussion and that readers will use e-letters to share their personal perspectives.

We all benefit from our teachers and mentors, particularly those with whom we work directly. Bob Usher is someone with whom I did not work directly, but he had a great influence on my thinking and development. It is a pleasure to present his contribution to the readers of *NeoReviews*.

Alistair G. S. Philip, MD, FRCPE, FAAP
Editor-in-Chief, NeoReviews

References

1. Usher R, Shephard M, Lind J. The blood volume of the newborn infant and placental transfusion. *Acta Paediatr Scand*. 1963;52:492–512
2. Usher R, Lind J. Blood volume of the newborn premature infant. *Acta Paediatr Scand*. 1965;54:419–431
3. Buckels LJ, Usher R. Cardiopulmonary effects of placental transfusion. *J Pediatr*. 1965;67:239–247
4. Usher RH, Saigal S, O'Neill A, Surainder Y, Chua L-B. Estimation of red blood cell volume in premature infants with and without respiratory distress syndrome. *Biol Neonate*. 1975;26:241–248
5. Scott KE, Usher R. Epiphyseal development in fetal malnutrition syndrome. *N Engl J Med*. 1964;270:822–824
6. Philip AGS. Fontanel size and epiphyseal ossification in neonates with intrauterine growth retardation. Preliminary communication. *J Pediatr*. 1974;84:204–207
7. Philip AGS. Neonatal mortality: is further improvement possible? *J Pediatr*. 1995;126:427–433

Development of Neonatology

I was asked to describe my approach in the unit I ran from the late 1950s until the turn of the century and to give a perspective on how neonatology has developed during this time, where it has gone astray, and the challenges I see for the future. I hope to share some sense of the excitement we have experienced as research has led to incredible progress in so many different areas.

RDS

Clinical Aspects

Arriving back in Montreal at the Royal Victoria Hospital (RVH) in 1957, I had a grant to do research on some aspect of newborn care. I chose hyaline membrane disease (later called RDS), which was then the major cause of neonatal death. At that time, RDS developed in 14% of infants weighing 1 to 2.5 kg, and 56% of them died. Their deaths accounted for 50% of the deaths of all infants of low birthweight. Even one third of infants who weighed 2 to 2.5 kg and had RDS died of the condition.

My studies described the 3-day clinical course of the disease, the development of the patent ductus arteriosus (PDA) murmur during recovery, and perhaps most importantly, the contribution of cesarean section delivery to the development of RDS, even if delivery was only 2 weeks prior to term. [1][2][3][4]

Hyperkalemia

My major finding then was the hyperkalemic electrocardiographic changes that developed in most infants after 12 hours of distress and often led to death. (5) This was associated with a catabolic state of acidosis and azotemia. (2) Remember that such distressed babies were not fed until their distress resolved several days later. A randomized, controlled trial of intravenous glucose and bicarbonate as a constant infusion was instituted to control this catabolic state and resulted in a reduction in mortality from 37% to 17% among affected infants weighing 900 to 2,500 g. (6) During the 1960s, such infusions became standard treatment. It was only at this time that microchemistry allowed capillary sampling and micro-butterfly scalp vein needles (designed by me and made by our instrument shop engineer) allowed continuous infusion by peripheral veins in even the smallest babies. Subsequently, intravenous fluids have been standard therapy, although bicarbonate now seldom is employed.

Respirators

The use of respirators was introduced in the mid-1960s by Paul Swyer. (7) Their benefit was tempered by a sharp increase in the risk of pneumothorax and chronic lung disease. The latter was described as bronchopulmonary dysplasia (BPD) by Northway, Rosan, and Porter (8) and occurred even in larger infants. A major development in the management of RDS occurred in the early 1970s when Gregory and associates introduced continuous positive airway pressure (CPAP). (9) This has become standard therapy in managing many cases of RDS as well as apneic spells without need for intubation or intermittent positive pressure ventilation (IPPV). Today, high-frequency ventilation and nitric oxide also are available. Their appropriate role now is being assessed.

Oxygen Monitoring

Continuous monitoring of blood oxygen tensions became feasible by 1980 with the introduction of transcutaneous (Tc)Po_2 measurements by the Huchs, and later $TcPco_2$ measurements. (10) It was only in the mid-1980s that the pulse oximeter was developed, which provided constant readouts of oxygen saturation. (11) We now await the development of a means of servocontrolling oxygen delivery

via the baby's oxygen saturation on pulse oximetry. This would avoid the wide variation in saturation that occurs frequently on ventilators when there are sudden drops in oxygen saturation, usually followed by an overshoot in arterial oxygen tension as the nurse corrects the hypoxemia.

Glucocorticoid Prophylaxis

Liggins in New Zealand was studying the role of glucocorticoids in the onset of preterm labor in the pregnant ewe when he noted that the preterm lambs so produced had much more mature lung function than naturally occurring preterm lambs. He showed in 1972 that when betamethasone was administered to mothers for at least 24 hours up to 7 days prior to preterm birth, the incidence of RDS was reduced by 50%. (12) By the 1990s, this became standard prophylaxis. At least 24 hours of therapy can be achieved in two thirds of births before 34 weeks' gestation.

Surfactant

In 1959, Avery and Mead found that lungs of babies dying of hyaline membrane disease had much less surfactant activity than those dying of other causes. (13) After several unsuccessful attempts to use exogenous surfactant, Fujiwara and colleagues in Japan in the early 1980s finally documented dramatic effects of endotracheal instillation of a calf lung surfactant. (14) Safety and efficacy subsequently have been proven in a multitude of studies through the 1980s. What remain as questions are not whether, but when and how to use surfactant. Prophylactically? If so, to whom? Therapeutically? If so, to all infants who have RDS or only to those in whom the condition is life-threatening? What is its role in the borderline viable infant who does not have RDS?

I pose these questions because we at the RVH were conservative in introducing surfactant therapy, using it only for therapy of moderate cases of RDS in extremely low-birthweight (ELBW) infants and for severe cases in infants weighing more than 1,200 g. With this policy during the 1990s, we had almost no losses from RDS among infants weighing more than 1,000 g, excellent

survival rates of infants born at 22 to 27 weeks' gestational age, and a lower-than-average incidence of bronchopulmonary dysplasia.

Fetal Malnutrition (IUGR)

Working in a maternity hospital during the 1960s, I found that 1 baby in 60 was born dead. Fetal malnutrition in our terminology (IUGR today) became a major area of interest in the 1960s. IUGR proved to be one of the most frequent causes of fetal death. Using our then primitive database, we found that predisposing factors included severe maternal hypertension, underweight mothers, and familial tendency shown by IUGR in siblings. (15) Unfortunately, at that time we did not record cigarette smoking on our charts, which soon proved to be the cause of 40% of cases of IUGR. By the 1970s, with a Quebec-wide database, we found that 44% of women smoked during their pregnancy. The incidence of IUGR doubled with moderate smoking of up to one pack per day, tripling in the 11% of mothers who smoked more than one pack per day. Because smoking also predisposed to preterm birth, the incidence of low birthweight in the province rose from 4% in nonsmokers to 13% in heavy smokers. (16)

Subsequently, suspected cases of IUGR were confirmed by fetal ultrasonography and carefully followed by nonstress tests and biophysical profiles. Over the last 30 years, IUGR as a cause of fetal death decreased from 1 in 400 to 1 in 1,400 births. (17) It remains, however, along with abruptio placenta, as one of the two leading causes of fetal death. We find routine mid- to late pregnancy ultrasonography screening to be useful in detecting IUGR. Infants who exhibit IUGR at birth should have their blood glucose measured in the first hours after birth. Cornblath and associates demonstrated in the 1960s that such infants may develop severe, potentially damaging or lethal degrees of hypoglycemia at this time. (18)

Bilirubin

Major breakthroughs in the 1960s included the introduction of Rh immunoglobulin prophylaxis for Rh-negative mothers (19) and the discovery of phototherapy to prevent dangerous levels of hyperbilirubinemia. (20)(21) Prior to 1967, the neonatologist spent much of his or her time performing exchange transfusions in term babies whose bilirubin concentrations rose to 20 mg/dL (342 mcmol/L) or in preterm infants who had lower levels of bilirubin. This potentially hazardous procedure now is needed so seldom that many trainees never have performed it. (22) How stringent a monitoring program is needed in the first week after birth? How safe or dangerous are high bilirubin levels in otherwise healthy term infants? (23) At our hospital, we test about one third of babies who have more-than-average jaundice on discharge at 36 hours (3 to 4 d for infants delivered by cesarean section) and request 10% of babies who have the most worrisome levels to return the next day for outpatient testing. About 10% of this 10% are readmitted for risk of developing hyperbilirubinemia at or above 18 mg/dL (308 mcmol/L). Such infants usually require phototherapy for only 24 hours.

The development of the Rh antibody prophylactic program in the late 1960s is probably the most important discovery of our time. (19) Prior to its initiation, 1 in 100 babies was affected with the disease and had a high risk of intrauterine death or neonatal hydrops. Many exchange transfusions were needed to prevent kernicterus. (22) With prophylactic Rh antibody injection after delivery, 95% of cases are prevented. This early injection, combined with a 28-week injection, has practically eliminated the condition. (24)

Regionalization

From a public health standpoint, regionalization has been one of the greatest accomplishments of our field. In 1967, the Quebec government, on the advice of a very politically active Professor of Obstetrics, Dr Roger Brault, became convinced that improvements in perinatal mortality could be achieved. They mandated perinatal mortality committees within each of the 140 hospitals to review their deaths and submit information on questionnaires to a central committee. This committee evolved into a very effective voluntary program of regionalization of high-risk pregnancy care in the province. (25)

By 1974, it had become apparent that among infants born in large hospitals in Quebec, neonatal mortality was markedly lower in hospitals providing neonatal intensive care. (26) Infants weighing 1 to 1.5 kg, for example, had a much higher neonatal mortality (45%) if they were born in hospitals that did not refer to pediatric centers. It was lower (25%) in hospitals that did so. It was lowest (15%) in institutions where neonatal intensive care was available from birth. Today, almost all infants of very-low-birth-weight (VLBW) born in Quebec are delivered in appropriate perinatal centers, often after maternal referral in preterm labor, sometimes after a flight of more than 1,000 miles from the Arctic Circle.

The Very Preterm Baby
Survival Rates

Prevention of preterm births has been the least successful aspect of perinatal research in my time. More than 7% of infants continue to deliver before 37 weeks' gestation, and almost 1% before 31 weeks' gestation. This 1% accounts for almost all of the nonmalformation-related neonatal deaths today.

Treatment of very preterm babies has been remarkably successful. A survival rate of 50% now is possible for infants born at 24 weeks' gestation or weighing 600 g. (27) compared with 28.5 weeks' gestation and 1,150 g birthweight in the 1960s. Neurologic handicaps now occur rarely in infants of 1,000 to 1,500 g as they did before; they are of major concern for the infant weighing less than 1,000 g at birth.

Care at Birth and Use of Surfactant

At the borderline of viability (which today is at 22 through 24 weeks' gestation), parental consent always is obtained before initiating intensive care. Staff neonatologists meet with the parents before the delivery to review immediate and long-term risks. (28) Intubation and ventilation necessary for survival are not instituted for such infants if parents decide against these procedures. Sometimes the parents leave the decision to the neonatologist, depending on the baby's condition at birth. Such deliveries always are attended by a staff neonatologist. Some 30% of

infants born at these gestational ages in our hospital during the 1990s were allowed to die quickly, untreated.

In a study of our experience of treated infants of 22 to 27 weeks' gestational age, survival was related to both administration of 24-hour antenatal steroid therapy and to a 1-minute Apgar score of 4 or greater. Because condition at birth is of such major importance in survival, it is imperative to attempt to understand which factors are important determinants of the immature baby's condition when born.

During the 1990s, our care in the delivery room for very preterm babies consisted of bag-and-mask ventilation as needed, using intubation only if the ventilation was not rapidly effective. Intubation was required in only 5% of the babies born at 28 to 31 weeks' gestation and 25% of those born at 25 to 27 weeks' gestation. Even at 22 to 24 weeks' gestation, 33% of those for whom we had parental approval to treat did not require intubation at delivery. Infants born before 28 weeks' gestation, although often not intubated at birth, required intubation in later hours to treat RDS or apneic spells. However, they had been allowed to establish ventilation on their own for the first hours after birth. Surfactant was used only later in the neonatal intensive care unit (NICU) for significant RDS. With this conservative approach to resuscitation, our mortality rates for very preterm infants were comparable or better than most published for this period of time. At 22 weeks' gestation, 22% of infants survived; at 24 weeks' gestation, 50% survived. Of the 35 infants of 22 to 24 weeks' gestation who survived, only nine had received surfactant therapy; it was used in almost all of the fatal cases that had more significant respiratory distress. (29)

Now we have begun using a more interventional approach. Extremely preterm infants are intubated and receive surfactant in the first minutes after birth. Does the benefit of such prophylactic management exceed the risks? Is the physiologic opening and aeration of the lungs at birth by the baby's own efforts (often supported by a few moments of bagging followed, at times, by nasal CPAP) more conducive to good pulmonary function than the IPPV provided by a machine through an endotracheal tube? This aspect of neonatal care needs further study with randomized, prospective, controlled trials.

Hypotension

Another common intervention that we have resisted is the treatment of hypotension in preterm infants early in their course using volume expansion or drugs. Our early studies in the 1950s showed that blood pressure, which was slightly lower in infants who had RDS, did not relate to survival and did not decrease prior to death in fatal cases. Not being convinced of the benefits compared with the risks, we have, therefore, not treated hypotension. (29) One concern is that volume expansion can produce intraventricular hemorrhage (IVH), of which we see little, or impair pulmonary function. The recent comparison of outcomes in various Canadian NICUs does not indicate that such treatment is associated with lower mortality, but rather the reverse. The multicenter randomized, controlled trial protocol being proposed by Dr. Keith Barrington to study the outcomes of volume, pharmacologic, or no specific treatment for hypotension is needed urgently.

Humidity

Humidity is very important for very preterm infants because there is a high rate of evaporative water loss, with heat loss through the very porous skin during the first few days after birth. The humidified incubator of the pre-1990s had a bath of water lying in a well underneath the tray on which the baby lay. Warm air passed over the water, picking up humidity. However, experience by the mid-1960s showed that the risk of acquired infection from water-borne bacteria, usually *Klebsiella* and *Pseudomonas* sp, was so great that most of us preferred to use dry incubators and simply provide high fluid intakes and higher ambient temperatures in the immediate postnatal period. Dehydration hypernatremia up to 150 to 160 mEq/L (150 to 160 mmol/L) was common. Fluid intakes of 200 mL/kg often were necessary during the first 2 or 3 days after birth.

It was only in the 1990s that new techniques became available to dispense humidity from fluid extruded very slowly from a sterile container and vaporized into the air as it left the container. With this safe form of humidity, fluid requirements after birth were reduced markedly. Hypernatremia no longer was a problem. Interestingly, the frequency of hyperkalemia also was reduced, perhaps due to lower catabolic rates with less energy loss. The fragile skin of these very preterm babies is maintained much better with humidity, and body temperatures are easier to maintain. Very preterm babies now are placed in 60% to 70% humidity in incubators by 1 hour after birth.

Nutrition, Intestinal

This is a major challenge for the very preterm infant. Intestinal tolerance often takes weeks and occasionally 1 to 2 months to develop. Abdominal distention, gastric residuals, and difficulty passing stools are the norm.

There now is general agreement that small milk intakes by gastric tube can be administered safely and may be beneficial from the first day or two after birth. The rate of increase often is scheduled at 10 to 15 kcal/kg per day, leading to full milk intake by day 7 to 10. Rare, however, is the very preterm baby who tolerates that schedule. (30)

Little is understood of the factors that determine intestinal capacity to acccept milk feedings. Some babies who have severe pulmonary disability have good milk tolerance or vice versa. Further, some babies tolerate rapidly increasing feedings for a number of days and then for no apparent reason, without any signs of necrotizing enterocolitis, become distended and need bowel rest. We offer 2-hour intermittent feedings by indwelling orogastric tube. We test gastric residuals before each feeding to avoid regurgitation if these start to increase. We use glycerin suppositories if there is any distention and no stools have been passed for 24 hours.

We had a remarkably successful experience in the 1990s using the intestinal motility agent cisapride in ELBW infants who had intractable problems of abdominal distention for at least 3 weeks after birth that prevented

any but minimal milk intake. (31) Unfortunately, cisapride has been withdrawn from the market because of potential adverse effects. Hopefully, some other pharmacologic therapy may be discovered for these infants' intestinal motility problems. We monitor intestinal tolerance by recording on our database the age at which full milk feedings were established and the number of days when milk feedings had to be stopped for intestinal intolerance. We recently switched from using mineral-enriched concentrated formula in most VLBW infants to human milk with added calorie- and mineral-enriched supplement. We are watching closely for signs of intestinal tolerance and hope to see a benefit. In any case, mothers and nurses are very happy with the change.

The need for mineral enrichment only became apparent in about 1980. Studies performed at our hospital and elsewhere in the early 1980s showed the need to use mineral enrichment to prevent demineralization and pathologic fractures, significant problems seen previously in the smallest infants as they grew.

Nutrition, Parenteral

Parenteral nutrition consisted of glucose, water, and electrolytes until the late 1960s, when Heird at Columbia and others began using amino acid solutions as well. (32) Energy intake always was insufficient because glucose tolerance was limited to about 40 kcal/kg per day. In 1971, we were willing to try the new, more tolerable type of fat solution, intralipid, now available using soybeans. It was immediately clear in our studies with Jeanne Duncan and then published work with Bill Cashore that intakes of 85 to 90 kcal/kg per day administered parenterally were well tolerated. They permitted normal intrauterine rates of growth in ELBW infants. (33)

With improved formulations, parenteral nutrition no longer causes cholestatic jaundice or metabolic acidosis. There remains, however, the danger of catheter-related sepsis if indwelling catheters are required. Our nurses have been able to find peripheral veins for up to 30 to 60 days in most ELBW infants, although peripherally inserted central catheter lines now are being initiated somewhat earlier. These provide more prolonged and secure access with less trauma, although with a greater risk of infection. (34)

With parenteral nutrition, the average ELBW infant requires 12 to 14 days to regain birthweight compared with the 20 to 30 days required for the smallest babies when they were fed only milk and intravenous glucose. However, maximum weight loss after birth in ELBW infants remains about 15% (sometimes 20%).

Growth

The ELBW infant on average drops from the 50th percentile of weight for age at birth to the 3rd percentile by the time birthweight is regained at 2 weeks of age. He or she grows well thereafter, but does not rise above the 3rd percentile growth channel and is discharged as a small-for-date baby. Not only are such infants underweight for age, but they have undersize heads at discharge because head circumference does not grow during periods of weight loss or growth arrest. It may be impossible to decrease the initial weight loss, but more vigorous feeding programs subsequently may enable infants to grow faster and may affect future neurologic function.

An exciting study reported by us to the Society for Pediatric Research recently described the use of "top-up" intravenous nutrition. (35) This involved a supplement of parenteral nutrition added to full milk feedings to enhance postnatal growth of infants born with extreme degrees of IUGR (below the 1st percentile of weight for date or more than 30% underweight for gestational age). Almost all of these severely IUGR infants showed above-normal intrauterine rates of growth, not only in weight, but in head circumference and length on this program. Can IUGR infants who are born extremely growth retarded or VLBW infants who become growth retarded after birth achieve catch-up growth while in the NICU? If so, can this be accomplished by top-up parenteral nutrition or by increasing the intestinal feedings?

Intrauterine Infection

Until recent years, intrauterine infection was considered the result of prolonged rupture of membranes, a common problem in very preterm births. It then became apparent that histologic chorioamnionitis, funisitis, and umbilical vasculitis often were associated with very early birth. This is unrelated to whether membranes had been ruptured for a long or short time before birth. Infants exposed to this intrauterine infection often have abnormal acute-phase reactant results, although usually negative blood cultures. This situation is present for 50% of infants born before 26 weeks' gestation.

Goldenberg and others now have clearly shown that ascending infection is not so much the result of, but rather the cause of, very preterm labor or rupture of membranes. (36) It still is too early to know whether this knowledge has therapeutic value in preventing preterm labor by use of antibiotics.

Rather than totally relying on blood cultures, which usually are negative, we have placed much reliance on the acute-phase reactants, the gastric aspirates at birth, and placental histology to diagnose what we term systemic infection of intrauterine origin. Our acute-phase reactant battery includes white blood cell count, manual differential count, C-reactive protein, and a microerythrocyte sedimentation rate technique that we developed 40 years ago. Such "infected" babies often are relatively asymptomatic. Our policy has been to treat them with antibiotics until acute-phase reactants are normal, covering at least the organisms that may have grown from the mother's vagina or the baby's gastric aspirate or from the endotracheal tube in intubated babies.

PDA

It was in the late 1960s that Peter Auld in New York and Bill Tooley in San Francisco recognized that the PDA I had described following RDS could cause left ventricular strain and failure by increased left ventricular flow load. Surgical closure was introduced in the late 1960s and 1970s. With the less sophisticated surgical and anesthetic techniques of that time, the hazards of operating on very tiny babies were great. It was Rudolph's group and Friedman and

colleagues (37)(38) in the 1970s that described the prostaglandin mechanism for PDA closure. They introduced indomethacin therapy, which now is the standard initial approach. Unfortunately, it is only 70% effective per trial. We usually try it three times before proceeding to surgery that today, when needed, is remarkably well tolerated. Success with indomethacin is greater with advancing gestational age. Infants born before 26 weeks' gestation often require surgery.

Chronic Lung Disease

Until the 1960s, pulmonary problems in preterm infants were considered to be restricted to the first postnatal week. With increasing survival of VLBW infants, Wilson and Mikity described a chronic respiratory problem in some. (39) This pulmonary dysmaturity or chronic lung disease of prematurity was unrelated to preexisting RDS or oxygen toxicity or barotrauma from respirators, which had not yet been developed.

By the late 1960s, Northway, Rosan, and Porter described a more severe, often fatal, form of chronic lung disease that followed prolonged ventilator use with high oxygen concentrations. (8) This BPD affected—and at times killed—infants of all sizes, including many weighing more than 1,500 g. It must be remembered that at that time, positive pressure ventilation for newborns was in its infancy. There was no understanding of the need for positive end-expiratory pressure, and ventilation attempted to achieve lower carbon dioxide tensions and higher blood oxygen levels than we now consider necessary. As a result, ventilatory pressures and ambient oxygen concentrations were higher than we now use. Philip's succinct title in reviewing this condition was "BPD=oxygen plus pressure plus time." (40)

Today, with gentler ventilation and lower oxygen goals, chronic lung disease almost is restricted to infants weighing less than 1,200 g. When it follows high ventilatory pressures and high oxygen need for the treatment of RDS, it is considered BPD. When chronic lung disease develops at this age without significant preexisting lung disease or significant ventilatory or oxygen need, it is considered to be of the usually milder Mikity Wilson variety. Fitzgerald and associates studied infants cared for in our unit and found no difference in pulmonary functions in BPD versus Mikity Wilson type. (41)

Chronic lung disease originally was defined as radiologic abnormalities and oxygen need for 28 days. It now is restricted to oxygen need for at least 28 days extending to 36 weeks of gestational age. Our experience with infants of 22 to 31 weeks' gestational age indicates that the 28-day definition includes some 40% of very preterm infants, adding 36 weeks to the definition reduces this to 14%, and restricting it to those still receiving oxygen at term includes only 3%. In only the latter group is the chronic lung disease of practical significance in delaying hospital discharge of the infant. Very preterm infants on average are ready to go home only when they reach full term.

It was in the late 1960s that we experienced dramatic improvement in pulmonary function by using the newly developed powerful diuretic ethacrynic acid in infants who had chronic lung disease of prematurity. With a sudden loss in weight and peripheral edema, the clinical and radiologic pulmonary disorder improved markedly. Prevention and control of fluid retention now is a cornerstone of management. The oral diuretics of the 1970s (hydrochlorothiazide and spironolactone) cause much less alkalosis and electrolyte depletion than do the rapid-acting diuretics. In some infants, we also have restricted fluid intake by administering very concentrated (100 kcal/100 mL) formula.

The late 1980s and 1990s saw a burst of enthusiasm for adrenal corticosteroids (dexamethasone) in the management of chronic lung disease. Oxygen need could be reduced rapidly, and the babies who were ventilator-dependent could be extubated. However, mortality and length of hospital stay were affected little. The doses needed were high, stopping growth for at least 1 week. They also caused glucose and fat intolerance, with a necessary duration of the weaning of up to 3 to 6 weeks. Fortunately, several randomized, controlled trials of dexamethasone use,

including long-term follow-up, had been performed. By the late 1990s, it was evident that steroid use was associated with a high frequency of cerebral palsy, estimated as a risk of 1 case per 4 infants treated. (42) Over the past 5 years, we have discontinued its use except for occasional infants who have severe laryngeal edema problems or repeated failed extubation attempts in whom a 1- to 2-day steroid course may be helpful.

We have been ventilating with permissive hypercapnia, allowing CO_2 levels to rise as long as pH is above 7.25, and permissive hypoxemia (using 88% to 92% oxygen saturation as our goal). With this approach, the amount of oxygen and pressure needed are reduced. It seems likely that the 88% arterial saturation limit that we have been using since the pulse oximeter became available may be even higher than necessary. Lung and eye injury may be lessened if the baby's organs can tolerate lower levels, perhaps 80% to 85%. Further randomized, controlled trials are needed, similar to one we performed 35 years ago to determine the lower limit of acceptable oxygen saturation in the preterm infant.

Sequelae

We now can save many infants as young as 24 weeks' gestation and probably soon those of only 22 weeks' gestation. With costs so high and outcomes of extremely preterm infants often uncertain, there is frequent criticism (epitomized by Bill Silverman) of our efforts to salvage them.

Blindness, deafness, and severe cerebral palsy have become very uncommon. On the other hand, cerebral injury with retarded development with or without intracranial hemorrhage or periventricular leukomalacia can be expected today in 33% of survivors born between 22 and 27 weeks' gestation. Surprisingly, the frequency of damage is not much greater at the lower end than the upper end of this spectrum. In addition, attention-deficit and hyperactivity disorders are frequent, even when there is normal mental development. Many of these children require special educational support in school.

However, we always must recognize, as shown by Saroj Saigal, that almost all of these NICU graduates who have problems can function independently in later life. The extreme forms of brain damage, as are found following severe birth asphyxia, are fortunately rare. Dr Saigal found in interviews that neither the children in later life nor their parents regretted that intensive care was provided at birth. (43) For every child who has some cerebral problem, there are at least one or two others who are developing normally.

We do not know what causes the cerebral injury and, therefore, how to prevent its occurrence. Studies relating perinatal events to long-term outcome are needed urgently if we are to make progress in preventing disability.

Conclusion

To close, I would like to express some of my thoughts on what I feel are the responsibilities of the neonatologist with regard to the parents:

1. Parents must be made fully aware from the start of the risks, both immediate and long-term, that their baby faces.
2. At the borderline of viability (now before 25 and perhaps 24 weeks' gestation), treatment never should be initiated without informed consent of the parents, at least verbally.
3. Parents should be informed of significant developments as they occur and told how they may influence outcome. In the event of complications that are likely to lead to severe handicap, withdrawal of treatment should be offered as an option.
4. At several times during the course of care, the neonatologist responsible for the baby's care at the time should sit down with both parents for a discussion of their questions, a review of the current situation, and an outline of the course expected until discharge. Parents need much moral support as they face so many uncertainties.
5. Adequate follow-up after discharge should be ensured, with support provided for any special needs that develop.

I hope that I have been able to communicate some of the fascination that neonatology has held for me throughout my career; that you always will be willing to challenge conventional wisdom when you have reason to doubt it; and that you will continue to search for answers to the questions such as those I posed in this personal view of neonatology in the late 20th century.

Robert Usher, MD
Professor of Pediatrics and of Obstetrics and Gynecology
McGill University
Montreal, Quebec, Canada

References

1. Usher R. Clinical investigation of the respiratory distress syndrome of prematurity, interim report. *N Y State J Med.* 1961; 61:1677–1696

2. Usher R. The respiratory distress syndrome of prematurity: clinical and therapeutic effects. *Pediatr Clin North Am.* 1961;8: 525–538

3. Usher R, McLean F, Maughan GB. Respiratory distress syndrome in infants delivered by cesarean section. *Am J Obstet Gynecol.* 1964;88:806–815

4. Usher RH, Allen AC, McLean FH. Risk of respiratory distress syndrome related to gestational age, route of delivery and maternal diabetes. *Am J Obstet Gynecol.* 1971; 111:826–832

5. Usher R. The respiratory distress syndrome of prematurity. I. Changes in potassium in the serum and the electrocardiogram and effects of therapy. *Pediatrics.* 1959;24:562–576

6. Usher R. Reduction of mortality from respiratory distress syndrome of prematurity with early administration of intravenous glucose and sodium bicarbonate. *Pediatrics.* 1963;32:968–975

7. Delivoria-Papadopoulos M, Swyer PR. Assisted ventilation in terminal hyaline membrane disease. *Arch Dis Child.* 1964; 39:481–484
   (*See also* Delivoria-Papadopoulos M. *Historical perspectives: forty years of mechanical ventilation: then and now.* NeoReviews. *2003;4: e335–e339. Available at: http://neoreviews.aappublications.org/cgi/content/ full/4/12/e335*)

8. Northway WH Jr, Rosan RC, Porter DY. Pulmonary disease following respirator therapy of hyaline membrane disease: bronchopulmonary dysplasia. *N Engl J Med.* 1967;276:357–368

9. Gregory GA, Kitterman JA, Phibbs RH, Tooley WH, Hamilton WK. Treatment of the idiopathic respiratory-distress syndrome with continuous positive airway pressure. *N Engl J Med.* 1971;284:1333–1340
   (*See also* Gregory GA. *Historical perspectives: continuous positive airway pressure (CPAP).* NeoReviews. *2004;5:e1–e4. Available at: http://neoreviews. aappublications.org/cgi/content/full/5/1/e1*)

10. Huch R, Huch A. Historical perspectives: transcutaneous blood gas measurement. *NeoReviews.* 2003;4:e223–e227. Available at: http://neoreviews. aappublications.org/cgi/content/full/4/9/e223

11. Peabody JL, Emery JR. Non-invasive monitoring of blood gases in the newborn. *Clin Perinatol.* 1985;12:147–160

12. Liggins GC, Howie RN. A controlled trial of antepartum glucocorticoid treatment for prevention of the respiratory distress syndrome in premature infants. *Pediatrics.* 1972;50:515–525
    (*See also* Liggins GC. *Historical perspectives: antepartum glucocorticoid treatment.* NeoReviews. *2002;3:e227–e228. Available at: http://neoreviews. aappublications.org/cgi/content/full/3/11/e227*)

13. Avery ME, Mead J. Surface properties in relation to atelectasis and hyaline membrane disease. *Am J Dis Child.* 1959;97: 517–523
    (*See also* Avery ME. *Historical perspectives: surfactant deficiency to surfactant use.* NeoReviews. *2002;3:e239–e242. Available at: http://neoreviews. aappublications.org/cgi/content/full/3/12/e239*)

14. Fujiwara T, Maeta H, Chida S, Morita T, Watabe Y, Abe T. Artificial surfactant therapy in hyaline-membrane disease. *Lancet.* 1980;i:55–59

15. Scott KE, Usher R. Fetal malnutrition: its incidence, causes and effects. *Am J Obstet Gynecol.* 1966;94:951–963

16. Usher RH. Clinical and therapeutic aspects of fetal malnutrition. *Pediatr Clin North Am.* 1970;17:169–183

17. Fretts RC, Boyd ME, Usher RH, Usher HA. The changing pattern of fetal death, 1961–1988. *Obstet Gynecol.* 1992; 79:35–39

18. Cornblath M, Wybregt SH, Baens GS, Klein RI. Symptomatic neonatal hypoglycemia: studies of carbohydrate metabolism in the newborn infant VIII. *Pediatrics.* 1964;33:338–402
    (*See also* Cornblath M. *Historical perspectives: transient symptomatic neonatal hypoglycemia.* NeoReviews. *2003;4:e1–e5. Available at: http:// neoreviews.aappublications.org/cgi/content/full/4/1/e1*)

19. Freda VJ, Gorman JG, Pollack W. Successful prevention of experimental Rh sensitization in man with an anti-Rh gamma 2 globulin antibody preparation: a preliminary report. *Transfusion.* 1964;4:26–32
    (*See also* Bowman JM. *Historical perspectives: prevention of Rh hemolytic disease of the newborn.* NeoReviews. *2002;3:e223–e226. Available at: http://neoreviews.aappublications.org/cgi/content/full/3/11/e223*)

20. Cremer RJ, Perryman PW, Richards DH. Influence of light on hyperbilirubinemia of infants. *Lancet.* 1958;i:1094–1098

21. Lucey JF, Ferreiro M, Hewitt J. Prevention of hyperbilirubinemia of prematurity by phototherapy. *Pediatrics.* 1968;41: 1047–1054
    (*See also* Lucey JF. *Historical perspectives: phototherapy.* NeoReviews. *2003;4:e27–e29. Available at: http://neoreviews.aappublications.org/cgi/ content/full/4/2/e27*)

22. Diamond LK, Pearson HA. The rise and fall of exchange transfusion. *NeoReviews.* 2003;4:e169–e174. Available at: http://neoreviews.aappublications. org/cgi/content/full/4/7/e169

23. Bhutani VK, Johnson LH. Kernicterus: lessons for the future from a current tragedy. *NeoReviews.* 2003;4:e30–e32. Available at: http://neoreviews. aappublications.org/cgi/content/full/4/2/e30

24. Bowman JM, Chown B, Lewis M, Pollock JM. Rh isoimmunization during pregnancy: antenatal prophylaxis. *Can Med Assoc J.* 1978;118:623–627
    (*See also* Bowman JM. *Historical perspectives: prevention of Rh hemolytic disease of the newborn.* NeoReviews. *2002;3:e223–e226. Available at: http://neoreviews.aappublications.org/cgi/content/full/3/11/e223*)

25. Usher RH. The role of the neonatologist. *Pediatr Clin North Am.* 1970;17: 199–202

26. Usher R. Changing mortality rates with perinatal intensive care and regionalization. *Semin Perinatol.* 1977;1:309–331

27. Horbar JD, Badger GJ, Carpenter JH, et al, Members of the Vermont-Oxford Network. Trends in mortality and morbidity for very low birth weight infants, 1991–1999. *Pediatrics.* 2002;110:143–151

28. Halamek LP. Prenatal consultation at the limits of viability. *NeoReviews.* 2003;4: e153–e156. Available at: *http://neoreviews.aappublications.org/cgi/content/full/4/6/e153*

29. Usher RH, Vallerand D, Willis D, Faucher D. Short term outcomes of conservative management of very premature infants. *Pediatr Res.* 2003; 53:422A

30. Berry MA, Abrahamowicz M, Usher RH. Factors associated with growth of extremely premature infants during initial hospitalization. *Pediatrics.* 1997; 100:640– 646

31. Kandil H, Hamilton R, Usher RH. Response of premature infants with prolonged feeding intolerance to cisapride. *Pediatr Res.* 1999;46:285A

32. Heird WC, Driscoll JM Jr. Historical perspectives: total parenteral nutrition. *NeoReviews,* 2003;4:e137–e139. Available at: *http://neoreviews.aappublications.org/cgi/content/full/4/6/e137*

33. Cashore WJ, Sedaghatian MR, Usher RH. Nutritional supplements with intravenously administered lipid, protein hydrolysate and glucose in small premature infants. *Pediatrics.* 1975;56:8–16

34. Chock V. Peripherally inserted central catheters in neonates. *NeoReviews.* 2004;5: e60–e62. Available at: *http://neoreviews.aappublications.org/cgi/content/full/5/2/e60*

35. Kandil HJ, Chartier L, Beaumier L, Kovacs L, Usher RH. Top-up parenteral nutrition (TPN) in the management of severe intrauterine growth retardation (IUGR). *Pediatr Res.* 2000;47:405A

36. Goldenberg RL, Culhane JF. Infection as a cause of preterm birth. *Clin Perinatol.* 2003;30:677–700

37. Friedman WF, Hirschklau MJ, Printz MP, Pitlick PT, Kirkpatrick SE. Pharmacologic closure of patent ductus arteriosus in the premature infant. *N Engl J Med.* 1976; 295:526–529
    (*See also Friedman WF. A look back: the clinical initiation of pharmacologic closure of patent ductus arteriosus in the preterm infant. NeoReviews. 2003;4:e259–e262. Available at: http://neoreviews.aappublications.org/cgi/content/full/4/10/e259*)

38. Heymann MA, Rudolph AM, Silverman NH. Closure of the ductus arteriosus by prostaglandin inhibition. *N Engl J Med.* 1976;295:530–533

39. Wilson MG, Mikity VG. A new form of respiratory disease in premature infants. *Am J Dis Child.* 1960;99:489–499

40. Philip AGS. Oxygen plus pressure plus time: the etiology of bronchopulmonary dysplasia. *Pediatrics.* 1980;55:44–50

41. Fitzgerald D, Mesiano G, Brosseau L, Davis GM. Pulmonary outcome in extremely low birth weight infants. *Pediatrics.* 2000;105:1209–1215

42. Halliday HL. The effect of post-natal steroids on growth and development. *J Perinat Med.* 2001;29:281–285

43. Saigal S, Pinelli J, Hoult L, Kim MM, Boyle M. Psychopathology and social competencies of adolescents who were extremely low birth weight. *Pediatrics.* 2003; 111:969–975

Historical Perspectives: Neonatology: The Long View
Alistair G. S. Philip and Robert Usher

NeoReviews 2005;6;e3-e11
DOI: 10.1542/neo.6-1-e3

Necrotizing Enterocolitis: An Inherited Or Acquired Condition?

David K. Stevenson, MD* Martin L. Blakely, MD†

Necrotizing Enterocolitis

Perhaps the least understood of the disorders of prematurity is necrotizing enterocolitis (NEC). Although it is not certain when this problem initially was observed, it was well described in 1964 by Berdon and coworkers at Babies Hospital in New York, (1) with amplification from the same group in slightly later publications. (2)(3) A group in Seattle also contributed important observations of a significant number of survivors in a comparatively large series (4) and an increased frequency of the disorder in the late 1960s. (5) The role of radiographic interpretation was emphasized in these later reports, with pneumatosis intestinalis considered the hallmark of the disorder. It subsequently was emphasized that a provisional diagnosis was required before pneumatosis was evident to allow for medical rather than surgical intervention. (6)

Even in the early reports, the very low-birthweight (VLBW) infant (<1,500 g) born before 32 weeks' gestation seemed to be particularly susceptible, although larger and more mature infants also could be affected. Both then and now, NEC was and is a disorder of uncertain etiology. (7)(8) The role of bowel ischemia seemed to be paramount, with bacterial infection and method of feeding being other important contributors. Although infection seemed to be important, it was not possible to isolate a responsible organism in many cases. Despite this, the periodicity of the disorder in nurseries and the ability to reduce the incidence by infection control measures (9) was highly suggestive of the potential importance of infection (possibly viral). The ability of human milk to protect against NEC in the VLBW infant is well established, (10) and minimal enteral nutrition over several days also has been shown to decrease the incidence of NEC in VLBW infants. (11)

At one point, the idea that NEC was a form of inflammatory bowel disease seemed most attractive. Data suggest that prenatal corticosteroid therapy may reduce the incidence of NEC, (12)(13) which would support this hypothesis. In addition, the possibility that oxygen free radicals (14) or increased concentrations of proinflammatory cytokines (15) might contribute to NEC also has been entertained. A recent report indicates that the protective effect of human milk may reside in the concentration of anti-inflammatory cytokines present. (16)

In this Historical Perspectives, David Stevenson provides a personal insight into this challenging disorder. His father was an important contributor to the early reports coming from Seattle, and father and son later combined their views in two additional contributions. (17)(18) The present contribution also provides surgical input from Martin Blakely.

Alistair G. S. Philip, MD, FRCPE, FAAP
Editor-in-Chief, NeoReviews

References

1. Berdon WE, Grossman H, Baker DH, Mizrahi A, Barlow O, Blanc WA. Necrotizing enterocolitis in the premature infant. *Radiology.* 1964;83:879–887
2. Mizrahi A, Barlow O, Berdon WE, Blank WA, Silverman WA. Necrotizing enterocolitis in premature infants. *J Pediatr.* 1965;66:697–705
3. Touloukian RJ, Berdon WE, Amoury RA, Santulli TV. Surgical experience with necrotizing enterocolitis in infant. *J Pediatr Surg.* 1967;2:389–398

4. Stevenson JK, Graham CB, Oliver TK, Goldenberg VE. Neonatal necrotizing enterocolitis: a report of twenty-one cases with fourteen survivors. *Am J Surg.* 1969; 118:260–272
5. Bell RS, Graham CB, Stevenson JK. Roentgenologic and clinical manifestations of neonatal necrotizing enterocolitis: experience with 43 cases. *Am J Roentgenol.* 1971;112:123–134
6. Bell MJ, Ternberg JL, Feigin RD, et al. Neonatal necrotizing enterocolitis: therapeutic decisions based upon clinical staging. *Ann Surg.* 1978;187:1–7
7. Kliegman RM, Fanaroff AA. Necrotizing enterocolitis. *N Engl J Med.* 1984;310:1093–1103
8. Kliegman RM, Walker WA, Yolken RH. Necrotizing enterocolitis: research agenda for a disease of unknown etiology and pathogenesis. *Pediatr Res.* 1993;34: 701–708
9. Book LS, Overall JC Jr, Herbst JJ, Britt MR, Epstein B, Jung AL. Clustering of necrotizing enterocolitis: interruption of infection-control measures. *N Engl J Med.* 1977;297:984–986
10. Lucas A, Cole TJ. Breast milk and neonatal necrotizing enterocolitis. *Lancet.* 1990;336:1519–1523
11. Berseth CL, Bisquera JA, Paje V. Prolonging small feeding volumes early in life decreased the incidence of necrotizing enterocolitis in very low birth weight infants. *Pediatrics.* 2003;111:529–534
12. Bauer CR, Morrison JC, Poole WK, et al. A decreased incidence of necrotizing enterocolitis after prenatal glucocorticoid therapy. *Pediatrics.* 1984;73:682–688
13. Halac E, Halac J, Begue EF, et al. Prenatal and postnatal corticosteroid therapy to prevent neonatal necrotizing enterocolitis: a controlled trial. *J Pediatr.* 1990;117:132–138
14. Saugstad OD. Oxygen toxicity in the neonatal period. *Acta Paediatr Scand.* 1990;79:881–892
15. Edelson MD, Bagwell CE, Rozycki HJ. Circulating pro- and counterinflammatory cytokine levels and severity in necrotizing enterocolitis. *Pediatrics.* 1999;103: 766–771
16. Fituch CC, Palkowetz KH, Goldman AS, Schanler RJ. Concentration of IL-10 in preterm human milk and in milk from mothers of infants with necrotizing enterocolitis. *Acta Paediatr.* 2004;93:1496–1500
17. Stevenson JK, Stevenson DK. Necrotizing enterocolitis in the neonate. *Surg Annu.* 1977;9:147–169
18. Stevenson DK, Graham CB, Stevenson JK. Neonatal necrotizing enterocolitis: 100 new cases. *Adv Pediatr.* 1980;27:319–340

*Department of Pediatrics, Division of Neonatal and Developmental Medicine, Stanford University School of Medicine, Stanford, Calif.
†Departments of Surgery and Pediatrics, University of Tennessee Health Science Center, Memphis, Tenn.

Introduction

NEC is not considered an inherited condition in the usual sense. In fact, all human conditions result from the interaction between our inherited biologic predispositions and environmental challenges – life literally hangs in the balance. Nonetheless, I (DKS) "inherited" this condition from my father, a general surgeon, who was among the first pediatric surgeons to confront surgically this terrible affliction with its predilection for the most immature and smallest of preterm infants. My "inheritance" was apparent even before my decision to become a physician, but became fully established during my training in medical school, in pediatrics, and subsequently in neonatology.

John Stevenson was one of the first of several pioneering pediatric surgeons to attempt a surgical solution to what was, at the time, a medical and almost hopeless diagnosis in the small preterm infant. NEC was (and still is) associated with a very high mortality rate in the most immature infants. In the context of usually fulminant and lethal disease in the neonatal intensive care nursery (NICU) at the University of Washington in the 1960s, my father's surgical approach was aggressive and radical. He proposed a two-stage technique that consisted of an early laparotomy and removal of any apparently dead bowel and a "second-look" laparotomy with removal of any additional dead intestine, often within several days of the first procedure. This approach, developed by a talented, dexterous, and gentle-handed surgeon, working in close collaboration with neonatologists at the University of Washington, reduced markedly the high mortality associated with such cases. The experience was reported in 1969. (1) At this time, I was in the middle of my undergraduate education at Stanford University, was primarily interested in philosophy and the humanities, and was not thinking much about NEC. In retrospect, I do recall my father talking about the condition, and that the name "necrotizing enterocolitis" had a foreboding sound of inflammation and death. I remember hearing my father express his perplexity about how such a condition could occur and how he felt that a surgical approach, although clearly mitigating once the condition had occurred, was not the right solution to the problem. Later, as I began to learn more about NEC during my pediatric residency training and on my rotation in neonatology, I began to appreciate more fully my father's perplexity and his frustration as a surgeon in addressing a problem that, by its nature, was already at "end-stage" when he confronted it

and the possibility of prevention or interruption of the process was already past.

In fact, the surgeon was faced with the difficult decision of weighing the risk of surgery and a necessary iatrogenic wound in a medically fragile patient against the need to remove already dead tissue threatening the patient's life. All too common was an intraoperative experience in which easy identification of clearly demarcated dead intestine was not possible and a simple resection was not an option because so much intestine was injured, resulting in unavoidable long-term morbidity with short gut syndrome or death. This dilemma for the pediatric surgeon, in fact, was best appreciated in the operating room after the intestine was exposed and it became apparent that a large portion was involved, with no segmental distribution but with patchy variation in injury ranging from frank necrosis and perforation to mild discoloration and hemorrhage into the bowel wall. Although I had learned that involvement of the distal ileum and proximal colon was typical, NEC could be encountered anywhere from the stomach to the rectum. Astutely, my father pointed out that the presence of serosa identified the part of the intestine that was vulnerable, using, as he often did, anatomy as a reference. I was also impressed with the dexterity of his hands, the size of which seemed enormous in juxtaposition to the tiny intestines of the very low birthweight (VLBW) infants such that the operation required use of simple magnifying lenses at a time when the use of robotic aids was not possible. He operated delicately and swiftly in a high-stakes surgical intervention to save a life.

To this day, the decision to operate on a preterm infant who has NEC remains difficult and unnerving because the surgeon is still joining the battle against this condition late in its course, with only the promise of creating another wound and removing obvious dead bowel if it is consistent with long-term survival in the context of uncertain and serious morbidities, and no promise of avoiding the condition that already has occurred. All in all, not much has changed in the 30 years since I first "inherited" this condition from my surgeon-father. Affirming this perspective requires only a revisit to our report of

100 new cases at the University of Washington from 1969 to 1976. (2)

Lew Barness invited us to share our experience. With my father deceased, I feel the need for a surgical companion to complete my commentary on this topic. My father would have agreed. This is not a journey that should be undertaken alone.

Epidemiology

NEC is one of the remaining scourges of the neonate, with most of the afflicted infants being preterm. The overall incidence is approximately 6% in VLBW infants (<1,500 g) and 8% in extremely low-birthweight (ELBW) infants (<1,000 g). (3)(4) For those ELBW infants needing surgery, the mortality approaches 50%. (5)(6)(7)(8)(9) In fact, the condition occurs more commonly in the smallest and most immature infants, with the incidence increasing inversely to gestational age and birth-weight among appropriately grown preterm infants. Ironically, mortality also increases in the same inverse relationship with gestational age and birthweight. The ELBW infant, thus, faces the greatest risk with respect to the occurrence of the condition, the need for surgical intervention, and the risks of complications and mortality.

Beyond the gastrointestinal morbidities, NEC is also the harbinger of neurologic deficits and developmental delay. (2)(10)(11)(12) Term and near-term infants who develop NEC (<10% of cases) almost always suffer profound asphyxia or catastrophic heart failure related to impaired cardiac output, as can be encountered in left-sided obstructive, ductal-dependent lesions that were not anticipated or recognized prior to birth. Furthermore, the role of infection in NEC remains uncertain. The condition has been variably understood as an unusual infectious disease or a type of intestinal injury that, when it occurs in the context of intestinal colonization, sometimes leads to opportunistic invasion of the bowel wall, blood stream, and brain. However, most infants do not have bacteremia or meningitis at the time of diagnosis.

NEC usually presents in the first two postnatal weeks after the initiation of formula feeding, but it can occur later or in the absence of enteral feeding. Human milk feeding is not a universal protection. The incidence varies from one NICU to another without apparent explanation, and the clinical condition itself varies from being fulminant and immediately life-threatening to insidious and fraught with uncertainty about its presence, allowing time for discussion and debate about whether the roentgenographic signs are really confirmatory of the diagnosis. Because the threat of injury or death is so great, enteral alimentation is usually suspended, even with only the slightest suspicion. In addition, broad-spectrum parenteral antibiotics, including anaerobic coverage, are started, and other nonspecific support is initiated for the infant who has nonspecific signs of illness consistent with the diagnosis. Not much has changed over 30 years.

Clinical Presentation and Diagnosis

The clinical syndrome associated with NEC is nonspecific. It involves abdominal distention, a relative increase in gastric residuals, and guaiac-positive stools. Importantly, scant stools or the complete absence of stools is also consistent with the adynamic ileus that occurs in the context of NEC. Thus, the classic clinical triad of abdominal distention, increased retention of gastric contents, and scant guaiac-positive stools or absent stools in the context of a nonspecific systemic illness, perhaps not even gastrointestinal in nature, is what most commonly confronts the neonatologist who often also is considering intestinal obstruction, neonatal sepsis or meningitis, and some inborn errors of metabolism in the differential diagnosis of an infant who presents with feeding intolerance, lethargy, apnea, bradycardia, and temperature instability. Refractory metabolic acidosis and hematologic changes, such as granulocytopenia and thrombocytopenia or complicating disseminated intravascular coagulation, and electrolyte abnormalities, such as hyponatremia, can be a part of the presenting picture. Nonspecific markers of inflammation, such as elevated C-reactive protein, are typical. Inflammation is central in the pathogenesis and contributing to the injury itself and associated morbidities.

The diagnosis continues to be made with the use of pathognomonic roentgenographic

signs. The earliest signs are nonspecific, yet often are sufficient motivation for initiating treatment in the context of the clinical syndrome. Increases in gaseous distention and gas fluid levels suggest adynamic ileus without anatomic obstruction. Thickened bowel walls are sometimes noted. However, the most specific signs, which still are the only "signs" that allow the diagnosis to be confirmed prior to surgical inspection of the intestine, are pneumatosis intestinalis (PI) in most cases (90%), hepatic portal venous gas (HPVG) in a minority of cases (30%), and pneumoperitoneum in a minority of cases (30%). A diagnosis requires one of the three roentgenographic findings or direct inspection of the intestine in the clinical context. Rarely now does the diagnosis await autopsy. Development of the roentgenographic signs can be rapid and obvious or insidious and indeterminate. They may occur together or alone. More recently, another clinical entity, isolated intestinal perforation, has been identified as possibly a separate condition to be distinguished from NEC with respect to its pathogenesis, which is still uncertain, and its treatment, which also is debated.

Radiologists often speculate about the severity of the condition based on the roentgenographic signs. However, it is important to remember that once air enters the subserosal plane of the intestine, it can dissect along this plane independent of where the injury has occurred. Thus, the roentgenographic presentation can appear extensive, with massive PI in association with very focal necrosis. Also, because the clinical syndrome may vary considerably in severity, it does not necessarily correlate with the roentgenographic presentation. The same reservations can be expressed with respect to identifying the location of intestinal injury based on roentgenography alone. Although some attempt to identify the involved part of the intestine often is made roentgenographically, the ability of gas to dissect along the subserosal plane makes it nearly impossible to be sure about the exact location of injury in most cases.

Gas in the bowel wall itself may be difficult to distinguish from gas intermixed with the contents of the intestinal lumen. The bubbly appearance of both is indistinguishable on a

flat plate of the abdomen (KUB). However, if the bubbles in the bowel wall are caught in a perpendicular projection in a complementary radiograph, the ability to identify the curvilinear lucencies that correspond to the apparent bubbles in the other projection may be enhanced. Thus, a KUB and a cross-table lateral radiograph, although perhaps not ideal for identifying free air, may be valuable in trying to identify PI. Of course, free air can, in fact, be identified on a KUB in the falciform ligament or in a cross-table film around the umbilical area, which is the highest point of the baby's abdomen, or sometimes as a large, often missed circular lucency, on a KUB. A lateral decubitus radiograph can be useful for identifying free air, but often allows the intestine to fall into another position, making interpretation of bowel wall gas more difficult or indeterminate.

Nonetheless, PI is observed most commonly in the right lower quadrant, reflecting injury in the distal ileum and proximal colon, but it can occur anywhere along the gastrointestinal tract from the stomach to the rectum. Also, the amount of PI on the roentgenograph does not correlate with the need for surgery. However, the presence of HPVG may indicate the extent of bowel wall injury and has been associated with a higher mortality and the need for surgery. Although perforation used to be an absolute indication for operation, there is an ongoing debate about whether a peritoneal drain can be used as a temporizing or permanent surgical approach to perforation occurring in the small infant who has NEC.

The source of the gas that contributes to the pathognomonic roentgenographic signs of NEC has always been intriguing. Although some gas in the intestine that escapes into the bowel wall, subserosal plane, or ultimately into the perineum may have been swallowed air, the gas contains a large amount of hydrogen (H_2). It is produced by microorganisms under the right conditions. Using semi-quantitative techniques for bacterial culture, it can be demonstrated that H_2 gas production correlates roughly with the magnitude of colonization by H_2-producing organisms in the intestine. If large amounts of H_2 gas diffuse into the circulation, the amount of H_2 gas excreted in breath would be expected to increase dramatically. Thus, H_2 gas in the breath of a baby can be a telltale sign of colonization by H_2-producing organisms, many of which are potential pathogens. In fact, H_2 gas detection in breath could be used in the context of serial testing to identify not only malabsorption relative to a roughly constant sugar substrate load, but also bacterial colonization by H_2-producing organisms. Large amounts of H_2 gas escaping through disrupted mucosa probably is the cause of HPVG. When I was introduced to the concept of HPVG, I (DKS) thought it was a static finding. However, my father instructed me that HPVG reflects a chance finding of gas in rapid, fleeting transit through the portal system, having coalesced from small bubbles in the mesenteric vascular bed. (13) Thus, it is not surprising that HPVG often has been associated with increased mortality because it probably reflects the increased load of H_2-producing bacteria colonizing the intestine, the extent of injury in the intestine, or disruption of mucosal surface and loss of intestinal integrity. In the context of broad-spectrum antibiotics, persistent H_2 in the breath implies resistant organisms or inaccessibility of the antibiotics to the organisms. The monitoring of H_2 gas production rates in preterm infants, with serial tracking of H_2 gas excretion, might provide information about the early stages of the pathogenesis of NEC prior to the obvious appearance of the hallmark roentgenographic features, such as PI or HPVG. (14)

Medical Treatment and the Decision to Operate

All infants in whom NEC is suspected should be treated medically, with immediate cessation of enteral feedings, if they have been initiated. The administration of broad-spectrum parenteral antibiotics to eradicate aerobic or anaerobic bacteria, but most often a single biotype of *Enterobacteriaceae*, is warranted. Gastric suction to decompress the intestine is needed, and appropriate fluid administration is required to address compromise of the intravascular volume related to "third space" problems caused by the inflamed and edematous intestine as well as to correct any hematologic or electrolyte

complications. If respiration is compromised because of abdominal distention or if apnea is occurring, assisted ventilation is necessary. The antibiotic course is usually 10 to 14 days, with the caveat that any injury to the mucosa of the intestine requires at least 7 to 10 days to recover in terms of reconstitution of the intestinal epithelium from the crypt to the tip of the villous, a time frame that is longer than in the adult. (15)

The decision to operate is the most difficult decision that the surgeon has to make in the context of NEC, and it is based usually on clinical, roentgenographic, and laboratory information. The overall condition of the infant is an important consideration and has led to the introduction of abdominal drains as a method of approaching perforation in the immature small and unstable preterm infant. Free intra-abdominal air, clear-cut evidence of peritonitis (such as edema and erythema of the abdominal wall), intractable acidosis, or respiratory insufficiency requiring ventilatory assistance may move the surgeon to initiate surgical intervention. The presence of PI or HPVG is not an indication for surgery in and of itself, although HPVG may suggest the severity or extent of mucosal disruption and bowel wall injury. The intraoperative challenge, of course, is that the integrity of the intestine is often difficult to evaluate with respect to viability. Because NEC is not segmental and may be patchy, resections need to be limited to obviously necrotic tissue, with exteriorization of proximal and distal stomas. The possibility of necrotic progression and postoperative anastomotic leaks make attempts at primary anastomosis in the context of NEC inadvisable.

As our patients have become less mature and smaller, the debate surrounding laparotomy and peritoneal drainage for NEC or isolated intestinal perforation has intensified. Although the debate has not been resolved to date, the relevance of the underlying pathogenesis that might differentiate NEC from isolated intestinal perforation is at the core of the decision about the appropriateness of laparotomy versus peritoneal drainage. The key is to apply the appropriate procedure to the particular diagnosis. To date there has been no way to identify with confidence the distinctive syndromes prior to operation.

Surgical Treatment

Much as my coauthor (DKS) feels that he has inherited the condition of NEC from his father, Dr John K. Stevenson, I (MLB) also feel somewhat "entitled" to this inheritance as one of the next generation of pediatric surgeons. I also have acquired the challenge of treating neonates who have NEC, in large part from my interaction with Dr David Stevenson and other neonatologists who comprise the National Institute of Child Health and Development's (NICHD) Neonatal Research Network.

As mentioned earlier, it seems that the surgical approach and management have not changed drastically since the time that the elder Dr Stevenson and others were reporting their results in the 1960s and 1970s. Although the overall postoperative mortality rate may not have changed significantly, a careful review of the surgical experience from 30 to 40 years ago does reveal considerable changes. In the series of patients reported by Dr Stevenson in 1969, and referred to previously, the median birthweight was 1,530 g and gestation was 32 weeks. (1). Of the 21 infants included, 12 had surgery, with 9 survivors. Remarkable features of this report include the finding that 5 of the 12 (42%) surgery patients had resection with anastomosis (no ostomies), there was a dedicated effort at long-term follow-up of these infants, and approximately 25% of the article is a discussion of potential etiologies for NEC that highlights the importance of searching for the cause of this disease. These features contrast with many recent reports (including some by MLB) that do not include follow-up beyond the neonatal period and devote one sentence to the cause of NEC remaining unclear.

One conclusion from this very early experience with surgical NEC was that early operative intervention should be considered and may allow a favorable outcome. In some infants who had very extensive disease, the authors questioned whether earlier surgical intervention might have been beneficial. This aggressive approach did produce surprisingly good results, with a survival rate of 67% in their series. It is interesting to note that in Dr Robert Gross' textbook of pediatric surgery from 1953, there is no mention of NEC, despite a very detailed description of a broad and high-volume surgical experience. (16) These references together remind us that the surgical treatment of NEC, and in fact the disease itself, has only been a practical problem for 40 to 50 years, which is a relatively short time compared with many human maladies.

In addition to the NEC surgical patient population becoming smaller and more immature, there is perhaps a new condition similar to NEC, but with distinct features and now known as isolated intestinal perforation. This "acquired" condition is associated with the resuscitation and treatment of more extremely preterm infants and with some of the medical therapies for these infants (eg, indomethacin for patent ductus arteriosus and steroids for respiratory pathology). Although controversial, most of us believe that isolated intestinal perforation and NEC are distinct pathologic entities. There is much overlap in their clinical presentations, and they are currently treated similarly, both medically and surgically. We attempted recently to distinguish NEC from isolated perforation prospectively in an observational study and found at least some ability to do so. (17) Babies experiencing isolated perforation are on average smaller at birth and more immature at delivery, have an earlier onset of the abdominal disease process, and have characteristic abdominal imaging findings (eg, no pneumatosis and often a "gasless" abdomen). This distinction appears to be important for several reasons. First, the prognosis after operation for isolated perforation is improved in most series. Second, whether a given patient has isolated perforation or NEC has implications for the choice of laparotomy or peritoneal drain placement. Many believe that the "biologic plausibility" of treating an isolated perforation with a peritoneal drain is more reasonable compared with treating true NEC with at least some segment of ischemic bowel. Others, of course, feel that a patient who has an isolated perforation is an ideal and perhaps lower-risk patient for a laparotomy. Lastly, because the prognosis is affected by the specific diagnosis (NEC versus isolated perforation), a distinction should be made when designing and reporting clinical trials and other studies. For example, if a randomized trial compared laparotomy with peritoneal drainage and no stratification by preoperative diagnosis were used, it is possible that the two treatment groups would not be balanced with regard to the preoperative diagnosis. Accordingly, if isolated perforation has a better outcome and one treatment group has an overrepresentation of this particular preoperative diagnosis, the outcome might be attributed erroneously to the treatment rather than correctly attributed to the starting diagnosis. Also, in comparing series between institutions, it seems important to report the exact composition of the study cohort with regard to the particular diagnosis of isolated perforation or NEC.

One of the most ubiquitous controversies surrounding the surgical management of babies who have NEC concerns the use of laparotomy or peritoneal drainage. When Dr Stevenson reported his series in 1969, the reports describing the use of peritoneal drain placement were approximately 1 year away. Because preterm infants who have NEC or isolated intestinal perforation are so desperately ill and such high surgical risks, a new surgical strategy was devised in the 1970s. This involved the placement of a Penrose drain into the abdomen via a small incision, which could be performed at the bedside under local anesthesia. The purported benefits of this procedure included lower physiologic stress to the compromised patient, lower risk of procedure-related bleeding, the potential to "temporize" the situation and allow for some improvement prior to laparotomy, and perhaps the avoidance of a laparotomy. Although originally devised as an adjunct to resuscitation, peritoneal drain placement has been used increasingly as an alternative to laparotomy and as a strategy of definitive treatment of NEC or isolated intestinal perforation. In our recent observational study of neonates weighing less than 1,000 g at birth who had NEC or isolated intestinal perforation, the initial surgical treatment performed most commonly was peritoneal drain placement. Two ongoing randomized surgical trials focusing on neonatal outcomes (survival) after drain or laparotomy represent the first trials examining this question despite 30 years of the use of peritoneal drainage and its firm acceptance into the surgical armamentarium for these diseases. In the author's opinion (MLB), each surgical therapy will remain useful, depending on a number of patient and disease characteristics. The other missing piece of needed information related to the choice of initial surgical therapy is the long-term follow-up assessment of these infants. There are obviously many examples of effective therapies in the early neonatal period that are not used because of deleterious long-term effects, especially neurodevelopmental impairment.

One aspect of the surgical management of NEC that is changing is the improved method of clinical research. Two multicenter, prospective, randomized clinical trials were designed to compare the use of laparotomy with drainage. One trial involves multiple United States centers, has been organized by Dr R. Lawrence Moss, and represents one of the first randomized trials within the field of pediatric surgery. The other trial originated in the United Kingdom and involves multiple centers in different countries. Both of these trials should provide a higher level of evidence than previously available and help to better inform our use of various surgical therapies. We have completed a relatively large observational study that points to potential important differences in neurodevelopmental outcome in neonates after laparotomy versus drainage. A trial focusing on the impact of neonatal surgical therapy on later neurodevelopmental outcome appears to be important and is being considered by the NICHD Neonatal Research Network.

Causes

As someone who sees these desperately ill neonates and provides surgical treatment at least on a weekly basis, the most frustrating aspect of this disease is the lack of understanding of its etiology, which in all likelihood has resulted in the lack of dramatic improvement in the outcome. In other fields of medicine, such as oncology, many of the most important and significant advances have occurred only after discoveries related to the etiology and biology of the particular disease process. One of the clearest examples of improved understanding of etiology

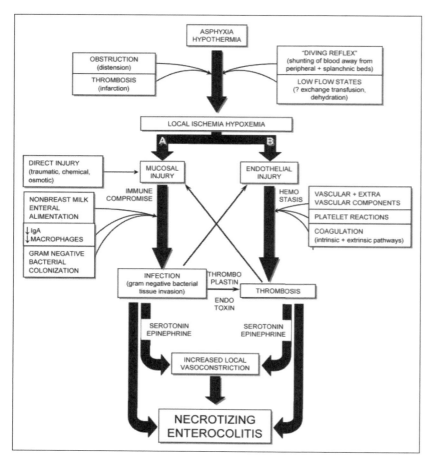

Figure 1. Scheme of the theories of the pathogenesis of necrotizing enterocolitis. This diagram was published in DK, et al. *Adv Pediatr.* 1980;27:319–340. Copyright Elsevier (1980).

leading to improved therapeutics is related to the development of the drug imatinib mesylate. This agent specifically inhibits tyrosine kinase, the enzyme that is causally linked to chronic myeloid leukemia and is the first drug approved by the United States Food and Drug Administration that targets an intracellular signaling molecule that is known specifically to cause a type of cancer. If the exact molecular pathology were determined for NEC or isolated intestinal perforation, specific targeted therapies might be developed to limit the disease, provide for earlier detection, or perhaps prevent the surgical form of these diseases.

Several features of the NEC disease process seem to have limited the understanding of its etiology. First, many of the animal models might not mimic the human condition in important ways and second, no large-scale attempts have been made to procure biologic specimens (eg, resected bowel, blood). Before substantial progress can be made in the

outcome of neonates who have NEC, significant strides will be required in our understanding of the biology of the disease process. One approach would be to attach "biology studies" to all clinical trials designed to evaluate various medical or surgical treatment options. As with studies performed within the Children's Oncology Group, essentially any clinical study of these patients also should consider studying various aspects of the biology of the disease. Tissue banks could be created at dedicated centers of excellence to explore various hypotheses.

Pathogenesis

Although not much has changed in 30 years with respect to our understanding of the causation of this life-threatening condition of the newborn, we do know more than we did. Based on animal experimentation, many hypotheses have been proposed for the mechanisms of injury in NEC. A general

scheme for the pathogenesis, incorporating various theories, was constructed more than 2 decades ago and conceptually remains not too far off the mark, according to more recent investigations into the pathogenetic concepts that might be relevant to this condition as it presents in the human newborn. The process of inflammation is central. Why inflammation leads to intestinal necrosis in some infants and not others suggests an interaction between the host and the environment. I (DKS) suspected this a long time ago, finding low C3 levels and lack of activation of complement in preterm infants who had NEC. Various animal models of NEC have helped inform newer etiologic hypotheses.

Caplan and associates (18)(19) have been at the forefront with respect to characterization of a proposed mechanism for the pathogenesis of NEC. It all begins with mucosal damage from some cause (eg, perinatal asphyxia or postnatal infection), followed by bacterial invasion of the damaged intestinal epithelium, which then begins to elicit endogenous production of platelet-activating factor (PAF), PAF-like phospholipids, and tissue necrosis factor (TNF). There may be various sources of PAF. Focal increases in intestinal epithelial permeability may lead to focal mucosal "leak" and local entry of bacteria or bacterial products, thus leading to a patchy type injury. I (DKS) also speculated about mechanisms to explain the patchy nature of the injury, focusing on local serotonin release and focal vasoconstriction. Interactions of PAF with lipopolysaccharides or TNF may trigger inflammatory cascades. The final result depends on the balance between the injurious mechanisms (inflammatory mediators, cytokines, ischemia) and the protective mechanisms (primarily inducible nitric oxide synthase) (Fig. 1). (2) A more recent detailed molecular analysis of the events, still hypothetical, differs very little from the overall conceptual scheme my father and I presented more than 20 years ago (Fig. 2). (19)

Prevention

Understanding the pathogenetic mechanisms for NEC is the best hope for preventing the condition, which when it is diagnosed, is accompanied by serious mortality and morbidity and the reactive dispositions of pediatricians and surgeons. Targeted approaches to interrupting various processes have been demonstrated in animal models, but none of these approaches is currently clinically available. Because of the apparent important role of bacteria in the pathogenesis of NEC, another approach to control the colonization patterns in the intestine has been suggested. (19) This probiotic approach remains investigational, and whether temporary alteration of the intestinal flora of the preterm infant in the context of the NICU will prevent the condition is unknown. That it will prevent NEC completely is unlikely; a variety of approaches probably will be necessary, reflecting the multifactorial initiation of what ultimately is the intersection of coalescing cascades of inflammation leading to permanent injury.

Concluding Comments

Although superficially it appears that the treatment of NEC (and isolated intestinal perforation) has not changed in the past 30 to 40 years, actually much has changed. The patient population has changed dramatically due to improvements in neonatal intensive care and the increased survival rate of smaller and more immature babies. The overall survival rates are similar, but the patient cohort is perhaps higher risk at the onset. A very important change is the improvement of research methods evaluating medical and surgical management. Due to currently ongoing randomized trials as well as potential biology studies, improvements in the management of this condition are highly likely within the next generation of neonatologists and pediatric surgeons.

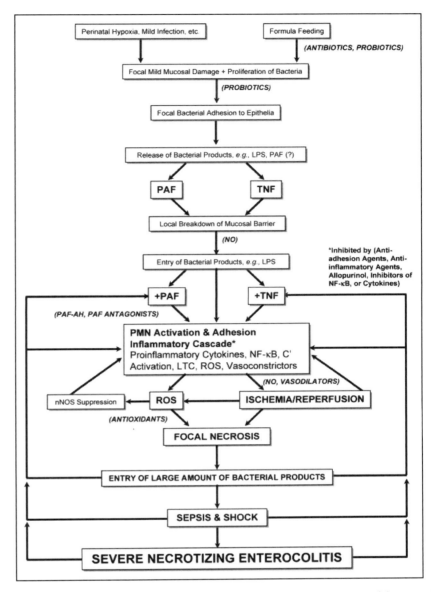

Figure 2. Flow diagram of the proposed pathogenesis of necrotizing enterocolitis (inhibitors are in italics and within parentheses). PAF = platelet-activating factor, LPS = lipopolysaccharide, TNF = tumor necrosis factor, PAF-AH = PAF acetylhydrolase, NO = nitric oxide, C' = complement, NF-κB = nuclear factor-κB, LTC = leukotriene C4, ROS = reactive oxygen species, PMN = polymorphonuclear leukocyte. Diagram from W. Hsueh, M. S. Caplan, X.-W. Qu, X.-D. Tan, I. G. De Plaen, and F. Gonzalez-Crussi, *Pediatric and Developmental Pathology*, vol. 6, no. 1, pp. 6–23, 2003, Society for Pediatric Pathologists, Allen Press, Inc.

References

1. Stevenson JK, Graham CB, Oliver TK Jr, Goldenberg VE. Neonatal necrotizing enterocolitis. A report of twenty-one cases with fourteen survivors. *Am J Surg.* 1969;118:260–272

2. Stevenson DK, Graham CB, Stevenson JK. Neonatal necrotizing enterocolitis: 100 new cases. *Adv Pediatr.* 1980;27:319–340

3. NICHD. ResearchNetwork NN. *Summary Tables of Generic Database.* 2003. Available at: http://neonatal.rti.org/

4. Uauy RD, Fanaroff AA, Korones SB, Phillips EA, Phillips JB, Wright LL. Necrotizing enterocolitis in very low birth weight infants: biodemographic and clinical correlates. National Institute of Child Health and Human Development Neonatal Research Network. *J Pediatr.* 1991;119:630–638

5. Cheu HW, Sukarochana K, Lloyd DA. Peritoneal drainage for necrotizing enterocolitis. *J Pediatr Surg.* 1988;23:557–561

6. de Souza JC, da Motta UI, Ketzer CR. Prognostic factors of mortality in newborns with necrotizing enterocolitis submitted to exploratory laparotomy. *J Pediatr Surg.* 2001;36:482–486

7. Ein SH, Shandling B, Wesson D, Filler RM. A 13-year experience with peritoneal drainage under local anesthesia for necrotizing enterocolitis perforation. *J Pediatr Surg.* 1990;25:1034–1036

8. Ricketts RR, Jerles ML. Neonatal necrotizing enterocolitis: experience with 100 consecutive surgical patients. *World J Surg.* 1990;14:600–605

9. Robertson JF, Azmy AF, Young DG. Surgery for necrotizing enterocolitis. *Br J Surg.* 1987;74:387–389

10. Chwals WJ, Blakely ML, Cheng A, et al. Surgery-associated complications in necrotizing enterocolitis: a multi-institutional study. *J Pediatr Surg.* 2001;36:1722–1724

11. Hintz SR, Kendrick DE, Stoll BJ, et al. Neurodevelopmental and growth outcomes of extremely low birth weight infants after necrotizing enterocolitis. *Pediatrics.* 2005;115:696–703

12. Stevenson DK, Kerner JA, Malachowski N, Sunshine P. Late morbidity among survivors of necrotizing enterocolitis. *Pediatrics.* 1980;66:925–927

13. Stevenson JK, Stevenson DK. Necrotizing enterocolitis in the neonate. *Surg Annu.* 1977;9:147–169

14. Stevenson DK, Shahin SM, Ostrander CR, et al. Breath hydrogen in preterm infants: correlation with changes in bacterial colonization of the gastrointestinal tract. *J Pediatr.* 1982;101:607–610

15. Cohn R, Sunshine P, De Vries P. Necrotizing enterocolitis in the newborn infant. *Am J Surg.* 1972;124:165–168

16. Gross RE. *The Surgery of Infants and Children: Its Principles and Techniques.* Philadelphia, Pa: WB Saunders Co; 1953

17. Blakely ML, Lally KP, McDonald S, et al. Postoperative outcomes of extremely low birth-weight infants with necrotizing enterocolitis or isolated intestinal perforation: a prospective cohort study by the NICHD neonatal research network. *Ann Surg.* 2005;241:984–989

18. Caplan MS, Jilling T. New concepts in necrotizing enterocolitis. *Curr Opin Pediatr.* 2001;13:111–115

19. Hsueh W, Caplan MS, Qu XW, Tan XD, De Plaen IG, Gonzalez-Crussi F. Neonatal necrotizing enterocolitis: clinical considerations and pathogenetic concepts. *Pediatr Dev Pathol.* 2003;6:6–23

Historical Perspectives: Necrotizing Enterocolitis: An Inherited Or Acquired Condition?

David K. Stevenson and Martin L. Blakely

NeoReviews 2006;7;e125-e134

DOI: 10.1542/neo.7-3-e125

Forty Years of Mechanical Ventilation ...Then and Now...

Artificial Ventilation in Respiratory Distress Syndrome

It is difficult to know with certainty who first applied assisted ventilation for the management of neonates who have respiratory distress syndrome (RDS), which was known more commonly as hyaline membrane disease (HMD) at the time of initial assisted ventilation use. However, Maria Deliveria-Papadopoulos and Paul Swyer definitely were among the first to use endotracheal tubes and positive pressure ventilation, and their successful use of this methodology is the choice for this 2003 Historical Perspective. In fact, as Dr. Deliveria-Papadopoulos indicates in her accompanying commentary, assisted ventilation may have been employed successfully on occasion a decade earlier. Undeniably it was used in some countries for infants who had neonatal tetanus, but these neonates had normal lungs, and early reports concerned the use of tracheostomy tubes. (1) Several groups embarked on the course of assisting ventilation in RDS (HMD) in the early 1960s. Some used positive pressure ventilation, including Strang and Reynolds in London, (2) Thomas and coworkers at Stanford, (3) and Heese and colleagues in Cape Town. (4) Others employed negative pressure ventilators, such as Stahlman and associates in Nashville (5) and Stern and colleagues in Montreal. (6) Indeed, negative pressure ventilation could have been used earlier. In 1889, Alexander Graham Bell "designed and built a body type respirator for use with newborn infants. Presented to the American Association for the Advancement of Science in Montreal, the invention met with little enthusiasm." (7) The design and device are preserved in a museum in Nova Scotia, Canada.

In 1969, a conference on assisted ventilation was organized in Paris by Professor Alex Minkowski, with representatives from France, Belgium, England, South Africa (data from Sweden), Finland, Canada, and the United States. (8) The big question was whether neonatologists should continue to provide assisted ventilation (perhaps more aggressively) or whether the possible complications outweighed the potential advantages. Bronchopulmonary dysplasia (or "respirator lung") had been described, (9)(10) and this complication proved to be a serious disadvantage for many years. Needless to say, assisted ventilation did not stop at that time.

Soon to follow was the realization that continuous distending pressure (particularly continuous positive airway pressure) was very beneficial in minimizing or preventing atelectasis in RDS. (11) This will be the featured topic in next month's Historical Perspective.

Alistair G. S. Philip, MD, FRCPE, FAAP
Editor-in-Chief, NeoReviews

References

1. Smythe PM, Bull A. Treatment of tetanus neonatorum with intermittent positive pressure respiration. *Br Med J.* 1959;2:107–113
2. Adamson TM, Collins LM, Dehan M, Hawker JM, Reynolds EOR, Strang LB. Mechanical ventilation in newborn infants with respiratory failure. *Lancet.* 1968;2:227–231
3. Thomas DV, Fletcher G, Sunshine P, Schafer IA, Klaus MH. Prolonged respirator use in pulmonary insufficiency of the newborn. *JAMA.* 1965;193:183–190
4. Heese H deV, Wittman W, Malan AF. Management of respiratory distress syndrome of newborn with positive-pressure respiration. *S Afr Med J.* 1963;37:123–126
5. Stahlman MT, Young WC, Gray J, Shepard FM. The management of respiratory failure in the idiopathic respiratory distress syndrome of prematurity. *Ann N Y Acad Sci.* 1965;121:930–941
6. Stern L, Ramos AD, Outerbridge EW, Beaudry PH. Negative pressure artificial respiration: use in treatment of respiratory failure of the newborn. *Can Med Assoc J.* 1970;102:595–601
7. Stern L. Description and utilization of the negative pressure apparatus. *Biol Neonate.* 1970;16:24–29
8. Symposium on artificial ventilation, Paris 1969. *Biol Neonate.* 1970;16:1–196
9. Northway W, Rosan R, Porter D. Pulmonary disease following respirator therapy of hyaline membrane disease. *N Engl J Med.* 1967;276:357–368
10. Hawker JM, Reynolds EOR, Taghizadeh A. Pulmonary surface tension and pathological changes in infants dying after respirator treatment for severe hyaline membrane disease. *Lancet.* 1967;2:75–77
11. Gregory GA, Kitterman JA, Phibbs RH, Tooley WH, Hamilton WK. Treatment of idiopathic respiratory distress syndrome with continuous positive airway pressure. *N Engl J Med.* 1971;284:1333–1340

Small Steps Toward Assisted Ventilation

The magnitude of the disastrous 1952 poliomyelitis epidemic in Europe had a major impact in the medical world. During the years of the epidemic, respiratory muscle weakness and bulbar respiratory failure often were treated successfully with tank-type negative pressure ventilators of the Drinker design or by continuous positive pressure delivered manually through an endotracheal tube or tracheostomy. Many affected children were weaned to a negative pressure chest cuirass or to a foot-tilt rocking bed as they improved. As a result of these revolutionary new treatments, mortality in spinobulbar poliomyelitis was reduced from 80% at the beginning of the epidemic to 25% with tracheostomy and manually controlled respiration.

In Greece, during the catastrophic 1958 poliomyelitis epidemic, the morbidity and mortality among children, including infants from 2 months of age, was so overwhelming that at the request of the Hellenic Red Cross, the World Red Cross sent to Athens a team of experts from Sweden consisting of physicians, nurses, and physiotherapists with the necessary equipment. I was recruited to work in the special polio unit established in Athens for the treatment of respiratory failure, and for the first time I faced the devastating effects of respiratory failure.

With initially elementary equipment (bag and oxygen mask), we could not sustain respiration in children who had polio; they were dying helplessly without the assistance of a mechanical ventilator. With the Swedish team, we began to use the Drager iron lung, the Freiberger, the Lundia Kifa positive pressure, and the "rocking bed" to assist children who had potentially fatal respiratory failure. (1) A number of children survived, but the 19 young infants who could not be saved stand out in my memory.

Concurrently, a number of positive pressure ventilators, usually volume-controlled, were designed and put into use in major medical centers throughout Europe, making the tank (iron lung) largely obsolete. By 1959, two such ventilators had been used on newborns—a volume-controlled ventilator (the Engstrom respirator) in Sweden and the East Radcliff pump, also a volume-controlled ventilator, in South Africa.

Success in Neonates

Upon starting my residency in the United States, I faced for the first time the high mortality of infants who had HMD and died from respiratory failure. The images of the young children from Greece who had bulbar polio came back vividly, and I began to want to attempt ventilating these babies who otherwise would have died.

In July 1962, at the Hospital for Sick Children in Toronto, I was allowed to intubate preterm babies who had HMD only after they were pronounced dead by the housestaff. For 6 long continuous months, our failure to sustain life in those intubated and ventilated babies was met with sadness and despair. However, perseverance, persuasion, and the agony of attempting to resuscitate babies who had died combined with the use of the Bird Mark VIII Respirator led to my first survivor, an 1,800-g infant of 34 weeks' gestation who had had complete cardiorespiratory arrest on January 9, 1963. The infant was discharged home on the 47th postnatal day with minimal perihilar infiltration radiologically, no abnormal symptoms or physical signs, and a weight of 2,800 g. Examination of the patient at 6 months of age disclosed no neurologic or other abnormality, and the chest radiograph was normal. I reported our results to the Society for Pediatric Research in May 1963 and published the paper with Paul Swyer entitled "Assisted Ventilation in Terminal Hyaline Membrane Disease." (2)

The first report describing the use of assisted ventilation in the treatment of atelectasis neonatorum was by Donald and Lord in 1953. (3) Subsequently, reports accumulated in the literature of the use of assisted ventilation in the treatment of newborn RDS. (4)(5)(6)(7)(8)

In those early days, we felt the risks of ventilation were so great that infants should not be mechanically assisted unless they could not otherwise survive. Consequently, the criteria used to select infants for ventilation were very rigorous: inability to restore respiration using bag and mask, sustained bradycardia of less than 60 beats/min for 1 minute or cardiac arrest of 3 minutes, pH of less than 7.0, Po_2 of less than 30 to 40 mm Hg in 100% oxygen, and $Paco_2$ of greater than 80 mm Hg. The hesitancy to use mechanical ventilation, especially in small preterm infants, was based on the significant hazards associated with this mode of therapy. Of particular concern were the small size of the endotracheal tube and its connections, the susceptibility of the preterm infant to infection, and the high pressures that often were required to achieve adequate gas exchange. In spite of the reluctance to ventilate babies, early reports did demonstrate a small but definite reduction in mortality among infants who weighed more than 1,800 g and who did not require ventilation before 24 hours after birth. (9)

From the milestones of the early 1960s, when mechanical ventilatory support was introduced in the management of newborn respiratory distress, until the end of the decade, little additional progress was made in reducing further the mortality of the critically ill infant, despite the introduction of various types of more sophisticated ventilators and various modes of using them for therapy. During this time, however, progress was made in understanding the nature of newborn RDS and the complexity of the pathophysiology of the immature lung. (10)

Continuous Distending Pressure

The 1971 introduction by Gregory and associates of continuous distending pressure (continuous positive airway pressure [CPAP]) using an endotracheal tube was a breakthrough in the treatment of newborn RDS. (11) They demonstrated dramatic improvement of oxygenation, presumably by recruiting narrowed terminal conducting airways and incompletely collapsed air spaces. The resultant increased lung volume following a given end-distending pressure improved gas exchange and reduced regional vascular resistance and right-to-left shunt in most infants. Subsequently, Rhodes and Hall (12) applied CPAP by face mask and showed a significant decrease in mortality among infants weighing more than 1,500 g who had RDS, and in 1973, Kattwinkel and associates (13) extended the use of CPAP in applying end-distending pressure using nasal catheters positioned in the midnares. These techniques left the trachea undisturbed and preserved the infant's grunt, but erosion of the nasal septum and gastric distension sometimes occurred. Subsequent studies (14)(15) following the original report by Gregory also documented significant reductions in oxygen requirements and oxygen exposure with the use of CPAP. Most studies indicated that early intervention with CPAP increased survival, presumably by stabilizing small air spaces, thereby preventing disruption of surfactant films and ameliorating the disease process. CPAP was found to be beneficial in the management of RDS when the patient required less than 60% oxygen to maintain a Pao_2 of 50 to 60 mm Hg. Optimal levels of CPAP may be titrated according to the level of inspired oxygen. Generally, a level of 5 to 6 cm H_2O is used initially and may be increased as the need for oxygen approaches 100%.

Although CPAP is one treatment currently used for RDS, it is not without adverse effects. Pathophysiologic consequences of CPAP, such as increased work of breathing, decreased lung compliance, and decreased tidal volume, may result from overdistention of the relatively normal air spaces. During recovery from RDS, there also may be increased transmission of pressure to the air spaces and an increased incidence of interstitial emphysema and pneumothorax. Additionally, cardiac output may be impaired due to compression of thoracic veins and pulmonary capillaries.

Intermittent Positive Pressure

Both intermittent positive pressure ventilation and intermittent negative pressure ventilation have been effective in correcting blood gas derangements of RDS and decreasing mortality. The use of intermittent negative pressure ventilation is limited in infants weighing less than 1,500 g and in those who have hypercapnia. (16)(17)(18)(19) Therefore, intermittent positive pressure ventilation has been used more extensively to treat RDS in infants of all birthweights.

Intermittent positive pressure ventilation initially was used with high flow rates during inspiration, a low inspiration-expiration ratio (I:E), and high frequencies, which were consistent with the infant's respiratory pattern. As a result, peak inflation pressures tended to be high. The emphasis on patient-triggered assisted ventilation did not improve oxygenation significantly. (20) The effects of independent variation of rate, I:E ratio, and peak inflation pressure indicated that ventilation improved with higher frequencies or higher peak inflation pressures, while oxygenation improved with lower frequencies or higher peak inflation pressures. (21)(22)(23)

Intermittent positive pressure ventilation also has been used with continuous distending pressure or, as it was formerly called, positive end-expiratory pressure. Because mean airway pressure has been shown to correlate with oxygenation, the use of positive end-expiratory pressure can decrease both peak inflation pressures and the fraction of inspired oxygen. (24) By maintaining constant mean airway pressure, either a square- or sine-wave pressure profile in the respiratory cycle may be used. By using the pressure plateau of square-wave ventilation, gas may enter areas of high resistance and provide better expansion of the open low-V/Q (ventilation-perfusion ratio) compartment. (25) Conversely, a sine wave produces less overdistention of more normal air spaces.

Sequelae

During the pioneering days of mechanical ventilation, associated chronic complications and sequelae did not become apparent because gravely ill infants succumbed. However, as the number of surviving infants increased due to ventilatory assistance, improved technology, and organized regional medical centers, so did the number of sequelae of ventilator treatments. In 1967, Northway and associates described the syndrome of bronchopulmonary dysplasia among infants surviving severe RDS who had required mechanical ventilation. (26) The incidence of bronchopulmonary dysplasia varied from 5% to 30%; the mortality rate was 38%. Its cause still is disputed, but factors such as elevated inspired-oxygen concentration, positive-pressure ventilation, endotracheal intubation, and duration of primary therapy have been implicated. (27)(28) Oxygen alone has been shown to produce vascular engorgement, edema, hemorrhage, and epithelial necrosis, although the incidence of bronchopulmonary dysplasia is lower in infants who do not receive endotracheal intubation and positive pressure.

Although the mortality rate for infants suffering from RDS has decreased with increasingly sophisticated use of mechanical ventilation, questions regarding the quality of life of the survivors have been raised. Initial follow-up studies revealed significant neurologic sequelae. Subsequent follow-up studies indicated, however, that the prognosis for even the most critically ill newborn is good if intervention is early enough to prevent profound hypoxia and acidosis, temperature is maintained, and nutrition is provided. Most of the morbidity centers around the extremely low-birthweight infant (<1,000 g). If optimal care is instituted during the perinatal period, the consensus is that a favorable prognosis on the quality of life of even these survivors can be anticipated.

Conclusion

In the last 40 years, we have seen exponential progress in the care of high-risk newborns from almost 100% mortality of a 1,500-g preterm infant who has cardiorespiratory, metabolic, and nutritional problems to an optimal survival rate close to 100%. The next frontier needs to be the elimination of neurologic sequelae. We need to continue investigating and elucidating the basic cellular mechanisms that will further enable us to maintain the optimal quality of life for our precious preterm babies.

Maria Delivoria-Papadopoulos
Professor of Pediatrics and Physiology,
Emeritus
University of Pennsylvania School of
Medicine
Philadelphia, PA

[To read the original article on intermittent positive pressure respiration to treat RDS written by Dr. Delivoria-Papadopoulos and colleagues in 1965, which was reprinted with permission from the BMJ Publishing Group, please go to: http://neoreviews.aap publications.org/cgi/data/4/12/e335/DC3/1]

References

1. Mangrioti S, Delivoria M. Management of poliomyelitis patients with respiratory failure. *Ann Clin Paediatr Univers Athen.* 1959;6:183–206

2. Delivoria-Papadopoulos M, Swyer P. Assisted ventilation in terminal hyaline membrane disease. *Arch Dis Child.* 1964;39:481–484

3. Donald I, Lord J. Augmented respiration: studies in atelectasis neonatorium. *Lancet.* 1953;1:9–17

4. Benson F, Celander O. Respirator treatment of pulmonary insufficiency in the newborn. *Acta Paediatr (Uppsala).* 1959;48(suppl 118):49

5. Benson F, Celander O, Haglund G, Nilsson L, Paulsen L, Renck L. Positive-pressure respirator treatment of severe pulmonary insufficiency in the newborn infant. A clinical report. *Acta Anesth Scand.* 1958;2:37

6. Donald I. Augmented respiration: an emergency positive-pressure patient-cycled respirator. *Lancet.* 1954;1:895

7. Donald I, Kerr MM, MacDonald IR. Respiratory phenomena in the newborn: experiments in their measurement and assistance. *Scot Med J.* 1958;3:151

8. Heese H de V, Wittmann W, Malan AF. The management of the respiratory distress of the newborn with positive-pressure respiration. *S Afr Med J.* 1963;37:123

9. Stahlman M, Young W, Payne G. Studies of ventilatory aids in hyaline membrane disease. *Am J Dis Child.* 1962;104:526

10. Chu J, Clements JA, Cotton EK, et al. Neonatal pulmonary ischemia. 1. Clinical and physiological studies. *Pediatrics.* 1967;40:709–782

11. Gregory G, Kitterman JA, Phibbs RH, Tooley WH, Hamilton WK. Treatment of the idiopathic respiratory distress syndrome with continuous positive airway pressure. *N Engl J Med*. 1971;204:1333–1340

12. Rhodes P, Hall R. Continuous positive airway pressure delivered by face mask in infants with idiopathic respiratory distress syndrome: a controlled study. *Pediatrics*. 1973;52:1–5

13. Kattwinkel J, Fleming D, Cha CC, Fanaroff AA, Klaus MH. A device for administering continuous positive airway pressure by the nasal route. *Pediatrics*. 1973;52:131–134

14. Allen L, Reynolds ER, Rivers RP, Le Soueff PM, Wimberley PD. Controlled trial of continuous positive airway pressure given by face mask for hyaline membrane disease. *Arch Dis Child*. 1977;52:373–378

15. Krouskop R, Brown E, Sweet A. The early use of continuous positive airway pressure in the treatment of idiopathic respiratory distress syndrome. *J Pediatr*. 1975;87:263–267

16. Ballard R, Kraybill EN, Hernandez J, Renfield ML, Blankenship WJ. Idiopathic respiratory distress syndrome: treatment with continuous negative-pressure ventilation. *Am J Dis Child*. 1973;125:676–681

17. Chernick V, Vidyasagar D. Continuous negative chest-wall pressure in hyaline membrane disease: one-year experience. *Pediatrics*. 1972;49:753–760

18. Fanaroff A, Cha CC, Sosa R, Crumrine RS, Klaus MH. Controlled trial of continuous negative external pressure in the treatment of severe respiratory distress syndrome. *J Pediatr*. 1973;82:921–928

19. Stern L. Description and utilization of the negative-pressure apparatus. *Biol Neonate*. 1970;16:24–34

20. Llewellyn MA, Swyer P. Assisted and controlled ventilation in the newborn period: effect on oxygenation. *Br J Anaesth*. 1971;43:926–931

21. Smith P, Schach E, Daily W. Mechanical ventilation of newborn infants: effects of independent variation of rate and pressure on arterial oxygenation of infants with respiratory distress syndrome. *Anesthesiology*. 1972;37:498–502

22. Klein M, Harrison V, Malan A. The effect of varying inspiratory-gas-flow rate. *Br J Anaesth*. 1969;41:370

23. Owen-Thomas J, Ulan O, Swyer P. The effect of varying inspiratory-gas-flow rate on arterial oxygenation during IPPV in the respiratory distress syndrome. *Br J Anaesth*. 1968;40:493–502

24. Boros S, Matalon SV, Ewald R, Leonard AS, Hunt CE. The effect of independent variations in inspiratory-expiratory ratio and end-expiratory pressure during mechanical ventilation in hyaline membrane disease: the significance of mean airway pressure. *J Pediatr*. 1977;91:794–798

25. McIntyre R, Laws A, Ramachandran P. Positive expiratory pressure plateau: improved gas exchange during mechanical ventilation. *Can Anaesth Soc J*. 1969;16:477–486

26. Northway W, Rosan R, Porter D. Pulmonary disease following respirator therapy of hyaline membrane disease. *N Engl J Med*. 1967;276:357–374

27. Nash G, Blennerhasset J, Pontoppidan H. Pulmonary lesions associated with oxygen therapy and artificial ventilation. *N Engl J Med*. 1967;276:1–7

28. Philip AGS. Oxygen plus pressure plus time: the etiology of bronchopulmonary dysplasia. *Pediatrics*. 1975;55:44–49

Historical Perspectives: Forty Years of Mechanical Ventilation ...Then and Now...

Alistair G. S. Philip and Maria Delivoria-Papadopoulos

NeoReviews 2003;4;335

DOI: 10.1542/neo.4-12-e335

Classification by Birthweight and Gestational Age

Introduction

This 2003 contribution by Dr. Battaglia draws attention to the importance of both birthweight and gestational age in determining neonatal morbidity and mortality. It is hard to imagine the language of neonatology without the terms SGA, AGA, and LGA (small, appropriate, and large for gestational age), but prior to 1967 it was unusual to combine birthweight with gestational age. As Dr. Battaglia points out, small babies were considered to have been born prematurely. It is also interesting to note the mortality statistics in that era. The figures in the original article from Colorado subsequently were revised in a chart that detailed birthweight/gestational age categories by 250 g/1 week groups. (1)

Alistair G. S. Philip, MD, FRCPE, FAAP
Editor-in-Chief, NeoReviews

Reference

1. Lubchenco LO, Searle DJ, Brazie JF. Neonatal mortality rate: relationship to birth weight and gestational age. *J Pediatr.* 1972;81:814–822

SGA, IUGR, FGR, and Everything In Between

Small for gestational age (SGA), a term that has become widely used and occasionally misused, originated in the 1960s. At that time, neonatal intensive care units (ICUs) were called "premature nurseries" because it was assumed that all babies admitted to those units were preterm infants. Consideration of the small baby born at term or even postterm had led to the use of the term "placental insufficiency syndrome," but scant attention had been paid to the heterogeneous population that was cared for in "premature nurseries" at that time.

Initial Birthweight/Gestational Age Distribution

Some years earlier, my colleagues and I at Johns Hopkins, Dr Hellegers and Dr Frazier, had published an article examining the outcome of teenage pregnancies. (1) That study alerted us to the fact that clinical problems could be missed with specific study restrictions. For example, if teenage pregnancies included 16- to 19-year-old women, the perinatal mortality rate was not increased compared with women ages 20 to 29 years. Pregnancies in the 16- to 19-year-old group were far more frequent than in girls younger than 15 years of age and masked the high perinatal mortality rate of the latter group. This prompted us to examine the birthweight/gestational age distribution for women delivering at the Johns Hopkins Hospital. (2) Lubchenco and colleagues had published a study of birthweight/gestational age distribution from Colorado involving both inborn and outborn infants. (3) The two studies, published within a few years of each other, showed remarkable agreement in the 10th percentile of the birthweight/gestational age plot, but differed markedly in the 90th percentile distribution. It is important to emphasize that there were no computers at that time, only sorting data by punch cards, a laborious and time-consuming enterprise. Once computers were available, numerous studies appeared that reported birthweight/gestational age distributions for many different populations. Both the Colorado and Baltimore studies were describing the distribution of a population, not attempting to identify infants who had intrauterine growth retardation.

At the time the Baltimore study was being submitted for publication, I moved to a faculty position at the University of Colorado. Dr Lubchenco and I began to talk about how the birthweight/gestational age data could be applied more widely clinically. It seemed that the agreement between the two studies for the 10th percentile could provide the foundation for a simple schema for use in nurseries, anticipating that future studies would support the validity of the 10th percentile, and there would be more variance in the 90th percentile. (4)

Gestational age was subdivided according to the variance of ± 2 weeks that obstetricians in the 1960s attributed to the estimate of gestational age based on the last menstrual period. Thus, we defined term as 38 to 42 weeks' gestation, preterm as fewer than 38 weeks', and postterm as more than 42 weeks'. The birthweight was subdivided into three groups with the 10th and 90th percentiles. This provided a simple but effective means of subdividing newborns into nine birthweight/ gestational age categories. The ease of application of this process led to increased recognition of SGA and large for gestational age (LGA) infants. Publications from many neonatal centers followed quickly, describing the clinical problems most frequently associated with SGA and LGA infants. Neonatal mortality rate data included in this first article were based on the largest series available at the time, that of Ehrhardt and associates. (5)

After publication of the article on classification, a number of authors introduced some variant form of this approach for subdividing newborns, such as small for dates (SFD) and light for dates (LFD). None of these became widely used, however, largely because all of these approaches soon were replaced by proper fetal growth curves determined by ultrasonographic fetal biometry.

A recent review of mortality rates conducted under the auspices of the National Institute of Child Health and Human Development Neonatal Research Network employed the approach of the original studies, using birthweight and gestational age data to construct mortality rates. (6) Unfortunately, the article did not present the data in a useable format that related mortality to both gestational age and birthweight. However, the only colored graph in the study suggested no difference for mortality at gestational ages older than 29 weeks whether the infants were LGA or SGA. The authors alluded to differences in mortality rates for fetal growth retardation (FGR) babies in the discussion, but the comparisons were weakened in terms of clinical usefulness by the inclusion of gender differences as well.

Abbreviations

AC:	abdominal circumference
FGR:	fetal growth retardation (restriction)
FL:	femur length
HC:	head circumference
ICU:	intensive care unit
LGA:	large for gestational age
SGA:	small for gestational age

Ultrasonographic Fetal Biometry

The next major change in assessing fetal growth stemmed from gradual improvements in ultrasonographic techniques that led to better criteria for estimating fetal weight. Population-based studies resulted in equations that related a number of fetal body measurements to fetal weight. The most commonly used involved head circumference, abdominal circumference, and femur length. Obstetric research pointed out that fetal growth curves constructed from ultrasonographic estimation of fetal size in normal pregnancies defined greater fetal weights at any given gestational age than the curves using birthweight data. This was to be expected because preterm birthweight data could not be considered as coming from perfectly normal pregnancies. Fortunately, obstetricians very effectively constructed fetal growth curves from ultrasonographic biometry for many different populations. Fetal growth curves based on ultrasonographic fetal biometry certainly represented a step forward from reliance on birthweight data alone. However, it is not clear that calculating an estimated fetal weight from population-based data of multiple fetal measurements is an improvement over using the measurements themselves to detect undersized infants. Comparisons of the range of error for an estimated fetal weight were not significantly different using abdominal circumference (AC) measurements alone compared with estimates that used head circumference (HC), AC, and femur length (FL). (7) In addition, in a recent study, we found that the reduction in umbilical blood flow that occurred in FGR pregnancies was more apparent when flows were expressed per unit HC or per unit AC than flow per kilogram of estimated fetal weight. (8)

If the primary objective is recognition of fetuses who truly have experienced growth retardation among SGA infants, then a further refinement can be the inclusion of maternal and paternal size. Several authors have encouraged the calculation of "expected" fetal weights from the inclusion of maternal and paternal size to discern FGR infants better among the SGA group. (9)(10)(11)

It seems more likely to me that, with the widespread use of Doppler techniques, physiologic data on the fetal circulation will be used to separate FGR infants from the "normal small" infants within the SGA group. In an earlier study aimed at categorizing SGA pregnancies into FGR of different clinical severity, the simple use of umbilical artery velocimetry and fetal heart rate monitoring established that two thirds of the infants had increased pulsatility in the umbilical artery, which would establish these pregnancies as FGR pregnancies. (12) The one third of infants who had normal velocimetry and heart rate represent a group containing FGR pregnancies and "normal small" pregnancies. One might ask if the latter group of babies all are "normal small," and the answer is that clearly they are not. Many in this group have been shown to have significantly reduced umbilical blood flows as well as reduced amino acid concentrations. (8) From a practical viewpoint, serial Doppler studies currently probably represent the best approach to detect FGR pregnancies among group 1 pregnancies and to detect those group 1 pregnancies that progress to group 2, using the classification established by Pardi and associates. (12)

Estimating Fat Concentrations

A word should be said about estimation of fat concentration. In animal studies, regardless of the model used, FGR fetuses are unable to deposit normal fat stores in late gestation. When FGR babies are examined after delivery, they show all the clinical signs of reduced fat stores. Thus, if fat concentration could be estimated fairly precisely during fetal life with ultrasonographic estimates of fat-to-lean ratios in various sites, this might help distinguish the "normal small" from the FGR fetuses in group 1. Such studies are underway at a number of centers.

Conclusion

We have learned a great deal about the problems associated with the recognition of FGR fetuses at different stages of gestation. The progression from the birthweight/gestational age data that formed the basis of the SGA classification to the current practice of using fetal growth curves derived from ultrasonographic estimates of fetal growth has been important.

The next few years should see the use of physiologic data to tighten further the separation of FGR from "normal small" among SGA infants and will lead to a more precise assessment of clinical severity. The collection of physiologic data will enable us to assess better those fetuses that have circulatory compromise or progressive deterioration in placental function.

Frederick C. Battaglia, MD
Professor of Pediatrics and Professor of
Obstetrics and Gynecology
University of Colorado School of Medicine
Denver, Colorado

[For the original article by Battaglia and Lubchenco on the classification of newborns by weight and gestational age, which was reprinted with permission of the *Journal of Pediatrics*, please go to: http://neoreviews.aap publications.org/cgi/content/full/4/4/e91/DC1]

References

1. Battaglia FC, Frazier TM, Hellegers AE. Obstetric and pediatric complications of juvenile pregnancy. *Pediatrics*. 1963;32:902–910

2. Battaglia FC, Frazier TM, Hellegers AE. Birth weight, gestational age, and pregnancy outcome, with special reference to high birth weight-low gestational age infants. *Pediatrics*. 1966;37:417–422

3. Lubchenco LO, Hansman C, Dressler M, Boyd E. Intrauterine growth as estimated from liveborn birth-weight data at 24 to 42 weeks of gestation. *Pediatrics*. 1963;32:793–800

4. Battaglia FC, Lubchenco LO. A practical classification of newborn infants by weight and gestational age. *J Pediatr*. 1967;71:159–163

5. Ehrhardt CL, Joshi GB, Nelson FG, Kroll BH, Weiner L. Influence of weight and gestation on perinatal and neonatal mortality by ethnic group. *Am J Public Health*. 1964;54:1841–1847

6. Lemons JA, Bauer CR, Oh W, et al. Very low birth weight outcomes of the National Institute of Child Health and Human Development Neonatal Research Network January 1995 through December 1996. *Pediatrics*. 2001;107:e1. Available at: www.pediatrics.org/cgi/content/full/107/1/e1

7. Creasy RK, Resnik R, eds. *Maternal-Fetal Medicine*. 4th ed. Philadelphia, Pa: WB Saunders Co; 1999

8. Ferrazzi E, Rigano S, Bozzo M, et al. Umbilical vein blood flow in growth restricted fetuses. *Ultrasound Obstet Gynecol*. 2000;16:432–438

9. DeJong CL, Gardosi J, Dekker GA, Colenbrander GJ, van Geijn HP. Application of a customised birthweight standard in the assessment of perinatal outcome in a high risk population. *Br J Obstet Gynaecol*. 1998;105:531–535

10. DeJong CL, Francis A, Van Geijn HP, Gardosi J. Customised fetal weight limits for antenatal detection of fetal growth restriction. *Ultrasound Obstet Gynecol*. 2000;15:36–40

11. Clausson B, Gardosi J, Francis A, Cnattingius S. Perinatal outcome in SGA births defined by customised versus population-based birthweight standards. *Br J Obstet Gynaecol*. 2001;108:830–834

12. Pardi G, Cetin I, Marconi AM, et al. Diagnostic value of blood sampling in fetuses with growth retardation. *N Engl J Med*. 1993;328:692–696

Historical Perspectives: Classification by Birthweight and Gestational Age

Alistair G. S. Philip and Frederick C. Battaglia

NeoReviews 2003;4;91

DOI: 10.1542/neo.4-4-e91

Phototherapy

Introduction

The story of how phototherapy started was documented eloquently some years ago by Dobbs and Cremer. How it came to be used in pre-term infants is equally eloquently presented by Jerold Lucey in the accompanying reminiscence. Learning how this staple of neonatal management came about makes for very interesting reading.

Alistair G. S. Philip, MD, FRCPE, FAAP
Editor-in-Chief, NeoReviews

Suggested Reading
1. Dobbs RH, Cremer RJ. Phototherapy. *Arch Dis Child.* 1975;50:833–836

Sculpins, Newborn Seals, Jaundiced Rats, and Phototherapy: A Study in Serendipity

The Uniqueness of Newborns

I first became interested in "newborns" in the summer of 1948 while working at the Mt. Desert Island Biological Laboratory conducting inulin clearance studies on sculpins with my college biology professor Roy Forrester of Dartmouth College. My first "significant (?)" contribution to science was devising a way to draw blood samples from fish and collect their urine over a 24-hour period. It was a challenging time for me. I remain to this very day probably the only person who knows the inulin renal clearance of the sculpin! It's a secret I cherish.

That same summer a very prestigious research group from New York University/Columbia/Yale and Johns Hopkins medical schools was studying renal blood flow in baby seals in the shed next to ours. They were studying the effect of the "diving reflex" on renal blood flow. Things were not going well. The precious baby seals, kept in a large pen in the ocean, were dying of starvation. They had apparently been separated from their mothers before they learned to catch and eat fish. The "prestigious" group decided to hand feed the seals. I volunteered to help. The seals wouldn't eat dead fish. It turned out to be impossible to push a live or dead fish down a baby seal's throat. I came up with the idea of using a blender to homogenize the fish and use a gavage tube for feeding. It worked. I smelled of seal vomit all that summer, but it

didn't matter. I realized for the first time how unique newborns were. I began to think I might go into research after medical school.

In my third year of medical school (1950) at NYU-Bellevue, we were allowed to take a few electives. Medical schools in that day were just beginning to allow such freedom. I took advantage of this to work for Dr. Henry Barnett at Cornell Medical School doing renal clearance studies on preterm infants. I volunteered to drink formula for 3 days and have my renal clearance compared to "a preemie." I beat "the preemie" at concentrating my urine. This experience played a major role in my decision to stay in academia and conduct research on preterm infants.

Following Bilirubin

I also took electives at Babies Hospital, Columbia Presbyterian Medical Center, where I first met Dr. William Silverman. I attended a lecture by Dr. Clement Smith from Harvard on the physiology of the preterm infant. He was a great speaker. I read his book, elected an extra month in the premature unit at Bellevue Hospital, and applied for a fellowship with Dr. Smith at Harvard. It was during my first year of residency at Babies Hospital (1953) that bilirubin entered my life. Dr. Silverman, who was in charge of the premature unit, was conducting a randomized trial of the efficacy of penicillin/sulfasoxazole versus oxytetracycline in preventing newborn infections. (1)

Dr. Ruth Harris, my attending, asked Dr. Bob MacLean and me to help her do a study to determine the normal levels of serum

bilirubin in "small" preemies (<2,000 g) during the first week after birth. We drew the blood and did the laboratory work, all after our regular "hours" as residents. Bob had trained in Vancouver, British Columbia. A few months into the study, he commented that infants rarely died of kernicterus in Vancouver. We had seen 19 die of kernicterus over a period of 7 months!

It was fortunate that Dr. Silverman's study was a randomized, controlled trial. We began to notice that kernicterus "seemed" to occur more often in the sulfasoxazole/penicillin-treated infants and that they had low levels of serum bilirubin. When the Silverman trial was completed, the results left no doubt that sulfasoxazole was related to kernicterus. Our study reported that kernicterus occurred with low levels of serum bilirubin. (2)

If Dr. Silverman had not been doing his randomized, controlled trial on these same infants, the association between sulfasoxazole and bilirubin would never have been discovered. It was remarkable that sulfasoxazole was widely used in premature nurseries at that time, yet no one had detected this unique lethal association, and no other "epidemics" ever were reported!

This experience made me an early convert to and believer in randomized, controlled trials. In looking back at the era (1950 through 1960), it's remarkable how few randomized trials (maybe one or two) were being conducted or had been conducted in neonatology. Dr. Silverman was indeed "a voice crying out in the wilderness." He became my idol.

Rat Tales

In 1955 through 1956, I took a fellowship in neonatology with Dr. Clement Smith in Boston. At that time, his group of "fellows" was studying pulmonary function in newborns, defining normal newborn lung parameters. I realized that I could not do that type of research in my new position in Vermont. I needed a small animal project I could do with the help of a technician. I began a literature search for a jaundice animal model and found that Dr. Gunn had first described the Gunn rat in 1944. (3) I tracked Dr. Gunn down on Prince Edward Island, Canada, where he was raising silver foxes. He informed me that Dr. Castle, a geneticist, maintained a small colony of Gunn rats to teach genetics to graduate students at the University of California, Berkeley. I contacted Dr. Castle, who kindly sent me a few rats, but warned me that they were difficult to raise because many of the jaundiced homozygous animals died in the newborn period. Being a geneticist, he had little interest in why they died! I thought, "Perhaps they are dying of kernicterus." He had also sent a starter colony to Dr. Rudi Schmid at the National Institutes of Health. Dr. Schmid used the Gunn rat to pinpoint the cause of their jaundice – an absence of hepatic glucuronyl transferase. (4) This very important study opened a whole new era of research in bilirubin metabolism.

I didn't have time or sufficient training in basic science to do solo research in Vermont. I had a lot of clinical responsibilities. I did examine a few rat brains. I thought they looked like they had kernicterus. The clinical picture of the deaths and the survivors that "wobbled" was also compatible with kernicterus.

Dr. Dick Day, my former attending at Columbia, and then Professor and Chairman at Downstate Medical School, heard that I had a small breeding colony. He and Dr. Lois Johnson were thinking along similar lines. I sent them a starter colony, and along with Dr. W. Blanc, they performed the proper studies to document that the high neonatal mortality rate among these animals was due to kernicterus. (5)

I subsequently sent starter colonies to several other research groups, including Drs. I. Arias in New York and L. Ballowitz in Berlin. The Gunn rat played a very important role as a research model in the study of neonatal jaundice. I'm very proud of the role I played in "saving them from their dull life in the world of genetics." These animals are now being used to test the effectiveness of gene

transplants to cure hyperbilirubinemia. In the early 1980s, Dr. Gunn wrote to me inquiring about whether I had "found" the Gunn rats. He was amazed to learn that the rats named in his honor had become such an important research tool.

Introducing Phototherapy

In 1958, I read the original article on phototherapy by Drs. Cremer, Perryman, and Richards in the *Lancet*. (6) I was intrigued but skeptical and unimpressed. I believed that the numbers of patients were small (nine infants), and the results needed to be confirmed. During the next several years, I didn't think much about phototherapy and apparently neither did the British or North Americans. There were no reports of its use in either country.

In 1965, I received an inquiry from Dr. Mario Ferreiro of Santiago, Chile. He wanted to come to Vermont to do a fellowship in newborn care. I warned him about our weather and that we had only a two-man department of pediatrics. He came anyway. After he had been in Burlington for a few weeks, he politely asked me, "Why aren't you using phototherapy?" I was surprised and asked, "Is anybody using it?" He replied, "Oh yes, we do in Santiago, and it seems to work." I was a bit arrogant. "How can you tell it works?" I asked. "I've seen no publications to support its use." Of course I hadn't because I rarely read the foreign literature! I sent Mario to the library. He found more than 20 articles, all in Spanish, Portuguese, Italian, or French, on the clinical use of phototherapy. (7) I was humbled, and ever since I've tried to keep up with the pediatric literature in other languages. However, because none of the studies was randomized and controlled, I remained unimpressed.

Mario needed a simple clinical research project that he could carry on when he returned to Santiago. We decided to conduct a randomized trial of phototherapy to test its effectiveness in preventing hyperbilirubinemia of prematurity. I secretly believed that

the trial would show that phototherapy was not effective and would provide evidence to stop the use of such a therapy.

We contacted Dr. Obes Polleri in Uruguay and Dr. Berzin in Brazil. (8) They kindly sent us the plans for the phototherapy devices that they were using, which we copied. Our randomized, controlled trial turned out to be a success, proving that phototherapy did work. (7) This was no surprise to many physicians in South America, France, and Italy, who had been using such therapy since the early 1960s. It was, however, a surprise to the British and North American physicians who also apparently had been unable or uninterested in reading the foreign literature.

Our study was confirmed by other randomized trials, and phototherapy was widely adopted over the next decade. Not everybody was enthusiastic. Dr. Gerard Odell of Johns Hopkins led the opposition to its clinical use. He raised many theoretical concerns about its effectiveness and safety. He banned its use at Johns Hopkins, and to this day, I think graduates of his program remain skeptical. I corresponded several times with Dr. Cremer, who generously thanked me for introducing the use of phototherapy in the United States and publicizing its effectiveness. He received a belated merit award in 1996 from the British Health Service for his work. Neither of us ever did understand why the English-speaking world hadn't done any studies on the use of phototherapy during the 1958 through 1968 decade.

Jerold F. Lucey, MD, FAAP
Wallace Professor of Neonatology
University of Vermont College of Medicine
Burlington, Vermont

[For the original article by Dr. Lucey and colleagues on the prevention of hyperbilirubinemia of prematurity by phototherapy, please go to: http://neoreviews.aappublications.org/cgi/content/full/4/2/e27/DC1 or http://pediatrics.aappublications.org/cgi/content/abstract/41/6/1047]

References

1. Silverman W, Anderson DH, Blanc WA, Crozier DN. A difference in mortality rate and incidence of kernicterus among premature infants allotted to two prophylactic antibacterial regimens. *Pediatrics*. 1956;18: 614–625

2. Harris RC, Lucey JF, MacLean JR. Kernicterus in premature infants associated with low concentrations of bilirubin in the plasma. *Pediatrics*. 1958;21:875–883

3. Gunn CK. Hereditary achlouric jaundice in the rat. *Can Med Assoc J.* 1944;50: 230–237

4. Schmid R, Axelrod J, Hammaker L, Swarm RL. Congenital jaundice in rats due to a defect in glucuronide formation. *J Clin Invest.* 1958;37:1123

5. Johnson L, Blanc W, Lucey JL, Day R. Kernicterus in rats with familial jaundice. [Abstract]. *AMA J Dis Child.* 1957;94:548

6. Cremer RJ, Perryman PW, Richards DH. Influence of light on hyperbilirubinemia of infants. *Lancet.* 1958;1:1094–1098

7. Lucey JF, Ferreiro M, Hewitt J. Prevention of hyperbilirubinemia of prematurity by phototherapy. *Pediatrics.* 1968;41: 1047–1054

8. Obes Polleri J. Phototherapy in neonatal hyperbilirubinemia. *Arch Pediatr Uruguay.* 1967;38:77–86

Historical Perspectives: Phototherapy

Alistair G. S. Philip and Jerold F. Lucey
NeoReviews 2003;4;27
DOI: 10.1542/neo.4-2-e27

Neurologic Maturation of the Neonate

Introduction

The article chosen for this month's Historical Perspectives is "Neurological Evaluation of the Maturity of Newborn Infants" by Claudine Amiel-Tison. (1) This paper previously was chosen for inclusion in the Ross series "Landmarks in Neonatology/Perinatology," at which time (August, 1982) Dr Amiel-Tison provided a commentary, which also is reproduced here.

Some of the maneuvers Dr Amiel-Tison described were incorporated into scoring systems for assessing gestational age, to which she raised several objections, but she described newer findings that have formed the basis for her continuing evaluation of not only the neonate, but also the infant and young child.

When I asked her to provide a personal reminiscence of how the paper came into being, I also asked her to put it into today's perspective. She prepared an overview of the evolution of her work over the past 40 years. Dr Amiel-Tison continues to emphasize the need for caution in interpreting the results of scoring systems for gestational age. She has maintained the great tradition of careful neurologic evaluation she inherited from Dr André Thomas and Dr Suzanne Saint-Anne-Dargassies. Because she has both trained and collaborated with many international investigators, her approach has been widely disseminated. This review provides some special insights that should be of interest not only to neonatologists but to all pediatricians.

Alistair G. S. Philip, MD, FRCPE, FAAP
Editor-in-Chief, NeoReviews

Reference

1. Amiel-Tison C. Neurological evaluation of the maturity of newborn infants. *Arch Dis Child*. 1968;43:89–93

The following commentary originally appeared in 1982 as one of a series published by Ross Laboratories entitled "Landmarks in Neonatology/Perinatology—Current Comment" and is reproduced with permission of Abbott Nutrition.

Commenting on Neurologic Assessment

While attending the clinic of Dr André Thomas at the Baudelocque Maternity Hospital in the early sixties, I came to understand Thomas' passion for the neurology of the newborn.

André Thomas was an old man by then, nearly blind and deaf. He concentrated all his strength on the examination of the infant before him, as he explained the reflexes and tone reactions he was eliciting to his few silent disciples. (1)

Dr Saint-Anne-Dargassies shared Thomas' passion, inherited his method of examination, and described the stages of development which characterize maturation between 28 and 40 weeks gestational age. (2) This neurologic approach has been invaluable help in determining gestational age and in determining and describing specific abnormal neurologic signs for a given gestational age.

This type of evaluation, however, was difficult to learn other than by direct observation and repeated practice. Having been taught by Saint-Anne-Dargassies, I tried to transmit her neurologic evaluation method to pediatricians. I selected the most important items from the examination, described precisely each maneuver involved, and illustrated, in table form, the normal responses according to six age groups. (3) As I gained personal experience, I came to feel that the maturational pattern of active tone in neck flexors and neck extensors could be better described and illustrated. (4)

The need to determine gestational age became increasingly evident with the growth of perinatology as a subspecialty. However, the extensive use of artificial ventilation and other accoutrements of newborn intensive care made it more and more difficult to perform the neurologic examination properly. The logical solution was to find other tools, such as external criteria. (5)(6) Another tendency was to simplify neurologic testing and to use it in conjunction with external criteria to create an even faster and easier evaluation. (7)(8)

I have three objections to such simplification of neurologic assessment:

1. One cannot call a sample of five passive muscle tone maneuvers a neurologic evaluation. The use of passive tone is certainly the most appealing; it can be quantitated, and one usually has access to infant's limbs, even in the most acute situation. However, active tone is more meaningful.

2. The adaptation into a score modifies the meaning of the maturational stages as they were first described. Maturation is a continuous process, and a conclusion can be reached only when the majority of the items are grouped in one of the 2-week stages described. This has been forgotten with these simplified methods. Providing a scoring system allows one to surmise a probable gestational age at any cost.

3. There are limitations to any method of defining gestational age, as reviewed by Finnstrom. (9) The 95% confidence limits calculated by Finnstrom vary from ±24 days for external criteria alone or neurologic evaluation alone to ±21 days for the addition of both. Factors limiting the accuracy of models used for estimating gestational age can be summarized in three parts:

   - There are limitations in the reproducibility of the methods. Reproducibility seems to be enhanced when several methods are combined.
   - The extent of a biologic variation in maturation is not known, but probably corresponds to at least ±1 week.
   - Standardization of any method has to rely on the date of the mother's last menstrual period.

Error in estimating gestational age from the mother's last menstrual period amounts to at least ±1 week, even if the dates are carefully verified.

Then, nice linear correlations showing that one score is better than another are perfectly all right as long as one decides to forget about the errors hidden behind the score.

Aside from these somewhat irritating distortions, and despite the difficulties and limitations described above, this neurologic approach to the newborn has been the basis of new research.

1. Neck extensor hypertonia may be detected by observing spontaneous posture and eliciting an abnormal pattern of head straightening. (10) This sign correlates with other signs of insult to the central nervous system and can be considered a symptom of raised intracranial pressure. The knowledge of maturational patterns in the neck muscles is clearly the preliminary basis of this detection.

2. Evidence of an advance in neurologic maturation can be shown following high-risk pregnancies in which there has been intrauterine stress. That was first described by Gould et al. (11)(12) Similar cases have been observed at Port-Royal. (13)

3. The observation of hypotonia in the upper part of the body is a common pattern in minimal birth trauma. (14) One can speculate on mechanisms of this transitory symptom. As if the last acquired capacities were the most fragile, the infant reverts to a previous pattern of maturation for a few days or weeks. This pattern is of no localizing value, and probably there is no cellular damage.

4. Neurologic maturation does not stop at 40 weeks. The prolongation of clinical observations of neurologic development within the first 3 postnatal months led Grenier to an elegant speculation. (14) It seems that many signs of the neonatal examination, such as the brisk primary reflexes in the upper extremities (Moro reflex, grasping reflex) and the anxiety brought by these brisk and uncontrolled reactions, are linked with neck impotence. This aspect changes dramatically when head control is acquired.

Therefore, if head control could be realized in the first weeks of life, a transformation of motor aptitude and behavior should be observed. In fact, one can observe these changes if the examiner patiently stabilizes the infant's neck.

These observations are of considerable theoretical interest, offering one way to show that upper structures are already functioning when lower structures are functionally suppressed temporarily.

Thus, the study of the evolution of tone and reflexes from fetal life through the first few months postnatally is one of continuing practical as well as theoretical value.

Claudine Amiel-Tison

References

1. Thomas A, Saint-Anne-Dargassies S. *Etudes Neurologiques sur le Nouveau-né etle Jeune Nourrisson.* Paris, France: Masson; 1952

2. Saint-Anne-Dargassies S. La maturation neurologique du prématuré. *Etudes Néo-natales.* 1955;4:71

3. Amiel-Tison C. Neurological evaluation of the maturity of newborn infants. *Arch Dis Child.* 1968;43:89

4. Amiel-Tison C. Neurological evaluation of the small neonate: the importance of head straightening reactions. In Gluck L, ed. *Modern Perinatal Medicine.* Chicago, Ill: Year Book Medical Publishers; 1974:347

5. Usher R, McLean F, Scott KE. Judgment of fetal age. II. Clinical significance of gestational age and objective method for its assessment. *Pediatr Clin North Am.* 1966;13:835

6. Farr V, Mitchell RG, Neligan GA, et al. The definition of some external characteristics used in the assessment of gestational age in the newborn infant. *Dev Med Child Neurol.* 1966;8:507

7. Dubowitz V, Goldberg C. Clinical assessment of gestational age in the newborn infant. *J Pediatr.* 1970;77:1

8. Ballard JL, Kazmaier-Novak K, Driver M. A simplified score for assessment of fetal maturation of newly born infants. *J Pediatr.* 1979;95:769

9. Finnstrom O. Studies on maturity in newborn infants. VI. Comparison between different methods for maturity estimation. *Acta Paediatr Scand.* 1972;61:33

10. Amiel-Tison C, Korobkin R, Esque-Vaucouloux MT. Neck extensor hypertonia, a clinical sign of insult to the central nervous system of the newborn. *Early Hum Dev.* 1977;1:181

11. Gould JB, Gluck L, Kulovich MV. The acceleration of neurological maturation in high stress pregnancy and its relation to fetal lung maturity. *Pediatr Res.* 1972;6:276

12. Gould JB, Gluck L, Kulovich MV. The relationship between accelerated pulmonary maturity and accelerated neurological maturity in certain neurologically stressed pregnancies. *Am J Obstet Gynecol.* 1977;127:181

13. Amiel-Tison C. Possible acceleration of neurological maturation following high risk pregnancy. *Am J Obstet Gynecol.* 1980;138:303

14. Amiel-Tison C, Grenier A, eds. *Evaluation Neurologique du Nouveau-né et du Nourrisson.* Paris, France: Masson; 1980:124

Clinical Assessment of Neurologic Maturation in the Neonate
First Steps

When, as a newcomer, I joined the clinical and research group of Alexandre Minkowski in 1962 in Paris, brain maturation in the fetus and the neonate was the central theme. Jupiter was well set indeed, with three ladies familiarly designated as "the three graces": Saint-Anne-Dargassies was the clinician, Dreyfus-Brisac the electrophysiologist, and Larroche the pathologist. They described typical maturation patterns on the one hand and specific types of brain damage in correlation with gestational age (GA) at birth on the other. Their pioneering work was rapidly and widely recognized.

As a clinician, I was taught by Saint-Anne-Dargassies. It was a permanent delight to observe her manipulating a "premie," but it took me years to determine how each maneuver could be analyzed and both typical and abnormal responses defined. I had to go from magic to analysis and synthesis. In this long process, I benefited from various effective supports. When I spent a few months as a fellow in Stanford in 1966, Marshall Klaus, with his usual communicative enthusiasm, strongly encouraged me to publish a simplified method that would be accessible to neonatologists. I was offered the help of the illustration department of Stanford University to elaborate the graphic representation, which resulted in the three tables included in my first paper. (1)

During the following years, due to the chronic lack of space in the research unit, my desk was in the pathology lab of Jeanne-Claudie Larroche. I was, therefore, participating in the lab life, with brains all over the place at various stages of pathologic processing from macroscopic inspection to serial slicing, coloration, microscopic analysis, and finally clinicopathologic conference. Each time Dr Larroche had an interesting slide under her microscope, she invited me to have a look ("Claudine viens voir"). This was such amazing training for a clinician that I was very well prepared for the imaging revolution that came in the early 1980s; anatomoclinical correlations were transposed with no surprise into clinicoradiologic correlations.

Anatomic and Physiologic Correlates

When Saint-Anne-Dargassies applied André Thomas' assessment of the term neonate (2) to 100 preterm infants born from 28 to 37 weeks' gestation, the approach was descriptive. (3) From these observations, organized at 2-week intervals, she brilliantly identified the upward (caudocephalic) progression of maturation during the last 3 months of fetal life. However, she did not elaborate on anatomic and physiologic correlates to understand the meaning of this caudocephalic progression. It was clear that most of the criteria used were dependent on brainstem activity, particularly primary reflexes that exerted such a fascination for adult neurologists such as Andre Thomas and many others.

At the same time, Peiper, a German pediatrician, described the downward (cephalocaudal) progression of maturation during the first 2 years after birth, depending on the cerebral hemispheres. (4) To illustrate the waxing and waning pattern, I proposed a graphic representation for both passive and active tone (Fig. 1). (5) Anecdotally, Heinz Prechtl did not like at all the upward progression of passive tone in flexion in the last 3 months of fetal life and sent me, with his kind regards, a reprint of his study in full contradiction of this upward progression. (6) In 1998, however, some support came from a fetal ultrasonographic study on prenatal development of arm posture that demonstrated a clear developmental trend toward increased flexion from 12 to 38 weeks' gestation. (7)

It was only in the 1980s, with the general review of Harvey Sarnat (8), that I began to feel comfortable about anatomophysiologic correlates (9) with two distinct neuromotor systems: the subcorticospinal (or "lower") system and the corticospinal (or "upper") system, including specific physiologic correlates and specific timing and direction of maturation. This new step resulted in a didactic representation (Fig. 2). Anti-gravity activity is dependent on the lower system. In contrast, the head passing forward in the raise-to-sit maneuver is the first neuromotor achievement under the control of the upper system, which can be demonstrated clinically from 34 weeks' gestation onward.

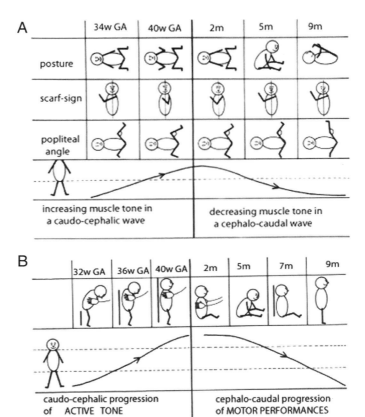

Figure 1. (A) Passive tone in upper and lower extremities. From 28 to 40 weeks' gestational age, muscle tone in flexor muscles increases in a caudocephalic progression, as indicated by posture, scarf-sign (evaluating extensibility in upper limbs), and popliteal angle (evaluating extensibility in lower limbs). Within the first year of life, muscle tone in flexor muscles decreases in a cephalocaudal progression to reach a global hypotonia maximum at 8 to 10 months. Reprinted with permission from Amiel-Tison C. Pediatric contribution to the present knowledge on the neurobehavioral status of infants at birth. In: Mehler J, Fox R, eds. *Neonate Cognition, Beyond the Blooming Buzzing Confusion.* Hillsdale, NJ: Lawrence Erlbaum and Associates Publishers; 1985. (B) Active tone in the axis. From 28 to 40 weeks' gestational age, when the infant is held in the upright position, a righting reaction first appears in the legs, later in the trunk, and finally in the neck and is maintained for a few seconds. Within the first year of life, head control is acquired first, later the sitting position; finally, around 9 months, the infant can stand up and maintain the standing position for a while. From about 4 to 7 months, no righting reaction Figure 1B Active tone in the axis. From 28 to 40 weeks' gestational age, when the infant is held in the upright position, a righting reaction first appears in the legs, later in the trunk, and finally in the neck and is maintained for a few seconds. Within the first year of life, head control is acquired first, later the sitting position; finally, around 9 months, the infant can stand up and maintain the standing position for a while. From about 4 to 7 months, no righting reaction is observed when the infant is held in the upright position, at the time when sitting position is being acquired. Reprinted with permission from Amiel-Tison C. C. Pediatric contribution to the present knowledge on the neurobehavioral status of infants at birth. In: Mehler J, Fox R, eds. *Neonate Cognition, Beyond the Blooming Buzzing Confusion.* Hillsdale, NJ: Lawrence Erlbaum and Associates Publishers; 1985.

These correlates shed light on clinical observations I made long ago on head straightening reactions (10) without fully understanding their meaning at the time: 1) When a term newborn or a preterm infant reaching 40 weeks' gestation is capable of showing identical activity in the neck flexor muscles (going forward in the raise-to-sit maneuver) and the neck extensor muscles (going backward in the sitting-to-lying maneuver), this is the best demonstration of an intact upper system. 2) In contrast, flexor muscles showing poor or no activity associated with a powerful response in the extensor muscles is one of the best early signs of damage in the upper system. 3) The association of hypotonic upper limbs with difficulties in oral feedings very likely indicates more severe damage reaching the lower structures (brainstem). These findings make sense, based on our knowledge that periventricular leukomalacia in the preterm infant typically is located in the upper structures; only in more severe cases are hypoxic-ischemic lesions also found at the lower level.

Ongoing Simplification for Routine Use

In my first paper, (1) passive tone criteria were overrepresented. In the following years, it became apparent that active tone is the most meaningful part of the assessment, both for assessment of maturation and for detection of neurologic signs. Passive tone is more contingent, within the first days, on many types of interference (eg, too much flexion in the limbs at birth due to restricted space in utero or hypotonia due to general condition). Primary reflexes also are not very helpful. At this stage, they simply have to be present to exclude central nervous system depression; therefore, their elicitation may be restricted to a few of them.

As a consequence, the next step has resulted in only one table (Fig 3) based on 10 criteria, including four passive tone items (popliteal angle, scarf sign, forearm recoil, dorsiflexion angle of the foot), three active tone items (righting reaction, neck flexor tone, neck extensor tone), and three primary reflexes (finger grasp and response to traction, crossed extension, sucking). Changes are described at 2-week intervals from 32 to 40 weeks' gestation, as originally proposed by Saint-Anne-Dargassies. Periods of rapid modification are highlighted, indicating the most discriminative period for each observation.

How to define the neurologic age of one infant from the responses obtained? A definite conclusion can be reached only if most of the responses are within the same age period, which is the case for most neonates in good general condition. However, responses can be scattered in some cases, with about 50% of them in one age period, a few in the "younger" interval, and a few in the "older" interval. For research purposes, the so-called "uniform pattern" is defined as 7 of 10 responses being in the same 2-week gestation period and the so-called "scattered pattern" as more than 3 responses being "out of line."

We attempted to discern the meaning of a "scattered pattern" by studying a few sets of twins who had discordant birthweights. We repeated the clinical assessment every 2 to 3 days until the "thin" (wasted) infant recovered from various degrees of undernutrition and under-hydration. The "thin" twin often exhibits a scattered pattern in the first postnatal week, reaching a uniform pattern with improvement in general condition, usually by the beginning of the second

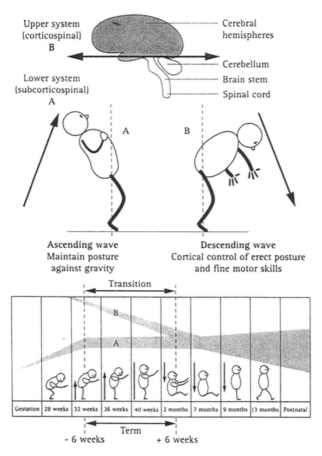

Figure 2. Maturation in motor control from fetal life through infancy. The subcortical pathways (lower system or extrapyramidal) derive from the brainstem, with myelination taking place between 24 and 32 weeks of gestation and proceeding upward, starting in the spinal cord. Their essential role is to maintain posture against gravity. The corticospinal pathways (upper system or pyramidal) originate in cerebral hemispheres. Their myelination starts around 32 weeks of gestation, proceeds downward from the pons to the spinal cord, reaching completion at about 2 years of age. They are responsible for control of erect posture and for movements of the extremities, including fine motor skills. From term onward, corticospinal controls take over, allowing development of mature head control, sitting, and walking. Reprinted with permission from Amiel-Tison C. Clinical assessment of the infant nervous system. This diagram was published in *Fetal and Neonatal Neurology and Neurosurgery,* 3rd ed. Levene MI, Chervanek FA, Whittle MJ, "Clinical Assessment of the Infant Nervous System," Amiel-Tison, C. 100, Copyright Elsevier (2001).

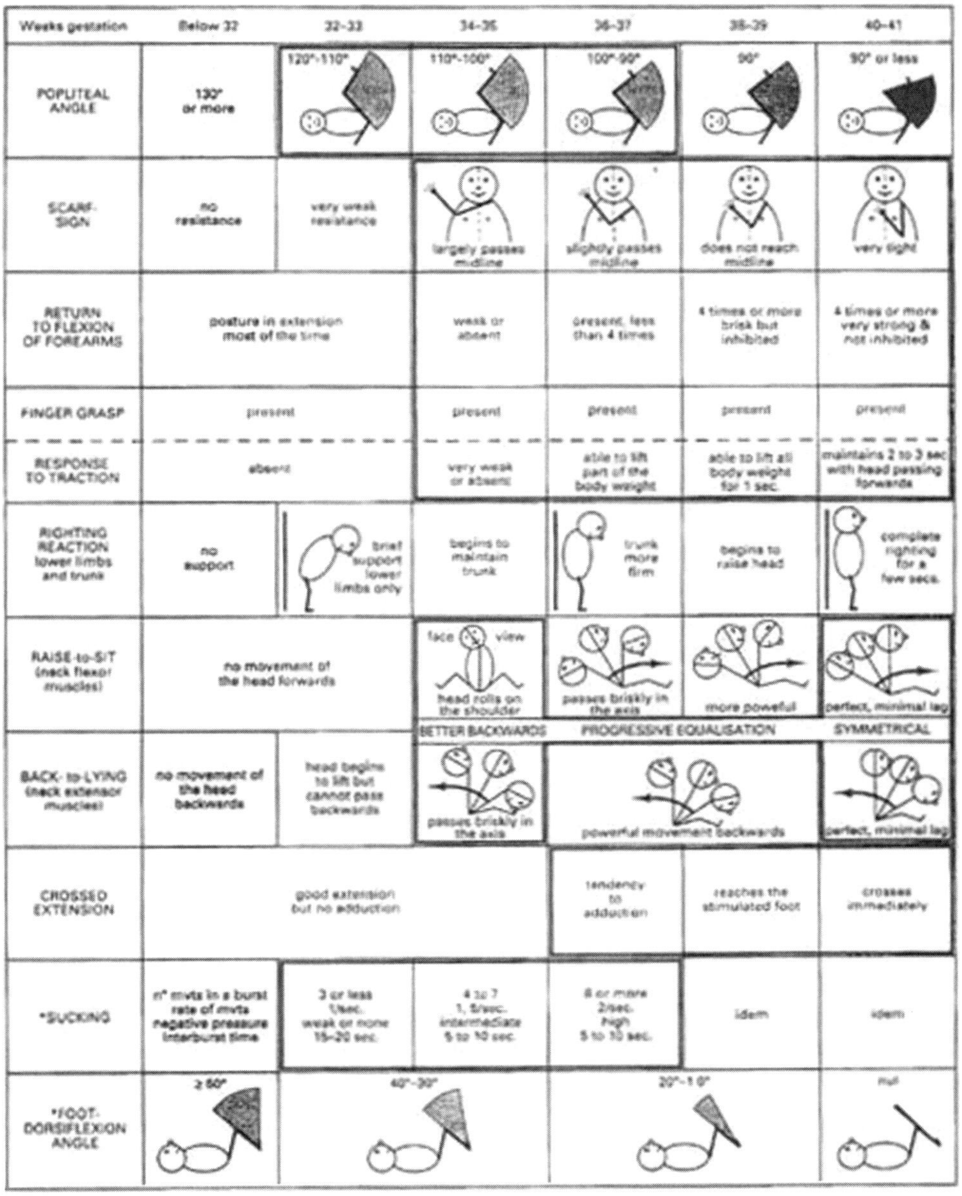

Figure 3. Neurologic criteria described at 2-week intervals from 32 to 40 weeks of gestation, without scoring. Periods of rapid modification are highlighted, indicating the most discriminative period for each observation. Asterisk indicates that the items are not appropriate for maturational assessment performed after several weeks of postnatal life: sucking is modified as a result of practice; the foot dorsiflexion angle remains as it was at the time of preterm birth. Reprinted with permission from Amiel-Tison C. Clinical assessment of the infant nervous system. This diagram was published in *Fetal and Neonatal Neurology and Neurosurgery*, 3rd ed. Levene MI, Chervanek FA, Whittle MJ, "Clinical Assessment of the Infant Nervous System," Amiel-Tison C. 110, Copyright Elsevier (2001).

postnatal week. In some of these infants, however, the maturation pattern remains scattered. These unpublished findings helped us to determine that: 1) Neurologic performances are not independent of the general condition of the neonate, which seems obvious to clinicians (asking active tone responses, such as response to traction or head straightening, of a very tired neonate is the equivalent of asking a convalescent adult to run a marathon) and 2) A uniform pattern, obtained immediately after birth or after convalescence, is a good marker for an intact brain. In contrast, a scattered pattern can suggest risk about transient or persistent brain dysfunction.

These examples illustrate how maturational profiles, derived from the "routine use" of Figure 3, can be an important part of the evaluation of the newborn brain. This is the opportunity for me to thank once more my sister, Annette Tison, who created most of the illustrations accompanying my didactic writing, particularly Figure 3. I have found that it is better for me not to ask her to produce a graphic representation of a maneuver still imprecise in my mind; she needs to understand before drawing, and she has no mercy for haziness. It is why her drawings are so sharp and helpful.

Flexibility Versus Clockwork Precision

There was a dogma in Port-Royal that brain maturation in utero is independent of unfavorable gestational circumstances and proceeds at the same speed ex utero. As a consequence of this independence, one can determine GA from the assessment of neurologic age at birth. At a time when GA was unknown in about one third of pregnancies, neurologic age was very helpful to separate small-for-gestational age (SGA) from appropriate-for-gestational age (AGA) babies, when early fetal measurements by ultrasonography (US) were not even a dream. However, being so confident in their abilities, pediatricians became somewhat arrogant and began to "correct" the GA calculated from last menstrual period or assessed on early fetal US. When assessing neonates whose GA was known precisely (based on temperature curve or stimulation of ovulation), I was puzzled by discrepancies of several weeks between GA and neurologic age, but I did not dare to challenge the dogma.

In 1972, Lou Gluck visited us in Paris on his way to the international pediatric meeting in Moscow. He was caught up in the excitement of his discovery concerning lecithin/ sphingomyelin ratio and lung maturation and observed that in a few abnormal pregnancies, the fetus showed accelerated maturation of both lung and brain. (11) He liked so much to share his enthusiasm that he announced to me when washing his hands before going into our neonatal unit: "Claudine, I know that maturation rhythm may vary with adverse gestational circumstances." He "knew" on the basis of five babies, a remarkable intuition, and a precious self-confidence. This was the trigger I needed to switch from the notion of immutability to the notion of flexibility of maturation speed.

From 1972 to 1978, I collected 32 cases in which the menstrual history was precise and neurologic assessment indicated a maturational advance of 2 or more weeks. Most of these 32 infants had abnormal pregnancies with causes similar to the cases published by Gluck and his group in 1977: placental insufficiency due to preeclampsia, multiple pregnancy, or uterine malformation. (12) As I gathered these data, the atmosphere was tense in the department because no one in Port-Royal really wanted to consider this flexibility. The electrophysiologists disagreed because they could not confirm an acceleration of maturation with electroencephalographic (EEG) criteria in the presence of clinical acceleration. (This disagreement is not surprising because EEG assesses primarily cortical activity, and clinical criteria at these ages primarily reflect brainstem activity.) Clinical criteria alone did not convince the editorial boards. Therefore, I had to follow the advice of Leonard Strang (on sabbatical in Port-Royal at this time) and sacrifice 50% of my cohort to concentrate the publication on the 16 cases in whom the acceleration was 4 weeks or more (ie, outside the 95% confidence limits). (13) From my initial cohort, however, I demonstrated that the adaptation was not an all-or-nothing phenomenon; rather, it was a progressive response of variable degree.

Confirmation of acceleration of maturation in stressed pregnancies came in 1985 from various horizons. Experimental data in intrauterine growth-restricted rats showed that the Na/K-ATPase activity was accelerated in the brainstem and delayed in the forebrain, cerebellum, and hippocampus. (14) At the same time, based on brainstem auditory evoked potentials, Alan Pettigrew found a significant decrease of mean brain-stem conduction among SGA infants compared with AGA infants. (15) When Pettigrew came on sabbatical to Paris, we enjoyed preparing together a general review on the topic. (16)

During all these years, the suggested physiopathologic mechanism of response to stress was adrenal stimulation, but the mechanism remained vague until the publications of Robert Denver, a biologist in Ann Arbor, Michigan, which came as a fantastic surprise to me. (17)(18) He reported that tadpoles of desert amphibians can accelerate metamorphosis as their pond dries, thereby escaping mortality in their larval habitat. This observation has been replicated in laboratory experiments, with tadpoles subjected to habitat desiccation exhibiting elevated hypothalamic content of corticotrophin-releasing hormone, precocious

Table 1. Clinical Criteria Defining Optimality of CNS Function Around Term

Observations or Tests	Optimal Responses	Signifies
(1) Head circumference . . . cm	Same range as birthweight	Adequate brain growth
(2) Cranial sutures	Edge-to-edge, squamous included	
(3) Visual pursuit	Easily obtainable	NO CNS depression
(4) Social interaction	Eager	
(5) Sucking reflex	Efficient, rhythmic	
(6) Raise-to-sit and reverse	Active flexor muscles (balance with extensor muscles)	Integrity of the upper motor control
(7) Passive tone in the axis	More flexion than extension	
(8) Passive tone in limbs	Within normal limits for gestational age and symmetric	
(9) Fingers and thumbs	Independent movements and abduction of thumbs	
(10) Autonomic control during assessment	No disturbance	Brainstem integrity

This article was published in *Fetal and Neonatal Neurology and Neurosurgery*, 3rd ed. Levene MI, Chervanek FA, Whittle MJ, "Clinical Assessment of the Infant Nervous System," Amiel-Tison C. 111, Copyright Elsevier (2001).

activation of the thyroid and inter-renal axes, and endocrine activation preceding morphologic changes by 3 days. Although endocrine mechanisms are probably not identical in amphibians and humans, sharing these adaptive processes with amphibians is a thrilling concept for those who are interested in the evolutionary aspects of maturation. A joint general review of the concept is in process. (19) Demonstration of fetal adaptation to the environment being shared with others in the animal kingdom at last may make this flexibility politically correct. If a convincing meta-analysis still is wanted, I am afraid it may have to wait for another 30 years!

Scoring Systems: A Disaster

Neonatologists certainly feel frustrated when considering the objectivity of the Gosner Table for staging anuran embryos and larvae based on morphologic changes. (17)(18) However, such frustration is not an excuse for scoring neurologic findings for several reasons. First, scoring systems such as the Dubowitz (20) and the Ballard (21) suggest a level of accuracy that really does not exist in these dynamic systems. Second, nearly exclusive use of passive tone criteria (easier to evaluate than active tone, but often misleading, as discussed previously) decreases the validity of the assessment, which hardly can be qualified as neurologic. Unfortunately, most neonatologists accept the use of scores, even if not accurate, because they want a GA at any price.

To me, this leveling is a real deprivation compared with identification of a maturational profile. As an example, it is typical for an infant born at 34 weeks' gestation to lie in a frog like position, to have a difficult response going forward in the pull-to-sit maneuver (head rolling on the shoulder), and to have a much more powerful response going backward. The same pattern at 40 weeks corrected age is definitely abnormal, indicating impaired control of the lower system by an impaired upper system. In other words, what is physiologic at 34 weeks must be interpreted as pathologic 6 weeks later. This identification of early neurologic signs is not a useless sophistication; it is a good reason to include a preterm newborn in a follow-up clinic, even if repeated head US studies within the first postnatal month did not show any sign of cerebral atrophy. (22)

Visual Attention and Cephalic Growth at 40 Weeks (Corrected)

The 10 criteria of Figure 3 test only neuromotor function and rely nearly exclusively on the lower (brainstem) structures. As discussed previously, only changes observed in neck flexor muscle reaction to the raise-to-sit maneuver are dependent on the upper system (motor cortex, corticospinal tracts, and basal ganglia). Because the brain damage due to perinatal hypoxia-ischemia generally is localized in the upper structures, absence of predictive value of the proposed maturational assessment is not surprising. For this reason, at around the corrected age of 40 weeks' gestation, we are using a more extensive assessment to define optimality of the central nervous system (Table). (9)(23) Other criteria are added to Figure 3, primarily in the domains of alertness and interaction (relying mostly on visual fix and track) and cephalic growth. Passive tone in the axis, independent movements of fingers, and abduction of thumbs are included as valuable criteria to define the integrity of cerebral hemispheres.

From my experience, typical responses at 40 weeks' gestation have a high predictive value for normal outcome; very deviant responses have a high predictive value for a poor outcome. Mild and moderate deviations do not have a good predictive value; they simply indicate the need for follow-up, even when imaging results are normal. Particularly in the "new survivors" group of neonates (22 to 26 wk), extreme immaturity at birth makes any prediction unwise. When tested at 40 weeks corrected gestational age, many of these infants are considered typical, based on tone and reflexes, but most demonstrate a poor visual ability to fix and track due to a short attention span. Generally, most will be able to walk independently by 18 months corrected age, but disorganization in many aspects of cerebral function will make their lives difficult. For this group of children, the clinical approach described previously is disappointing for prediction. New technologies to evaluate cerebral function are more promising, including cortical mapping or diffusion tensor magnetic resonance imaging.

Conclusion

Who should assess brain maturation of the neonate? The neonatologist can do it and is in the best situation for interpreting the results according to the general status of the neonate. Moreover, this clinical approach is indispensable to developmental pediatrics, and I strongly believe that any pediatrician has to be a "developmentalist."

Which neonates should be assessed? Everyone. It is clear, however, that active tone in particular cannot be assessed in a sick newborn or in a very immature newborn. In these neonates, the assessment will be completed later, when full stabilization is achieved, which may take months when the GA is 27 weeks or less. Using corrected age and assuming that maturation has been progressing at about the same speed as in utero, the type of assessment discussed previously will provide a valuable baseline for evaluation of further maturational steps and possible brain damage.

Can a single instrument be used from birth through childhood? Yes, it seems highly desirable because any deviation in clinical methodology makes conclusions uncertain (or epidemiologists unhappy). It is for the sake of a collaborative research project that I recently have tried with Julie Gosselin to adapt the same methodology through the maturational flow from birth to 6 years of age. With criteria similar to those described for assessing maturation up to 4 weeks, we developed a semiquantitative assessment scored 0, 1, and 2 from 40 weeks (23) to 6 years. (24) We used the same concept of "neurologic age," but as maturation slows, the 2-week assessment periods up to 40 weeks become 3-month periods up to 1 year and subsequently 6-month periods and finally 12-month periods up to 6 years. We persist in our refusal to assign a total score, using instead clusters to define various types of deviations, just as in the neonatal period.

The fluidity of maturation is comparable to the fluidity of water, and as the Greek philosopher Heraclite asserted, we cannot swim twice in the same river, and similarly we cannot assess the same neonate twice. One of Heraclite's disciples, more extremist than his mentor, claimed that we cannot even swim once in the same river because water flows constantly. In any case, brain maturation proceeds very rapidly, and we have to try hard not to get lost in the stream.

Claudine Amiel-Tison, MD
Emeritus Professor of Pediatrics
Port-Royal Baudelocque Hospital
University of Paris, France

[For the original article by Amiel-Tison regarding neurologic evaluation of maturity in newborns, which was published in 1968 in *Archives of Disease in Childhood,* and which was reprinted with permission, please go to: http://neoreviews.aappublications.org/cgi/data/4/8/e199/DC1]

References

1. Amiel-Tison C. Neurological evaluation of the maturity of newborn infants. *Arch Dis Child.* 1968;43:89–93

2. Thomas A, Saint-Anne-Dargassies S. *Etudes Neurologiques sur le Nouveau-né et le Jeune Nourrisson.* Paris, France: Masson; 1952

3. Saint-Anne-Dargassies S. La maturation neurologique du prématuré. *Etudes Néonat.* 1955;4:71

4. Peiper A. *Cerebral Function in Infancy and Childhood* [translation of the 3rd revised German edition]. New York, NY: Consultants Bureau; 1963

5. Amiel-Tison C. Pediatric contribution to the present knowledge on the neurobehavioral status of infants at birth. In: Mehler J, Fox R, eds. *Neonate Cognition, Beyond the Blooming Buzzing Confusion.* Hillsdale, NJ: Lawrence Erlbaum and Associates Publishers; 1985

6. Prechtl HFR, Fragel JW, Weinmann HM, Bakker HH. Postures, motility and respiration of low-risk pre-term infants. *Dev Med Child Neurol.* 1979;21:3–27

7. Ververs IAP, Van Gelder-Hasker MR, Devries JIP, Hopkins B, Van Geijn HP. Prenatal development of arm posture. *Early Human Dev.* 1998;51:61–70

8. Sarnat HB. Anatomic and physiologic correlates of neurologic development in prematurity. In: *Topics in Neonatal Neurology.* New York, NY: Grune and Stratton; 1984:1–24

9. Amiel-Tison C. Clinical assessment of the infant nervous system. In: Levene MI, Chervenak FA, Whittle M, eds. *Fetal and Neonatal Neurology and Neurosurgery.* 3rd ed. Edinburgh, Scotland: Churchill Living stone; 2001:99–120

10. Amiel-Tison C. Neurologic evaluation of the small neonate: the importance of head straightening reactions. In: Gluck L, ed. *Modern Perinatal Medicine.* Chicago, Ill: Year Book; 1974:347–357

11. Gould JB, Gluck L, Kulovich MV. The acceleration of neurological maturation in high stress pregnancy and its relation to fetal lung maturity. *Pediatr Res.* 1972;6:276

12. Gould JB, Gluck L, Kulovich MV. The relationship between accelerated pulmonary maturity and accelerated neurological maturity in certain chronically stressed pregnancies. *Am J Obstet Gynecol.* 1977;127:181–186

13. Amiel-Tison C. Possible acceleration of neurological maturity following high risk pregnancy. *Am J Obstet Gynecol.* 1980;138:303–306

14. Chanez C, Flexor MA, Hamon M. Long lasting effects on intrauterine growth retardation on basal and 5-HT stimulated Na + K + ATPase in the brain of developing rats. *Neuro chem Int.* 1985;2:319–329

15. Pettigrew AG, Edwards DA, Henderson-Smart DJ. The influence of intrauterine growth retardation on brainstem development of preterm infants. *Dev Med Child Neurol.* 1985;27:467–472

16. Amiel-Tison C, Pettigrew AG. Adaptative changes in the developing brain during intrauterine stress. *Brain Dev.* 1991;13:67–76

17. Denver RJ. Environmental stress as a developmental cue: corticotropin-releasing hormone is a proximate mediator of adaptive phenotypic plasticity in amphibian metamorphosis. *Hormones Behav.* 1997;31: 169–179

18. Denver RJ. Hormonal correlates of environmentally induced metamorphosis in the western spadefoot toad. *Gen Compar Endocrinol.* 1998;110:326–336

19. Amiel-Tison C, Cabrol D, Denver R, Jarreau PH, Papiernik E, Piazza PV. Fetal adaptation to stress. Part I: Acceleration of fetal maturation and earlier birth triggered by placental insufficiency in humans. Part II: Evolutionary aspects. Stress-induced hip-pocampal damage. Long-term effects on behavior. Consequences on adult health. Submitted to *Brain and Development*

20. Dubowitz LM, Dubowitz V. *Gestational Age of the Newborn.* London, England: Addison-Wesley; 1977

21. Ballard JL, Khoury JC, Wedig K, Wang L, Eilers-Walsman BL, Lipp R. New Ballard score, expanded to include extremely premature infants. *J Pediatr.* 1991;119: 417–423

22. Stewart A, Hope PL, Hamilton P, et al. Prediction in very preterm infants of satisfactory neurodevelopmental progress at 12 months. *Dev Med Child Neurol.* 1988;30: 53–63

23. Amiel-Tison C. Update of the Amiel-Tison Neurologic Assessment for the term neonate or at 40 weeks corrected age. *Pediatr Neurol.* 2002;27:196–212

24. Amiel-Tison C, Gosselin J. *Neurologic Development from Birth to 6 Years.* Baltimore, Md: Johns Hopkins University Press; 2001

Historical Perspectives: Neurologic Maturation of the Neonate
Alistair G. S. Philip, Claudine Amiel-Tison and Claudine Amiel-Tison
NeoReviews 2003;4;199
DOI: 10.1542/neo.4-8-e199

Monitoring the Newborn for Apnea

Cardiopulmonary Monitoring

Among the factors considered "standard operating procedure" in neonatal intensive care units today, the presence of monitors is key. Bedside monitoring almost defines neonatal intensive care. It is difficult to recall that it is less than 40 years ago that cardiopulmonary monitors were introduced into routine intensive care. Prior to their introduction, the bedside nurse was responsible for taking vital signs at intervals dictated by the severity of illness of the baby.

This 2005 contribution comes from Dr Joe Daily, who describes the early attempts to incorporate electronic monitoring into the care of premature (preterm) infants who had apnea. The technique involved the use of transthoracic impedance, which can detect both respiration and heart rate activity. At the time it was introduced, the application of electrodes to the chest seemed rather "invasive," and subsequent attempts were made to use other types of monitoring devices that did not require attachment to the baby's chest. As indicated by Dr Daily, our major concern at the time was the detection of apnea, and air mattresses were used in some nurseries for a while because they could detect breathing movements. However, other types of motion artifact (particularly seizure activity) could trigger the sensors for breathing and produce "false-negatives."

Not long after the apnea monitor was introduced, it became evident that monitoring of heart rate could provide additional useful information. Consequently, cardiopulmonary monitoring became the norm, to be followed by blood pressure monitoring (see *NeoReviews*, May 2003), transcutaneous blood gas monitoring (see *NeoReviews*, September 2003), and oxygen saturation monitoring.

In providing this recollection, Dr Daily was quick to point out to me that many people, over a long period of time, were involved in the evolution of the technology that led to the first apnea monitors used at Stanford.

Alistair G. S. Philip, MD, FRCPE, FAAP
Editor-in-Chief, NeoReviews

Introduction

Now 35 years ago, Daily, Klaus, and Meyer (1) published the first clinical report (in the United States) involving the use of an electronic monitoring technology that had an incorporated alarm circuit to detect apneic episodes in a series of preterm infants. As in all such reports, a significant preceding history of information generation enabled us to undertake that study. That history, in relation to apnea in preterm infants, is ancient, and the history and technology ultimately used to create these first electronic monitors now is nearly a century old.

Observing newborns for sudden, unexpected respiratory distress dates to antiquity; the earliest monitoring techniques consisted of continuous visual observation of the newborn, often associated with near continuous human contact. About 1200 AD, the Jewish physician/philosopher Moses-ben-Maimon described a device for monitoring neonatal activity consisting of a string attached to an extremity of the newborn passed over a pulley and connected to a simple bell-ringing mechanism. (2) Whether this system was used to monitor apnea through monitoring of neonatal activity or for other reasons is unknown. Subsequently, Mercurialis clearly suggested an association between irregular respiratory patterns and the occurrence of apnea. Renewed interest in the pathophysiology and mechanisms involved in neonatal apnea most likely dates to the work of Blystad, (3) Miller and coworkers, (4) and Deming and Washburn (5) early in the era of neonatal care.

Background

Technological interest in electrical signals derived from the thorax and associated with breathing was described initially by Cremer in 1907. (6) However, incorporation of these transthoracic impedance signals into monitoring of breathing patterns in newborns awaited the development of appropriate technologies in the early 1960s and the incorporation of an alarming device for the detection of apnea of varying durations (with or without simultaneous heart rate monitoring) in 1967 by Pacela and associates (7)(8) and by Domingues (personal communication, July 1996). The first apnea monitor used in our studies did not incorporate a heart rate monitor/alarm circuit–the IMI apnea monitor (Industrial Medical Instruments, Newport Beach, Calif). This monitor included both signal sensitivity and alarm delay adjustments of 0 to 30 seconds. Shortly thereafter, Beckman Medical Instruments developed a device that included both respiration and heart rate monitoring with adjustable alarm circuits–the Vital Signs Monitor 100 (VSM-100).

The development of the IMI and VSM-100 monitors at Stanford was possible only after prior, more basic engineering and clinical work in Sweden between 1964 and 1967, where significant research had been undertaken to develop a more complex, tetrapolar impedance plethysmographic system at the University of Gothenberg Children's Hospital and the Research Laboratory of Medical Electronics of the Chalmers University of Technology, Gothenberg, Sweden. These indepth studies of both engineering technology and the application of transthoracic impedance monitoring to the evaluation of neonatal pulmonary function provided both technological development and correlation with various aspects of neonatal pulmonary physiology and formed the basis for the development of the first clinical apnea alarm monitors. Both the technological and clinical scope of these studies was summarized in reports presented at the European Society for Pediatric Research in 1966 (9)(10) and more extensively in the report of Olsson and Victorin in *Acta Pediatrica Scandinavia* in 1970. (11)

Early Studies

As mentioned previously, sporadic reports of the use of impedance plethysmography to assess respiratory patterns in adults and children were published in the mid-1960s. (12)(13)(14)(15)(16) More intense investigations of the use of this technology were undertaken in Sweden and at Stanford during the fellowship of this author between 1964 and 1967. Clinical studies commenced in 1964 and involved the simultaneous evaluation of a number of physiologic and electrophysiologic parameters in newborns. In the course of these investigations, studies were undertaken related to the variation of blood volume and breathing patterns in term newborns and of pulmonary mechanical properties and their association with simultaneously measured thoracic electrophysiologic changes. Some early investigations of the effects of temperature on respiratory pattern also were undertaken.

Analysis of Tetrapolar Impedance During Breathing at Fixed Lung Gas Volumes

The transthoracic impedance electrophysiologic characteristics evaluated at multiple periods of zero lung volume change during pulmonary compliance measurements in term newborns were described as "electrophysiologic compliance loops," indicating differences in the timing of conducting fluid volume movement and gas movement within the lung. (11) These studies were interpreted to indicate that tetrapolar impedance signals, when coupled with simultaneous measurement of pulmonary compliance, could be interpreted possibly to describe some characteristics of pulmonary blood volume/flow. Data obtained during predetermined blood volume changes accomplished in the course of exchange transfusion in stable, term infants who had physiologic hyperbilirubinemia were consistent with this hypothesis. (9)(10)(11)

Thus, evidence from 2 years of combined engineering and clinical physiologic investigation of newborns using tetrapolar impedance plethysmography suggested that tetrapolar technology could be employed to assess patterns of pulmonary blood volume change and correlated with directly measured characteristics of lung compliance. Further, respiratory patterns could be modified by alterations in blood volume, and the electrophysiologic characteristics of the lung fields studied in the term newborn were related to respiratory pattern changes that attended temperature variations within the thermal neutral zone.

It was these background studies that led to the association between the United States biomedical engineering firms (IMI, Beckman Medical Instruments) and the Center for Premature Infants at Stanford University Hospital that began in 1966. The initial studies used bipolar, transthoracic impedance monitoring and incorporated simultaneous separate external heart rate monitoring. The studies initially undertaken in Sweden using the tetrapolar technique were expanded at Stanford to include the specific study of periodically breathing, small, preterm infants and to characterize some physiologic and clinical changes that attended apneic intervals of varying durations. Also incorporated in that study was an evaluation of the effect of temperature on the breathing patterns of preterm infants. In the small number of infants studied, apnea was more frequent at the high end of thermal neutrality (ie, breathing *pattern* was altered) in contrast to the change in breathing *rate* noted in term infants in similar studies in Sweden.

During the course of these studies, the first monitor developed (IMI) linked respiration monitoring to an alarm system that was intended to alert caretaking staff of otherwise unobserved apneic events prior to the occurrence of heart rate/cardiovascular/neurologic changes that attended such episodes in the preterm infants studied. The incorporation of a 0- to 30-second variable time delay alarm system into the IMI apnea monitor and, ultimately, the Beckman VSM 100 Heart Rate Respiration Monitor constituted the first reported use of an electrophysiologic detection system for otherwise unanticipated events that might place the infant at risk.

Subsequently, studies of predetermined blood volume changes were undertaken during exchange transfusion in preterm and term infants by White and colleagues (17) Findings from these studies confirmed earlier observations that alterations of blood volume potentially outside of the "physiologic range" (65 to 120 mL/ kg, as determined in this study) were associated with alterations of periodic breathing patterns in preterm infants and respiratory rate in term infants. An incidental but not reported observation was grunting respiratory patterns beyond both the upper and lower limits of blood volume (ie, <65 or >120 mL/kg). This observation further suggested that cardiovascular events within the lung per se might relate significantly to breathing patterns and lung function in newborns.

Additional studies were undertaken regarding the effects of alteration of inspired oxygen and carbon dioxide concentrations (at constant inspired O_2) on breathing patterns in periodically breathing infants. Increased carbon dioxide concentrations decreased periodic breathing only in some infants; the effect was not consistent. The effects of oxygen on periodic breathing essentially confirmed the earlier reports of Miller and associates. (4) Other forms of apnea or bradycardia not associated with periodic breathing were not studied, although occasionally they were observed, including inspiratory apnea, apnea following prior onset cardiodeceleration/bradycardia, and rarely, episodes of cyanosis followed by bradycardia and apnea.

As emphasized in our original paper, the ability of the monitors to vary the time from detection of apnea (or bradycardia ultimately) to alarm was believed to be particularly important. This point was emphasized by the varying individual tolerance of infants for specific apneic durations, most particularly in small preterm infants, some of whom developed bradycardia, cyanosis, and neurologic state change as rapidly as 5 seconds after the onset of apnea. The implication of this recommendation was that the tolerance of individual infants for apnea of varying durations and for bradycardia should be determined carefully and the alarm delay times set within the limits of tolerance for each infant. In this manner, it was hoped that monitors might function more in a mode of prevention than of detection of already abnormal changes. The mechanisms related to the rate of onset of desaturation and hypoxemia continue to be defined. (18)(19)

Conclusion and Comment

No further investigations have been undertaken by the authors after the conclusion of these studies at Stanford in the early 1970s. Significant advances have occurred in monitor complexity and technologies as well as other technologies related to evaluation of neonatal pulmonary function, most particularly for infants receiving ventilatory support. Significant advances also have occurred in the pharmacologic treatment of neonatal apnea. However, the specific effects of medications in individual infants who have different breathing patterns or patterns of apnea per se may require additional research. More in-depth studies of the association between blood volume, environmental temperature, and neonatal respiratory patterns, pulmonary function, and pulmonary blood flow remain to be translated into technologies applicable to clinical practice.

One wonders whether the suggestive findings of early tetrapolar impedance studies with regard to pulmonary blood volume/flow now might be evaluated in a more sophisticated manner and correlated with advanced technologies for measurement of lung compliance, tidal volume, gas flow, and inspiratory/expiratory gas composition. Is it possible that current engineering and computer technologies might make the clinical measurement of the timing of pulmonary blood volume/flow and lung function an easily and immediately available parameter for the evaluation of neonatal breathing disorders and their treatment in newborn special care units?

William J. R. Daily, MD
Neonatology Associates, Ltd.

Phoenix, Ariz.
Chairman
District VIII Perinatal Section
American Academy of Pediatrics

Acknowledgments

These studies in Sweden and at Stanford would not have been possible without the input and support of Norman Kretchmer, MD, PhD (dec), and Philip Sunshine, MD, at Stanford and of Professor Petter Karlberg at the Gothenburg Children's Hospital, Sweden.

[To read the original article on electronic monitoring for apnea written by Daily and colleagues and published in *Pediatrics* in 1969, please go to: http://neoreviews.aap publications.org/cgi/data/6/5/e207/DC1   OR http://pediatrics.aappublications.org/cgi/content/abstract/43/4/510]

References

1. Daily WJR, Klaus M, Meyer HBP. Apnea in premature infants: monitoring, incidence, heart rate changes and an effect of environmental temperature. *Pediatrics.* 1969;43:510–518

2. Daily WJR, Cave-Smith P. Mechanical ventilation of the newborn infant – part I. *Curr Probl Pediatr.* 1971;1:3–14

3. Blystad W. Blood gas determinations on premature infants. III. Investigations on premature infants with recurrent attacks of apnea. *Acta Paediatr Scand.* 1956;45: 211–221

4. Miller HD, Behrle FC, Smull, NW. Severe apnea and irregular respiratory rhythms among premature infants: a clinical and laboratory study. *Pediatrics.* 1959;23: 676–685

5. Deming J, Washburn AH. Respiration in infancy: a method of studying rates, volume and character of respiration with preliminary report of results. *Am J Dis Child.* 1935;49: 108–124

6. Cremer M. Ueber des Saitenelektrometer und seine Anwendung in der Elektrophysiologie. *Munchen Med Wochnschr.* 1907;54:505–507

7. Pacela AF, Miller CE, Daily WJR, Savaglio FJ. Impedance technique for monitoring the newborn infant. *Digest of the 7th International Conference on Medical and Biological Engineering.* Stockholm, Sweden, August 1967

8. Savaglio FJ, Pacela AF Daily WJR. Monitoring respiration of newborn infants with an impedance plethysmograph. Presented at the *20th Annual Conference, Engineering in Biology and Medicine.* Boston, Massachusetts: November 1967

9. Daily WJR, Karlberg P, Olsson T, Thomsen A, Victorin JLH. A preliminary report of changes in transthoracic impedance and blood gases in relation to the mechanics of breathing in the newborn infant. *Proceedings of the European Society for Pediatric Research.* Athens, Greece; 1966:250

10. Karlberg P, Victorin L, Daily WJR, Olsson T. Transthoracic impedance variations in newborn babies with special regard to early and late clamping of the umbilical cord. *Proceedings of the European Society for Pediatric Research.* Athens, Greece; 1966:252

11. Olsson T, Victorin L (in collaboration with Daily WJR, Kjellmer I). Transthoracic impedance, with special reference to newborn infants and the ratio of air-to-fluid in the lungs. *Acta Paediatr Scand.* 1970: 207(suppl):1–90

12. Allison R. Stroke volume, cardiac output and impedance. *19th Annual Conference, Engineering in Biology and Medicine.* 1966:53

13. Allison R, Holmes EL, Nyboer J. Volumetric dynamics of respiration as measured by electrical impedance plethysmography. *J Appl Physiol.* 1964;19:166–173

14. Farman JV, Juett DA. Impedance spirometry in clinical monitoring. *Br Med J.* 1967;4:27–29

15. Hill PL, Schwan AP. Observations on four electrode impedance measurements. *19th Annual Conference, Engineering in Biology and Medicine.* 1966:57

16. Reid DHS, Mitchell RG. Recurrent neonatal apnoea. *Lancet.* 1966;1:786–788

17. White R, Browning E, Mesel E, Daily WJR. Impedance plethysmography as a qualitative guide to pulmonary blood flow [abstract]. *Clin Res.* 1970;18:219

18. Poets CF, Southall, DP. Patterns of oxygenation during periodic breathing in preterm infants. *Early Human Dev.* 1991; 26:1–12

19. Wilkinson MH, Berger PJ, Blanch N, Brodecky V. Effect of venous oxygenation on arterial desaturation rate during repetitive apnea in lambs. *Resp Physiol.* 1995;101: 321–331

Historical Perspectives: Monitoring the Newborn for Apnea
Alistair G. S. Philip and William J. R. Daily
NeoReviews 2005;6;e207-e210
DOI: 10.1542/neo.6-5-e207

Direct Blood Pressure Measurement

In today's neonatal intensive care unit, it would be inconceivable not to be able to accurately measure blood pressure (the fourth vital sign). However, as noted by Dr Roderic H. Phibbs in this 2003 article, until umbilical artery catheters became the primary method to assess arterial oxygen tension, blood pressure measurement was quite primitive. The initial report by Kitterman et al (18) in 1969 was limited to infants with birthweights greater than 1,000 g. The pace of change in neonatal intensive care is demonstrated by the fact that 12 years later, data from the same institution were extended down to birthweights as low as 610 g (Versmold et al, 1981) (19).

Nevertheless, it is difficult to know what constitutes a "normal" extremely low-birthweight (ELBW, <1,000 g) infant and therefore what constitutes "normal" blood pressure in such infants (1). While the method of blood pressure measurement, using a central catheter, has changed little over the ensuing years, there has been considerable debate on what constitutes a blood pressure that requires therapeutic intervention. It is now understood that an individualized approach that evaluates tissue perfusion, as well as blood pressure, may be necessary.

Alistair G. S. Philip, MD, FRCPE, FAAP
Editor-in-Chief, NeoReviews

Reference

1. Weindling AN, Subhadar NV. The definition of hypotension in very low birth weight infants during the immediate neonatal period. *NeoReviews.* 2007;8:e32–e43.

"The experimental hypothesis, in short, must always be based on prior observation." —Claude Bernard (1)

Aortic Blood Pressure in "Normal" Newborns

Modern adult intensive care started in Denmark in 1952 in response to the high mortality from the respiratory complications seen with a devastating epidemic of poliomyelitis. Anesthetists and physiologists created a new discipline when they collaborated to make sequential measurements of cardiorespiratory variables, then aggressively corrected abnormal conditions. (2) When modern neonatal intensive care emerged a decade later, it followed the same philosophy.

The start of modern neonatology was stimulated in large part by an expanding understanding of: 1) the circulatory and respiratory physiology of adaptation to extrauterine life, 2) how those adjustments could fail, and 3) the pathophysiology of hyaline membrane disease. (3)(4)(5)(6)(7)(8)(9)(10) (The monograph by Dawes (3) gives an excellent overview of the relevant animal research). This research had reached a point where it could be applied to clinical care if the necessary physiologic measurements could be made in newborns. To this end, investigators began to catheterize the umbilical arteries of newborns to measure blood gas tensions and pH, with several investigators also measuring aortic pressures. (9)(11)(12)(13) Such invasive techniques were highly controversial initially, but they gradually became the accepted methodology for monitoring the sick neonate. (12)

The use of oxygen in preterm infants who had cardiorespiratory distress was an important component of this change in approach to the sick infant. The standard had been to use no more than 40% oxygen to prevent retrolental fibroplasia (retinopathy of prematurity). However, it was obvious that this approach would be insufficient to relieve hypoxia in some infants and would produce hyperoxia in others. Avery and Oppenheimer (13) observed an increase in deaths due to hyaline membrane disease (respiratory distress syndrome) in pre-term infants following the implementation of these standards. The new approach, which was gaining popularity in the 1960s, was to administer sufficient oxygen to maintain the Pa_{O_2} in the normal range.

However, this could be achieved only by frequent measurements of P_{O_2} in arterial blood, which required the placement of an umbilical arterial catheter. At this time, the technique for placing and maintaining peripheral arterial catheters had not been perfected, and reliable transcutaneous monitoring was in the distant future. Thus, placement of umbilical arterial catheters became standard practice in most of the few neonatal intensive care units (NICUs) that existed at the time. Prior to this, clinicians rarely used umbilical arterial catheterization. Although umbilical venous catheters had been in use for years for exchange transfusions in infants who had erythroblastosis fetalis, clinicians rarely took advantage of them for physiologic measurements.

Using Indwelling Umbilical Arterial Catheters

In 1964, we started placing umbilical arterial catheters in infants who had respiratory distress in the NICU at the University of California at San Francisco (UCSF). Later that year Bill Tooley (who started the NICU at UCSF and for whom the current NICU is named) and I asked ourselves, "Why not measure blood pressure in every infant with an indwelling umbilical arterial catheter?" It appeared possible with little, if any, added risk to the infant, so why ignore physiologic information that was used routinely in critically ill adults and older children? Attempts to measure blood pressure by indirect methods in neonates had had limited success and because many infants who had respiratory distress had been shown to have reduced peripheral perfusion (as noted below), the then available methods for indirect measurements were unlikely to be accurate or broadly applicable to the care of sick infants. (14)(15)

In addition to the philosophical argument, there were three specific reasons to measure pressures through the umbilical arterial catheter. First, studies had shown that peripheral perfusion was subnormal in preterm infants with respiratory distress syndrome, (16) and Neligan and Smith (17) had found that blood pressure might be useful in monitoring the

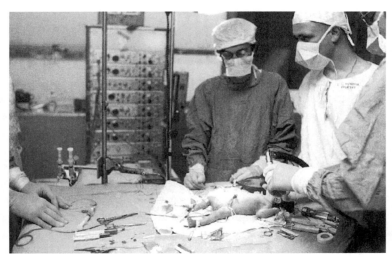

Figure 1. A Grass polygraph being used to measure and record aortic blood pressure through a catheter that has just been passed through the umbilical artery into the descending aorta of a newborn. The catheter is connected to a pressure transducer, which is at the level of the baby's heart, just above the pair of hands on the left. The transducer is connected to the polygraph recorder, the large silver machine with the black knobs behind the doctor in the center of the photograph. The paper on which the recording is made can be seen running across the bottom of the machine.

course of hyaline membrane disease. Second, such measurements could be used for the early detection of clot formation in the catheter. The type of catheter in use at this time was very prone to clot formation in the tip because it was made of polyvinyl chloride and only had a side hole near the tip. A clot often could be detected early by damping of the blood pressure wave form before other signs of clot formation (some of them disastrous) appeared. The third reason to measure pressures

through the umbilical arterial catheter was to monitor for an adverse effect of acetylcholine, which sometimes was used at that time for treating severe hyaline membrane disease, but which occasionally produced a sudden marked drop in systemic blood pressure. (11)

The system and routine for making these measurements was familiar to us because it was used regularly in the clinical and animal laboratories of the Cardiovascular Research Institute at UCSF. We employed a Grass

polygraph that recorded on paper and Statham strain gauges (Fig. 1).

Teresa Poirier, the highly creative head nurse of the NICU, was party to our conversation about measuring blood pressure in all infants with umbilical arterial catheters. Management of indwelling umbilical arterial catheters in neonates already had been made a nursing routine. Teresa insisted that if blood pressure monitoring was to be done well, it too must be in the hands of nursing, so she developed the nursing routine. It was added to the vital signs that the nurse recorded. The nurse recorded a 10- to 15-second strip of phasic pressure that provided systolic and diastolic pressures and heart rate, then reduced the frequency response to record mean pressure for another 10 to 15 seconds. The nurse wrote on the recorder paper the date and time, the infant's name, and comments about the infant's condition at the time (Fig 2), as well as entering the information in the bedside nursing record. Recordings were made hourly and could be made more frequently or even continuously if the infant's condition was changing rapidly. We saved all of these recordings.

Determining "Normal" Pressures

We noticed that some patients had blood pressures that were much lower than we were used to seeing. Some of them appeared to be in shock due to acute blood loss that probably had occurred during the intrapartum period. Although following an individual baby's changes in blood pressure was useful, it was obvious that we needed to define the range of normal blood pressure for the newborn to make the best use of the information. We also believed that "normal" probably would be lower in smaller, more preterm infants because studies in animals suggested that blood pressure increased with gestational age. (3) The problem was how to obtain data in truly normal infants, and the simple answer was that it could not be done. After struggling with this problem for some time, we realized that we did have data on two groups of patients who, although not normal, at least were healthy and that this information might provide a close approximation of normal.

Where did these "normal" data come from? By 1965 we had begun placing

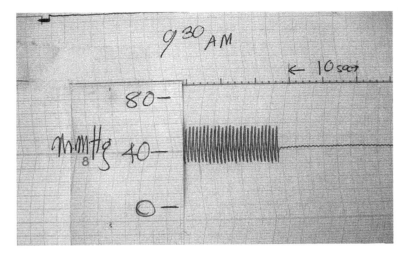

Figure 2. Tracing of an infant's aortic blood pressure on the paper record made by the polygraph. The first part of the tracing is phasic blood pressure and the second part is the mean pressure. The numbers on the left (0, 40, and 80) indicate the alibration of the pressure measurements in millimeters of mercury. The upper tracing marks the time in seconds.

umbilical arterial catheters soon after birth in preterm infants at high risk of developing respiratory distress. The need to measure arterial P_{O_2} when providing high concentrations of oxygen to a preterm infant was noted previously. The earlier an attempt was made to catheterize the umbilical artery, the more likely it would succeed because the umbilical arteries constrict soon after birth. The desire to avoid the situation of needing to administer oxygen to an infant in whom we no longer could pass a catheter led to the practice of early catheter placement in high-risk preterm infants. A few of these infants never developed respiratory distress syndrome, and when the outcome was clear, the catheters were removed. Among other infants who had cardiorespiratory symptoms at birth and had been catheterized quickly, some improved rapidly, and the catheters were removed when it was clear that the infants would do well. In each of these situations, there was a period when blood pressure was recorded in infants who were "healthy," and we decided to analyze these data to attempt to define "normal" blood pressure. Because of the circumstances of the data collection, we could examine the pressures only in the first 12 hours after birth. In a 30-month period, there were 45 "normal" infants among the 230 in whom umbilical arterial catheters were placed.

Dr. Joseph Kitterman, at the time a research fellow in the Cardiovascular Research Institute, analyzed the data. He divided the infants into three weight groups and compared blood pressures measured during the first 12 postnatal hours. Systolic, diastolic, and mean pressures increased with increasing birthweight with each of the 12 time periods. However, there was little variation in the average pressures within each group over the 12 hours. That highlighted the need to use different normal values for newborns of different birth-weights and indicated that "normal" for a particular weight was constant over the first 12 hours after birth. (18)

Our experience with these measurements convinced us that mean pressure was the most useful measurement. Although the other pressures also were helpful, mean pressure best reflected perfusion pressure, and this single value made it easier to follow trends in an individual. Accordingly, Kitterman performed a more detailed analysis of mean pressure versus birthweight to create a graph of normal values for use by clinicians (Figure 4 in the original 1969 article). He found that a parabolic regression best fit the relationship. After publication, this figure was reproduced in several textbooks and came into common use.

Epilogue

With time, one of the limitations of this research became a pressing problem. The "normal" data stopped at 1,000 g birthweight. At the start of this work, infants smaller than this weight usually died quickly and hardly fit even the loosest definition of "healthy." However, over the next decade, survival increased at lower birthweights. Dr. Hans Versmold (then from the University of Munich and now at the Free University of Berlin) spent 1977 and 1978 as a visiting scientist at the Cardiovascular Research Institute and the Department of Pediatrics at UCSF and reviewed the experience with these smaller infants. Among 202 infants who had birthweights less than 1,000 g in whom umbilical artery catheters were placed, he identified 16 who were appropriate to add to the previous pool of "normal" data. He repeated the analysis of pressure versus birthweight for mean, systolic, diastolic, and pulse pressures. With this analysis, the best correlation was achieved with linear regressions for each of the pressures. (19) These were shown in Figure 4 of the 1981 paper, and that figure of "normal" blood pressure also has been widely reproduced in textbooks. A pharmaceutical company made it into a colored poster to be hung up in NICUs.

Roderic H. Phibbs, MD
Department of Pediatrics and Cardiovascular
Research Institute
University of California San Francisco

Acknowledgments

Teresa Poirier, RN, John Clements, MD, and Joseph Kitterman, MD, gave me very helpful advice with this history.

[For the original article by Kitterman, Phibbs, and Tooley on aortic blood pressure in normal newborns, please go to: http://neoreviews.aappublications.org/cgi/data/4/5/e113/DC1 or http://pediatrics.aappublications.org/cgi/content/abstract/44/6/959]

References

1. Bernard C. *An Introduction to the Study of Experimental Medicine.* Green HP, trans. New York, NY: Dover Publications Inc; 1957

2. Wackers GL. Modern anaesthesiological principles for bulbar polio: manual IPPR in the 1952 polio-epidemic in Copenhagen. *Acta Anaesthesiol Scand.* 1994;38:420–431

3. Dawes GS. *Foetal and Neonatal Physiology.* Chicago, Ill: Yearbook Medical Publishers; 1968

4. James LS, Weisbrot IM, Prince CE, Holiday DA, Apgar V. The acid-base status of human infants in relation to birth asphyxia and the onset of respiration. *J Pediatr.* 1958;52:379–394

5. James LS, Weisbrot IM, Prince CE, Holiday DA, Apgar V. Acid-base homeostasis of the newborn infant during the first 24 hours of life. *J Pediatr.* 1958;52:395–403

6. Avery ME, Mead J. Surface properties in relation to atelectasis and hyaline membrane disease. *Am J Dis Child.* 1959;97:517–523

7. Strang LB, McLeish MH. Ventilatory failure and right to left shunt in newborn infants with respiratory distress. *Pediatrics.* 1961;28:17–27

8. Burnard ED, James LS. Atrial pressures and cardiac size in the newborn infant. *J Pediatr.* 1963;62:815–826

9. Rudolph AM, Drorbaugh JE, Auld PA, et al. Studies of the circulation in the neonatal period. The circulation in the respiratory distress syndrome. *Pediatrics*. 1961;27:551–566

10. Nelson NM, Prod'hom LS, Cherry RB, Lipsitz PJ, Smith CA. Pulmonary function in the newborn infant: the alveolar-arterial oxygen gradient. *J Appl Physiol*. 1963;18:534–538

11. Chu J, Clements JA, Cotton EK, Klaus MH, Sweet AY, Tooley WH. Neonatal pulmonary ischemia, part 1: clinical and physiological studies. *Pediatrics*. 1967;40(suppl):709–782

12. Stahlman M. Treatment of cardiovascular disorders of newborns. *Pediatr Clin North Am*. 1964;11:363–400

13. Avery ME, Oppenheimer EH. Recent increase in mortality from hyaline membrane disease. *J Pediatr*. 1960;57:553–559

14. Young M. Blood pressure in the newborn baby. *Br Med Bull*. 1961;17:154–159

15. Celander O. Blood flow in the foot and calf of the newborn. *Acta Paediatr*. 1960; 49:488–502

16. Kidd L, Levison H, Gemmel P, Aharon A, Swyer P. Limb blood flow in the normal and sick newborn. *Am J Dis Child*. 1966;112:402–407

17. Neligan GA, Smith CA. The blood pressure of newborn infants in asphyxial states and in hyaline membrane disease. *Pediatrics*. 1960;26:735–744

18. Kitterman JA, Phibbs RH, Tooley WH. Aortic blood pressure in normal newborn infants during the first 12 hours of life. *Pediatrics*. 1969;44:959–968

19. Versmold HT, Kitterman JA, Phibbs RH, Gregory GA, Tooley WH. Aortic blood pressure during the first 12 hours after birth in infants with birth weight 610 to 4220 grams. *Pediatrics*. 1981;67:607–613

Historical Perspectives: Direct Blood Pressure Measurement

Roderic H. Phibbs

NeoReviews 2003;4;113
DOI: 10.1542/neo.4-5-e113

Parents in the Preterm Nursery and Subsequent Evolution of Care

Introduction

When my elder daughter was born 40 years ago, I was the pediatric resident "on service" for the delivery room. However, as the prospective father, I was excluded from the delivery room. In that era, too, it was the norm for parents to view their pre-term (premature) infants through glass – either of the door or windows opening onto the "premature nursery." Nurseries that housed preterm infants were the domain of the nursing staff, and even the doctors were allowed to enter somewhat reluctantly. Caps, gowns, masks, and overshoes were standard and contributed to the aura that this was a very private place that required limited access.

How things have changed! Fathers now not only are encouraged to be in the delivery rooms, even for cesarean sections, but also (like mothers) to participate in skin-to-skin contact with their preterm infants. Rather than being exclusionary, the number of visitors to neonatal intensive care units (parents, grandparents, siblings, therapists of different types, subspecialists, medical students) can make them very crowded places at times. Much of this change comes from the work of Drs. Marshall Klaus and John Kennell, who describe in this 2004 article how parent-infant interaction has evolved over the last 40 years.

Alistair G. S. Philip, MD, FRCPE, FAAP
Editor-in-Chief, NeoReviews

Opening the Preterm Nursery to Parents

The first study to investigate the feasibility of permitting parents into the preterm nursery began in December 1964, at Stanford University, California. Barnett and associates (1) questioned whether parents of pre-term infants suffered from severe deprivation because of separation from their hospitalized infants. For a 2-year period, we studied the practicality of allowing mothers (total of 44) into the nursery soon after birth, first to handle and then to feed their infants while they were still in incubators. The mothers, because of state rules, wore masks and gowns, and the nurses in the unit instructed them in handwashing procedures. Initially, the nurses accompanied the mothers and stood by them while they handled their babies through the portholes and incubators. On subsequent visits, a nurse remained nearby to answer questions. When the babies could be fed easily by nipple, the mothers were encouraged to assume this task.

The threat of infection had been a formidable deterrent to permitting parents to enter the nursery. To evaluate the possibility that parents would bring pathogenic agents into the preterm unit, cultures were taken weekly from the umbilicus, skin, and nares of each infant and from the nursery equipment for the entire period that mothers were allowed into the unit. Investigators observed that mothers washed more frequently and more thoroughly than both the nurses and house officers. The results of these cultures, as well as the results of studies performed by Williams and Oliver (2) and Silverman and Sinclair (3) showed no increase in potentially pathogenic organisms resulting from the mothers' presence in the nursery.

In fact, at Stanford University, the number of positive cultures actually declined between 1964 and 1965. It has been speculated that infants may pick up nonpathogenic bacteria from their mothers that offer some protection against pathogenic hospital organisms, resulting in a decrease in the number of positive cultures. According to the Barnett investigation,

no staphylococcal, hemolytic streptococcal, or upper respiratory viral disease was documented in the charts of infants during the time that the mothers went into the nursery. The investigators concluded that these initial data suggested that the presence of mothers in the nursery did not increase the risk or the occurrence of infection. (1)

These researchers observed important behavioral differences between the mothers allowed into the nursery and those who were excluded. Those who had entered the nursery showed increased commitment to the infant, more confidence in their mothering abilities, and greater stimulating and caretaking skills.

When mothers initially are permitted to touch their preterm babies, they typically begin by circling the incubator and touching the baby's extremities with the tips of their fingers. (4) These reactions differ from those of the parents of term infants, who by the end of the first visit, are stroking the infants' trunks with the palms of their hands. Mothers of term infants align their heads with their babies' heads in the *en face* position for a substantially longer period of time than do mothers of preterm infants (Fig. 1).

Two long-term studies on the effects of early mother-infant separation as a result of special care nursery policies—one at Stanford University and the other at Case Western Reserve University, Ohio—have been completed (Table 1). (5) The hypothesis in each study was that if human mothers are affected by this period of separation, altered maternal attachment and mothering behavior may become apparent during the first weeks and months after birth in separated as opposed to nonseparated mothers, and subsequent differences in later infant development may be seen.

In the Stanford University study, three groups of mothers from similar socioeconomic backgrounds were observed. One group of mothers was given "contact" with their preterm infants in the intensive care unit in the first 5 days after birth, a second group

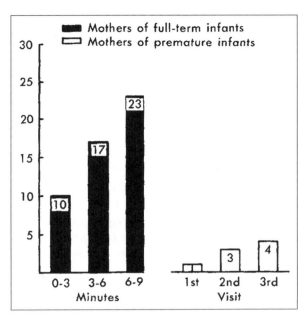

Figure 1. The percentage of *en face* position recorded during the first visit of 12 mothers of term infants and the first three visits of nine mothers of preterm infants. Reprinted with permission from Klaus MH, Kennell JH, Plumb N, Zuehlke S. *Pediatrics*. 1970;46:187–192.

of mothers was "separated" from their preterm infants with only visual contact for the first 21 days, and a third group of mothers of term infants had routine contact with their infants at feedings during a 3-day hospitalization. When the separated infants reached a weight of 2,100 g, at ages ranging from 3 to 12 weeks, they were transferred to a discharge nursery where their mothers were allowed to be with them as much as they desired for the 7 to 10 days until discharge at a weight of 2,500 g.

The interactions between the mothers and their own infants were observed three times: just prior to discharge and 1 week and 1 month after discharge. The behavior of the mothers of term infants was not the same as that of the mothers of pre-term infants. The former group smiled at their infants more and had more ventral contact with their infants. No striking differences were found between the behaviors of the separated and contact mothers of preterm infants. However, the primiparous mothers in the noncontact group showed significantly less self-confidence in their ability to care for their infants. (6) Sameroff (7) interpreted this finding as suggesting that the previous successful childbirth experience of multiparous mothers served to "insulate" them from the debilitating effects of

separation from their current preterm infants. The initial lack in self-confidence among mother who were allowed to visit in the preterm care nursery decreased by the time their infants were ready to go home. In contrast, only one of the mothers in the separated group showed such an increase in self-confidence. It would appear from these data that allowing mothers, especially those who are primipara, to be in contact with their preterm infants reduces their feelings of inadequacy. (7)

Leifer and colleagues (8) also reported an important set of clinical findings that had not been anticipated. Only 1 of 22 mothers in the contact group divorced during the period of the study, in contrast to 5 of 22 mothers in the separated group. It should be noted that a prerequisite for admission into the study was that the parents planned to keep and raise their babies. Surprisingly, in two cases in the separated group, neither parent wanted custody of their babies, who subsequently were given up for adoption.

In the Case Western Reserve University study, 53 mothers of preterm infants were assigned, on the basis of when the baby was born, to two groups: "early contact" and "late contact." (5) Mothers in the early contact group were allowed to come into the preterm nursery to handle and care for their infants 1 to 5 days after birth. The late contact group of mothers was not permitted to enter the nursery until 21 days after birth. For the first 3 weeks, these mothers had only visual contact with their infants through the nursery windows.

Time-lapse movies of both groups of mothers feeding their infants were obtained just before discharge and 1 month later. In addition, to determine whether early contact influenced maternal behavior that subsequently affected infant development, Bayley Developmental Scales were administered just before discharge and at 9, 15, and 21 months of age, and a Stanford-Binet test was administered at 42 months of age.

The mothers who had early contact spent significantly more time looking at their infants during the first filmed feeding. Additionally, there was a correlation between the amount of time that mothers looked at their

Table 1. Studies of Early and Late Maternal Contact in the Preterm Nursery

	Stanford University*	Case Western Reserve University
Early contact	22†	27 (1,537 g) ‡
Late contact	22†	26 (1,428 g) ‡
Number of married mothers	44	42
Socioeconomic status	Middle class	Wide range
Hollingshead Index	3	1 to 5
Length of follow-up (mo)	22	42

*Also included 24 term infants and mothers.
†Range of birthweights: 890 to 1,899 g.
‡Mean weight.

babies during the second filmed feeding and the infants' intelligence quotient (IQ) scores on the Stanford-Binet test at 42 months of age. Infants of mothers who had early contact had higher IQs ($r = 0.71$), with a mean of 99 for early contact children compared with a mean of 85 for late contact children ($P < .05$). Interestingly, Bayley Developmental Scores for the two groups of infants were not significantly different for the first 21 months after birth. (9)

Several problems associated with each of these studies should be mentioned. Both investigations were continued for 2 years, during which there were changes of procedure and personnel. Eighteen patients were lost from the Case Western Reserve University study during the follow-up period. Had these patients been included in the testing, the final results may have been altered.

Studies of preterm mother-infant dyads are especially difficult because of problems that occur during the long and stressful period of hospitalization, combined with the almost impossible task of obtaining a homogenous population for both groups with respect to parity; gender, birthweight, and gestational age of infant; religion; cultural background; and socioeconomic status. It also is difficult to control for the early life experiences of the mother as well as for home stresses. Neither group of investigators found it possible to run the early and late contact groups in the nursery simultaneously. Each study had a 3-month period of late contact followed by a 3-month period of early contact to prevent late-contact mothers from observing early-contact mothers in the nursery.

As part of the Stanford University study, the parents were interviewed seven times before the infant was discharged. This tended to bring both the early- and late-contact mothers into the hospital, possibly increasing the number of visits that the late-contact mothers made to the hospital. It is surprising that in this study, the early-contact mothers visited only an average of once every 6 days. We observed that the parents washed their hands more than young resident doctors. The rate of infection did not increase when parents entered the intensive care nursery. The increased rate of divorce and the two

infants given up for adoption in the late-contact group suggests one possible advantage of early visiting. This was the first study that began 40 years of work on the "bonding" early- and late-contact research and studies of doula observations.

The Mourning Response of Parents to the Death of a Newborn

Several physicians asked Dr Kennell and myself whether it was best to keep the parents out of the preterm nursery until clinicians were certain the baby would live (implying that parents do not become bonded if there is no contact) or whether it was "better to have loved and lost than never to have loved at all." With this question in mind, we studied all of the parents whose infants died at Babies and Children's Hospital in Cleveland in 1 year, including stillborn infants if they had no congenital malformations. We talked to them three times—on the day of the death of the baby, at the end of 7 to 10 days, and at 3 months after the death. The results of this study (10) could be summarized as follows: all parents experienced a period of mourning and grief that lasted 6 to 14 months whether the baby was 6 months' gestation, weighed 560 g, and lived for only 10 minutes; the baby weighed 3,000 g, was term, and lived for 12 days; or the baby was a preterm stillborn who weighed 1,000 g. It is the responsibility of the neonatal unit that cared for the baby to meet with parents twice or three times to find out how the parents are doing. An interview at 3 to 4 months can check for pathologic grief. It is best for the mother not to become pregnant again until the grief is nearly finished. If the mother becomes pregnant almost immediately, the new baby can be the repository for the many concerns she had for the dead infant. These findings suggest that every parent at birth has begun the bonding process and needs to be helped to complete the grieving process if the baby dies.

Human Maternal Behavior at the First Contact with Her Young

Although no studies have yet defined which neonatal characteristics elicit maternal touching, three independent observers have described a characteristic touching pattern that mothers use in the first contact with

their newborns. Rubin (11) noted that human mothers show an orderly progression of behavior after birth while becoming acquainted with their babies. Klaus et al (4) observed that when 13 nude infants were placed next to their mothers a few minutes or 1 hour after birth, most mothers touched them in a pattern of behavior that began with fingertip touching of the infant's extremities and proceeded in 4 to 8 minutes to massaging, stroking, and encompassing palm contact of the trunk. In the first 3 minutes, mothers maintained fingertip contact 52% of the time and palm contact 28% of the time. In the last 3 minutes of observation, however, this was reversed. Fingertip contact had greatly decreased, and palm contact increased to 62% of the total scored time. Rubin (11) observed a similar pattern but at a much slower rate. In her study, mothers usually required about 3 days to complete the sequence, but the infants were dressed, which may account for the difference. Rodholm and Larsson (12) have noted similar touching sequences in fathers.

Mothers of healthy preterm infants who were permitted early contact followed a similar sequence of touching their infants in the incubator but at an even slower rate; even at the third visit, mothers of preterm infants were not using their palms. (4) Much more progress in tactile contact occurred in mothers of term infants in just 10 minutes. On the mothers' fourth or fifth visits with small preterm infants, they often continued to touch the extremities with their fingertips. Further exploration of this area suggested a possible reason for continuing this behavior. Approximately 2 to 3 months later, after they learned how to care for their baby, they were asked what the baby looked like initially to them. Shortly following birth, they reported that the baby looked like a small animal: a mouse. Surprisingly, 60% to 70% of mothers suggest that the small preterm infant looks like an animal, both in the United States and in Europe (personal communication with the mothers).

Studies Supporting the Hypothesis of a Sensitive Period

From 1970 to 1981, 17 separate studies have focused on whether additional time for

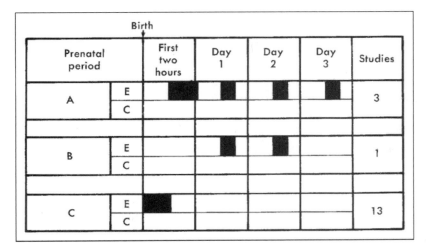

Figure 2. Time patterns and number of three types of controlled studies in which one group of mothers had additional contact (E) with their infants compared with another group who had routine contact (C).

close contact of the mother and term infant in the minutes, hours, and days after birth alters the quality of the maternal-infant bond. Figure 2 illustrates the timing of the contact in these studies. In three studies (A) the extra time was added not only during the first 2 hours after birth, but also during the next 3 days. In one study (B), the additional contact was added on postnatal days 1 and 2. In 13 studies (C), the additional mother-infant contact occurred only in the first hour after birth. We have detailed these differences because the results of these investigations have stimulated extensive discussion about the significance of contact during these early hours. Because hospital practices have been altered based on these 17 studies, it is essential to explore in depth their design, ecology, and outcome measures as well as their strengths and weaknesses.

Group A Studies

Some of the most intriguing and thoughtful observations about the effect of early contact have been made by Siegel and colleagues, (13) who assessed 202 patients in a beautifully designed investigation. The aim of the study was to explore the effect on maternal attachment of early and extended contact as well as the influence of home visits by well-trained paraprofessionals. Observations were made at 4 and 12 months after birth. There were no significant effects due to the home visit interventions. However, early- and extended-contact mothers showed differences in attachment variables, such as acceptance of the infant and consoling of the crying infant at 4 months, as noted in a home visit. These mothers also had significantly increased positive versus negative infant behaviors in the home at 12 months.

A most important contribution of this study was the exploration of the variance contributed by the interventions or, to put it more simply, the power of early and extended contact to influence maternal attachment behavior. The investigators calculated that 2.5% to 3% of the variance could be explained by the early and extended contact, whereas between 10% and 22% of the variance was explained by background variables such as the mothers' economic status, race, housing, education, parity, and age. The study participants were low-income mothers who were primarily multiparous and lived in a rural area of North Carolina. It should be noted that there was no significant difference between the experimental and control groups in the reports of child abuse and neglect in the first year after birth. The Siegel study emphasizes the contribution of background variables that are not changed easily. It also shows that some significant and advantageous parental and infant behaviors are changed by extra contact. Although early and extended contact contributes less variance than might be expected, it can be arranged for all parents at no additional cost.

Group B Studies

It is useful to compare the one study in this group by O'Connor and associates (14) with the large study by Siegel and associates. The Siegel investigators did not note any difference in parenting disorders, finding 10 in the control group and seven in the extended contact groups. On the other hand, O'Connor's group noted significant differences in parenting disorders, child abuse, neglect, abandonment, and nonorganic failure to thrive at 17 months, finding 10 in the control group compared with two in the extended-contact group (Table 2). O'Connor also noted that mothers who were given 12 additional hours of contact in the first 2 days after birth had significantly lower hospital admission rates for their infants and fewer accidents and poisonings. Thus, there is disagreement about whether additional early contact prevents or alters parenting failures. It should be noted that only primiparous mothers were included in the O'Connor study compared with the primarily multiparous mothers in the

Table 2. Child Abuse or Neglect

Study	Total Number	Abuse or Neglect (Number)
O'Connor et al, 1980		
Extended contact	134	2
Control	143	10*
Seigel et al, 1980		
Extended contact	97	7
Control	105	10
*P<.05.		

Siegel study. The income level of the parents in both studies was low, but families in the O'Connor study were from the inner city of Nashville, and Siegel's families came from the rural countryside.

Group C Studies

Thirteen separate studies have examined the effect of an additional mother-infant contact in the first hour after birth on breastfeeding, with contact following this period being similar in both the experimental and control groups. All but four of the studies documented a significant difference between the control and experimental groups.

Two recent studies focus on the questions raised by this research. Widstrom and colleagues (15) observed that mothers keep their infants in their rooms 100 minutes longer in the first 3 days after birth if the infant's lips touched the mother's nipples during a breastfeeding in the first hour after birth.

Kramer and associates (16) answered the question about the effects of early breastfeeding and the Baby Friendly Hospital Initiative (BFHI) on more than 17,000 mother-infant pairs in Belarus. The patients were randomized into two groups: traditional breastfeeding as practiced in Belarus or BFHI (all 10 steps), including breastfeeding in the first hour after birth and rooming-in. The BFHI group breastfed significantly more over the first year after birth than the other cohort. The BFHI is based firmly on this study but was stimulated by the 13 studies in Group C.

The Effects of a Doula on the Mother and Infant at Birth, 6 Weeks, and 2 Months

A number of studies show that humane, sensitive, and individually appropriate practices, including continuous physical, emotional, and social support for mothers during labor and birth, keeping the mother and baby together from the start with rooming-in, suckling in the first hours (with infants deciding when they should take the first drink), demand feeding, and the father holding and learning about his infant in the early period, have surprising benefits and multiple

advantages for the mother and infant. They have resulted in decreasing rates of infant abandonment, (17) increased father involvement in the first months, (18) and increased breastfeeding.

In addition, a comparison of mothers who received a cloth infant carrier to use on their chests in the first months of the infant's life with control mothers who received a plastic infant seat documented improved mother-infant interaction at 3 months by blinded observers and, at 13 months, an increased incidence of secure attachment of 83% in the experimental group versus 38% in the controls. (19)

The first doula study showed subtle but distinct differences in how mothers perceived or responded to their infants after being supported or not supported emotionally and physically in labor. Two groups of mothers were observed through a one-way mirror with their infants in a standardized situation in the first 25 minutes after leaving the delivery room. The observers were blinded to the care the mothers received during labor. The mothers who had been supported by a doula showed more affectionate interaction with their infants, with significantly more smiling, talking, and stroking than the controls. (20)

Hofmeyr and colleagues (21) at the University of Witwatersrand in Johannesburg, South Africa, and Wolman and associates (22) studied 189 women having their first babies. The patients were Indian urban mothers who were familiar with the hospital. The doulas in this study were laywomen (with a short weekend of training), who were asked to remain with the laboring women and used touch and verbal communication focusing on three primary factors: comfort, reassurance, and praise.

Although the mothers who had doulas experienced less pain than the controls, there were no differences in length of labor; use of medication, oxytocin, or forceps; and cesarean sections from controls at birth. However, there were significant differences at 6 weeks in anxiety, self esteem, and depression from controls (Table 3). Maternal perceptions at 6 weeks of the babies and themselves also were very different (Table 4).

Table 3. Psychological Outcome at Six Weeks

	Control	Doula
Anxiety	40%	28%*
Self-esteem	59%	74%*
Depression	23%*	10%*

*Highly significant.

In a study of 104 mothers over several months, healthy women expecting their first babies were assigned randomly to either a doula support or narcotic or epidural analgesia group. (23) To evaluate later mother-infant interaction, observers were specially trained in home observations. The observers did not know the labor experience of the mothers. When each of the infants reached 2 months of age, a home visit was made to test infant development and to observe the mother's interaction with her infant. The interaction was scored on a scale of one to seven based on the mother's physical contact, visual attention, and affectionate behaviors toward the infant. The mother's interaction with her baby was rated on five occasions during the visit: 1) when the examiner entered the mother's house, 2) while a developmental test was being set up, 3) while the test was being scored, 4) during a feeding, and 5) while the mother changed the baby. Scores on the developmental test were not related to the social support or analgesia that the mother received during labor.

The mother's interaction scores showed significant differences. The doula-supported mothers' scores were significantly higher than the score of the no-doula group mothers ($P<.001$). These results indicated that mothers who had the support of a doula had a remarkably positive level of affectionate interaction with their babies compared with the other mothers. This suggests that giving support continuously through labor with a doula may make a significant change in the mother when the infant is 6 weeks and 2 months of age.

Mothers Living in the Preterm Nursery

When we visited the High Wycombe unit in England, (24) where mothers are allowed to live in the neonatal intensive care unit, the

Table 4. Maternal Perception at Six Weeks

Perception	Control Group	Doula-supported Group
Of Baby:		
Cries less than others	17%	55%*
Special	71%	91%*
Easy to manage	27%	65%*
Clever	47%	78%*
Beautiful	67%	89%*
Regards baby as a separate, sociable person by 6 weeks	80%	100%*
Of Self:		
Feels close to baby	80%	97%*
Pleased to have baby	65%	97%*
Managing well	65%	91%*
Communicates well	68%	91%*
Becoming a mother was easy	11%	45%*
Can look after baby better than anyone else	31%	72%*
*Highly significant		

staff said that parents move more quickly to assume caregiving tasks, are less jealous of the staff and more chatty, and adapt more readily to the birth of a sick infant than previously, when mothers could not live in. The High Wycombe model has been examined closely and, in some cases, followed in part by high-risk nurseries in the United States.

In several countries, including Argentina, (25) Brazil, Chile, (26) South Africa, (27) Ethiopia, (28) and Estonia, (29) mothers of preterm infants live in a room adjoining the preterm nursery or they room-in. This arrangement appears to have multiple benefits. It allows the mothers to continue producing milk, permits them to care for their infants more easily, greatly reduces the care-giving time required of the staff for the infants, and allows a group of mothers of preterm infants to gain from discussion and mutual support.

We have studied the experience of mothers who are permitted to live in with their infants before discharge, a practice we have termed "nesting." As soon as babies reached 1.6 to 2 kg, each mother provided all caregiving in a private room with her baby. Impressive changes in the behavior of these women were observed. Even though the mothers had fed and cared for their infants in the intensive care nursery on many occasions before living in, eight of the first nine mothers were unable to sleep during the first 24 hours of the nesting experience. Most of the mothers closed the door to the room, completely shutting out any chance of observation, often to the consternation of the nurses, who felt a strong responsibility for the infants' well-being. It was interesting to observe that the mothers rearranged the furniture, crib, and infant supplies. However, in the second 24-hour period, the mothers' confidence and caregiving skills improved greatly. At this time, mothers began to make preparations at home for the baby's arrival. Several insisted on taking their infants home earlier than planned. The babies seemed to be quieter during this living-in period. Some mothers experienced physical changes, such as increased breast swelling accompanied by some milk secretion. The mothers were not satisfied with the living-in nesting procedure until we established unlimited visiting privileges for the fathers and provided them with comfortable chairs and cots.

Kangaroo Care

In South America, the United States, and Europe, mothers and fathers have found that holding the preterm infant skin-to-skin is uniquely helpful in developing a tie with their infants. At the first experience, the mother usually is tense, so it is best for the nurse to stay with her to answer questions and make any necessary adjustments in position and measures to maintain warmth such as blankets. However, most mothers discover that the experience is especially pleasurable. After the "kangaroo" contact, some mothers have mentioned timidly that they began for the first time to feel close to their babies and feel that the babies were theirs. Without prompting, one mother said that she was feeling much better because she was now doing something for her baby that no one else could do.

It is our belief that skin-to-skin care is useful in helping parents develop closer ties to their infants. Properly detailed observations have noted that the infant's heart rate, temperature, and respiratory rate are stable with kangaroo care, and there is no increase in apnea during the daily 1- to 1.5-hour experience. (30) With kangaroo care, the preterm infant has long periods of deep sleep. Brain wave patterns show 2 to 4 periods of "delta brush/ hour" not seen in the incubator. Delta brush occurs with synapse formation. Additionally, significant increases in milk output and an increase in the success of lactation have been documented with skin-to-skin care.

Feldman and colleagues (31)(32) (33) conducted a very useful and valuable study in Israel of kangaroo care that included a 6-month follow-up period. A total of 146 preterm infants weighing 530 to 1,720 g were matched for gender, birth-weight, gestational age, and medical risk. All families were middle class. Seventy-three infants had kangaroo care, and 73 were controls. At 31 to 34 weeks' gestation, the study group received at least 1 h/d for 2 weeks of kangaroo care, and they were evaluated at 37 weeks', 3 months', and 6 months' corrected age.

At 6 months, infants who had received kangaroo care had longer durations and shorter latencies to mother-infant shared attention and infant-sustained exploration in a toy session. The mothers were more sensitive and warm in their interactions, and infants had higher scores on the Bayley

Neonatal Developmental Index (kangaroo care mean, 96.39; control mean, 91.81) and the Psychomotor Developmental Index (kangaroo care mean, 85.57; control mean, 80.53). The authors underscored the importance of the role of early skin-to-skin contact of the mother in the maturation of the infant's psychological, emotional, and cognitive regulatory capacities. These findings suggest that kangaroo care probably should be used for every preterm infant at the critical time of 31 to 34 weeks' gestation.

Marshall Klaus, MD
Professor
University of California at San Francisco

John H. Kennell, MD
Emeritus Professor

Case Western Reserve University
Cleveland, Ohio

[To read the groundbreaking study on the feasibility of permitting parents into the preterm nursery published in 1970, please go to: http://neoreviews.aappublications.org/cgi/data/5/10/e397/DC1 or http://pediatrics.aappublications.org/cgi/content/abstract/45/2/197]

References

1. Barnett CR, Leiderman PH, Grobstein R, Klaus MH. Neonatal separation: the maternal side of interactional deprivation. *Pediatrics.* 1970;45:197–205

2. Williams CP, Oliver TK Jr. Nursery routines and staphylococcal colonization of the newborn. *Pediatrics.* 1969;44:640–646

3. Silverman WA, Sinclair JC. Evaluation of precautions before entering a neonatal unit. *Pediatrics.* 1967;40:900-901

4. Klaus MH, Kennell JH, Plumb H, Zuehlke S. Human maternal behavior at first contact with her young. *Pediatrics.* 1970;46:187–192

5. Klaus MH, Kennell JH. *Maternal-Infant Bonding.* St. Louis, Mo: CV Mosby; 1976:112–115

6. Seashore MH, Leifer AD, Barnett CR, Leiderman PH. The effect of denial of early mother-infant interaction on maternal self-confidence. *J Pers Soc Psychol.* 1973;26:369–378

7. Sameroff A. Psychologic needs of the mother in early mother-infant interaction. In: Avery CB, ed. *Neonatology.* Philadelphia, Pa: JB Lippincott; 1975:1023–1042

8. Leifer AD, Leiderman PH, Barnett CR, et al. Effects of mother-infant separation on maternal attachment behavior. *Child Dev.* 1972;43:1203–1218

9. Kennell JH, Klaus MH Wolfe H. Nesting behavior. In: Stetson J, ed. *Current Concepts of Neonatal Intensive Care.* St. Louis, Mo: Green Inc; 1975:245–351

10. Kennell JH, Slyter H, Klaus MH. The mourning response of parents to the death of a newborn infant. *N Engl J Med.* 1970;283:344–349

11. Rubin R. Maternal touch. *Nurs Outlook.* 1963;11:828–381

12. Rodholm M, Larsson K Father-infant interaction at the first contact after delivery. *Early Hum Dev.* 1979;3:21–27

13. Siegel E, Bauman KE, Schaefer ES, et al. Hospital and home support during infancy: impact on maternal attachment. Child abuse and neglect and health care utilization. *Pediatrics.* 1980;66:189–190

14. O'Connor S, Vietze PM, Sharrod KB, et al. Reduced incidence of parenting inadequacy following rooming-in. *Pediatrics.* 1980;66:176–180

15. Widstrom AM, Wahlberg V, Matthiesen AS, et al. Short-term effects of early suckling and touch of the nipple on maternal behavior. *Early Hum Dev.* 1990;21:153–163

16. Kramer MS, Chalmer B, Hodnett ED, et al. Promotion of Breastfeeding Intervention (PROBIT): a randomized trial in the Republic of Belarus. *JAMA.* 2000;285:413–420

17. Lvoff NM, Lvoff V, Klaus M. Effect of Baby Friendly Initiative on infant abandonment in a Russian hospital. *Arch Pediatr Adolesc Med.* 2000;154:474–477

18. Rodholm M. Effects of father-infant post partum contact on their interaction 3 months after birth. *Early Hum Dev.* 1981;5:79–85

19. Anisfeld E, Casper V, Nozy W, Cunningham N. Does infant carrying promote attachment? An experimental study of increased physical contact on the development of attachment. *Child Dev.* 1990;61:1617–1627

20. Sosa R, Kennell J, Klaus M, et al. The effect of a supportive companion on perinatal problems, length of labor and mother interaction. *N Engl J Med.* 1980;303:597–600

21. Hofmeyr GJ, Nikodem VC, Wolman WL, et al. Companionship to modify the clinical birth environment: effects on progress and perception of labour and breastfeeding. *Br J Obstet Gynecol.* 1991;98:756–764

22. Wolman WL, Chalmers B, Hofmeyr GJ, et al. Post-partum depression and companionship in the clinical birth environment: a randomized, controlled study. *Am J Obstet Gynecol.* 1993;168:1380–1393

23. Landry SH, McGrath SK, Kennell JH, et al. The effects of doula support during labor on mother-infant interaction at 2 months [abstract]. *Pediatr Res.* 1998;43:13A

24. Garrow DH. Special care without separation: High Wycombe, England. In: Davis JA, Richards MPM, Robertson NRC, eds. *Parent-Baby Attachment in Premature Infants.* New York, NY: St. Martins; 1983:223–231

25. Kennell JH, Klaus MH. The perinatal paradigm: is it time for a change? *Clin Perinatol.* 1988;15:801–813

26. Torres Pereyra J. The Sotero Del Rio Hospital, Santiago, Chile. In: Davis JA, Richards MPM, Robertson NRC, eds. *Parent-Baby Attachment in Premature Infants.* New York, NY: St. Martins; 1983:243–253

27. Kahn E, Wayburne S, Fouche M. The Baragwanath Premature Baby Unit: an analysis of the case records of 1000 consecutive admissions. *South Afr Med J.* 1954;28:453–456

28. Tafari N, Sterky G, Sleath K. Early discharge of low-birth-weight infants in a developing country. *Environ Child Health.* 1974;20:73–76

29. Levin A. The mother-infant unit at Tallinn Children's Hospital, Estonia: a truly baby friendly unit. *Birth.* 1994;21:39–45

30. Whitelaw A, Heisterkamp GK, Acolet D, et al. Skin to skin contact for very low-birth-weight infants and their mothers: a randomized trial of "kangaroo care." *Arch Dis Child.* 1988;63:1391–1401

31. Feldman R, Eidelman A, Sirota L, Weller A. Comparison of skin to skin (kangaroo) and traditional care: parenting outcomes and preterm infant development. *Pediatrics.* 2002;110:16–26

32. Feldman R, Weller A, Sirota L, Eidelman A. Skin to skin contact (kangaroo care) promotes self-regulation in premature infants: sleep-wake cyclicity, arousal modulation, and sustained exploration. *Dev Psychol*. 2002;38:191–207

33. Feldman R, Eidelman A. Skin to skin contact (kangaroo care) accelerates autonomic and neurobehavioral maturation in preterm infants. *Dev Med Child Neurol*. 2003;45:274–286

Suggested Reading

Klaus M, Kennell JH, Klaus PH. *Bonding: Building the Foundations of Secure Attachment and Independence*. Reading, Mass: Addison-Wesley Publishing; 1995

Klaus M, Kennell JH, Klaus PH. *The Doula Book*. Cambridge, Mass: Perseus Publishing; 2002

Klaus MH, Klaus, PH. *Your Amazing Newborn*. Cambridge, Mass: Perseus Publishing; 1998

Historical Perspectives: Parents in the Preterm Nursery and Subsequent Evolution of Care

Alistair G. S. Philip, Marshall Klaus and John H. Kennell

NeoReviews 2004;5;e397-e405
DOI: 10.1542/neo.5-10-e397

Prenatal Assessment of Fetal Lung Maturity

Introduction

In this 2004 article, we recognize one of the most important contributions of one of the pioneers of neonatology, Dr. Louis Gluck. (1) One of his coauthors, Dr. William Spellacy, provides the historical perspective. In addition to this contribution, it should be noted that Dr. Gluck was one of the first people to introduce the concept of neonatal intensive care, in a unit at Yale University, that included a specially designated social worker. After spending some time in Miami, he moved to San Diego and was one of the first to expand the concept to include "high-risk mothers" in a perinatal center. (2)

As mentioned by Dr. Spellacy, the idea that the lung might contribute to amniotic fluid probably was proposed initially by Reynolds in 1953, (3) but in the featured article, Dr. Gluck drew attention to the important article by Forrest Adams and colleagues, who described the sphincteric mechanism of the larynx, with periodic discharge of fetal lung fluid, using cineradiography in sheep. (4) Based on this information, he reasoned that evaluation of amniotic fluid could allow prenatal assessment of fetal lung maturity. With his primary coworker in this area (Marie Kulovich), he wrote an excellent review of work until that time in 1973. (5) Subsequently, his group documented the importance of phosphatidylglycerol (6) and the observation of accelerated fetal maturation in certain stressed pregnancies. (7) (8)

This was by no means the only area of interest for Lou Gluck, but this "imaginative pathfinder in neonatal medicine," (9) who died in 1997, is best known for his contributions in this field.

Alistair G. S. Philip, MD, FRCPE, FAAP
Editor-in-Chief, NeoReviews

References

1. Gluck L, Kulovich MV, Borer RC Jr, Brenner PH, Anderson GG, Spellacy WN. Diagnosis of the respiratory distress syndrome by amniocentesis. *Am J Obstet Gynecol.* 1971;109:440–445
2. Gluck L. Design of a perinatal center. *Pediatr Clin North Am.* 1970;17:777–791
3. Reynolds SRM. A source of amniotic fluid in the lamb: the nasopharyngeal and buccal cavities. *Nature.* 1953;172:307–308
4. Adams FH, Desilets DT, Towers B. Control of flow of fetal lung fluid at the laryngeal outlet. *Respir Physiol.* 1967;2:302–309
5. Gluck L, Kulovich MV. Fetal lung development: current concepts. *Pediatr Clin North Am.* 1973;20:367–379
6. Hallman M, Kulovich M, Kirkpatrick E, Sugarman RE, Gluck L. Phosphatidylglycerol in amniotic fluid: indices of lung maturity. *Am J Obstet Gynecol.* 1976;125:613–617
7. Gould JB, Gluck L, Kulovich MV. The relationship between accelerated pulmonary maturity and accelerated neurological maturity in certain chronically stressed pregnancies. *Am J Obstet Gynecol.* 1977;127:181–186
8. Obladen M, Merritt TA, Gluck L. Acceleration of pulmonary surfactant maturation in stressed pregnancies: a study of neonatal lung effluent. *Am J Obstet Gynecol.* 1979;135:1079–1085
9. *AAP Perinatal Section News.* 1998;23(1):28

The Development of the Lecithin/ Sphingomyelin (L/S) Ratio Test

Historically, a major concept in the management of severe fetal disease associated with maternal medical problems such as Rh sensitization, diabetes mellitus, or hypertension has been early delivery of the infant. The problem that existed for years was how to determine if the fetus was mature enough to survive in the nursery after the early delivery. To convert a fetal death into a neonatal death by early delivery obviously would have no effect on perinatal mortality.

To determine potential neonatal survival, many perinatologists began to develop tests of fetal organ maturity. One of the first was a radiograph of the uterus (fetogram). It was known that bone ossification centers developed at different times in the fetus. Thus, the radiographs were used to look for ossified centers of the fetal knee. The distal femoral epiphysis may be visualized at about 36 weeks' gestation and the proximal tibial epiphysis at about 38 weeks' gestation; the presence of both predicted a birth-weight of at least 2,500 g in 98% of cases. (1)

As ultrasonography became widely used in obstetrics, it provided more accurate pregnancy dating in women who had uncertain menstrual dates, but only if the examination occurred early in the pregnancy.

Ultrasonography also allowed precise localization of amniotic fluid pockets in the uterus and the introduction of safe amniocentesis for fluid sampling. This was used initially by Liley to evaluate the severity of fetal Rh sensitization, (2) and the success of these studies opened a new area for research on the composition of amniotic fluid as a measure of the maturity of fetal systems. Liley demonstrated that amniotic fluid bilirubin concentrations, as determined by the optical density at 450 nm (delta OD450), decreased in normal pregnancy. Mandelbaum and associates (3) extended these observations to show that amniotic fluid bilirubin was nonconjugated and that fetal liver maturity could be evaluated by measurement of amniotic fluid bilirubin because the level reached 0 at about 36 weeks' gestation when the liver was "mature" and had the capacity to conjugate bilirubin, which was passed into the gut and mother. Fetal kidney function also was studied. Pitkin and Zwirek (4) measured creatinine in the amniotic fluid, and when the renal clearance of creatinine was "mature," at about 37 weeks' gestation, amniotic fluid creatinine content increased to 2 mg/dL or more.

While all of these tests were being developed, it became clear that the principal clinical problem for the immature neonate was inadequate pulmonary function. Preterm neonates were not dying because of their immature bones, livers, or kidneys; they were developing respiratory distress syndrome (RDS) and dying from hypoxia. Many investigators had shown that maturation of the fetal lung depended on the ability of the type II pneumocyte to secrete surfactant into the alveolar space, thereby reducing surface tension. (5) (6) Good evidence from animal studies documented that fetal lung secretions were a major component of the amniotic fluid. (7) Gluck and associates (8) analyzed the

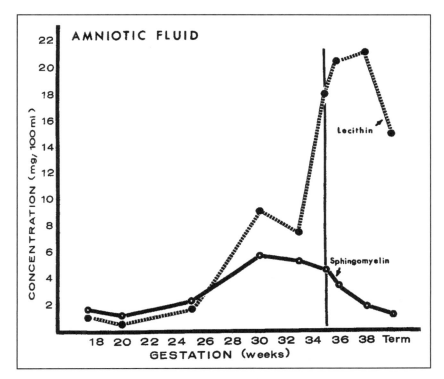

Figure 1. Mean concentrations in amniotic fluid of sphingomyelin and lecithin during gestation. The acute rise in lecithin at 35 weeks marks pulmonary maturity. This diagram was published in: *Am J Obstet Gynecol.* Feb 1;109(3):440–445. Gluck L, Kulovich MV, Borer RC Jr, Brenner PH, Anderson GG, and Spellacy WN. "Diagnosis of the Respiratory Distress Syndrome by Amniocentesis." Copyright Elsevier (1971).

surface alveolar lining and demonstrated that lecithin concentrations, a major component of surfactant, reflected alveolar stability.

Lou Gluck had become Professor of Pediatrics at the University of Miami School of Medicine in the late 1960s, and I was in the Department of Obstetrics and Gynecology. I was studying amniotic fluid hemoglobin disappearance rates when Lou told me of his theory that measurement of amniotic fluid lecithin might be a method of determining if the fetus was producing adequate alveolar surfactant to have normal respiratory function as a neonate. I began to supply amniotic fluid samples to Lou's laboratory for these analyses. The original report involved 302 amniotic fluid samples. The lipids were extracted from these samples after centrifugation with chloroform, and the lecithin was concentrated by precipitation in cold acetone. The lipids were identified with thin layer chromatography. The results showed the lecithin (L) levels increased at about 35 weeks' gestation, but sphingomyelin (S) levels did not (Figure). (9) To make the assay easy to carry out and to avoid problems with amniotic fluid volume changes affecting the laboratory result, they began to use the L/S ratio of amniotic fluid to predict fetal lung maturity. Further studies on 190 samples from 140 women showed that when the ratio was greater than 2, there was no significant RDS related to lung maturity; when the ratio was less than 2, there was some risk of RDS. (10) These data soon were confirmed in many centers, and the test became a common and very useful assessment of fetal lung maturity and the potential for neonatal RDS in pregnancies to be delivered before term.

Subsequently, additional tests of surfactant in amniotic fluid have been introduced. Hallman and associates (11) found that phosphatidylglycerol (PG) was a unique phospholipid of lung surfactant that increased in amniotic fluid. The absence of PG suggested that surfactant might not be mature. Other tests of fetal lung maturity included the lamellar body count (LBC) and the shake foam test. (12) The simultaneous analysis of amniotic fluid L/S, PG, LBC, and shake test showed excellent correlations, with high positive predictive values as well as good correlation with amniotic fluid creatinine and delta OD450. (10) (12) (13) Although all of these tests are of lesser clinical importance today, with the availability of neonatal surfactant inhalation treatments, they still command a significant place in management decisions about early delivery in high-risk pregnancies. They also opened a new chapter in the understanding of fetal development and the pathophysiology of common neonatal problems.

William N. Spellacy, MD
Professor of Obstetrics and Gynecology
University of South Florida
Tampa, FL

[To read the original article on use of the L/S ratio to predict fetal lung maturity written by Dr Gluck and colleagues in 1971, which was reprinted with permission from the American Journal of Obstetrics and Gynecology and the Mosby Corporation, please go to: http://neoreviews.aappublications.org/cgi/content/full/5/4/e131/DC1]

References

1. Schreiber MH, Nichols MM, McGanity WJ. Epiphyseal ossification center visualization: its value in prediction of fetal maturity. *JAMA.* 1963;184:504–507

2. Liley AW. Liquor amnii analysis in the management of the pregnancy complicated by Rhesus sensitization. *Am J Obstet Gynecol.* 1961;82:1359–1370

3. Mandelbaum B, LaCroix GC, Robinson AR. Determination of fetal maturity by spectrophotometric analysis of amniotic fluid. *Obstet Gynecol.* 1967;29:471–474

4. Pitkin RM, Zwirek SJ. Amniotic fluid creatinine. *Am J Obstet Gynecol.* 1967;98:1135–1139

5. Clements JA. Surface tension of lung extracts. *Proc Soc Exp Biol Med.* 1957;95:170–172

6. Avery ME, Mead J. Surface properties in relation to atelectasism and hyaline membrane disease. *Am J Dis Child.* 1959;97:517–523

7. Reynolds SRM. A source of amniotic fluid in the lamb. The naso-pharyngeal and buccal cavities. *Nature.* 1953;172:307–308

8. Gluck L, Sribney M, Kulovich MV. The biochemical development of surface activity in mammalian lung. *Pediatr Res.* 1967;1:247–265

9. Gluck L, Kulovich MV, Borer RC Jr, Brenner PH, Anderson GG, Spellacy WN. Diagnosis of the respiratory distress syndrome by amniocentesis. *Am J Obstet Gynecol.* 1971;109:440–445

10. Spellacy WN, Buhi WC. Amniotic fluid lecithin/sphingomyelin ratio as an index of fetal maturity. *Obstet Gynecol.* 1972;39:852–860

11. Hallman M, Kulovich M, Kirkpatrick E, Sugarman RG, Gluck L. Phosphatidyl-inositol and phosphatidylglycerol in amniotic fluid: indices of lung maturity. *Am J Obstet Gynecol.* 1976;125:613–617

12. Shephard B, Buhi W, Spellacy W. Critical analysis of the amniotic fluid shake test. *Obstet Gynecol.* 1974;43:558–562

13. Poggi SH, Spong CY, Pezzullo JC, et al. Lecithin/sphingomyelin ratio and lamellar body count: what values predict the presence of phosphatidylglycerol? *J Reprod Med.* 2003;48:330–334

Historical Perspectives: Prenatal Assessment of Fetal Lung Maturity

Alistair G. S. Philip and William N. Spellacy

NeoReviews 2004;5;e131-e133

DOI: 10.1542/neo.5-4-e131

Continuous Positive Airway Pressure (CPAP)

Although the principle might better be called "continuous distending pressure," continuous positive airway pressure (CPAP) was introduced before continuous negative pressure, a term that is rarely used. As noted by Dr George A. Gregory in this 2004 column, application of CPAP was initially with a head box, but proved to be much more reliable using an endotracheal tube. The system developed by Gregory et al was described in 1971 and was quickly followed in 1973 by a system that used nasal prongs (1), which tends to be the preferred method of application because it can avoid endotracheal intubation. Although some centers preferred to use negative pressure ventilators, their success was limited in infants with birthweights less than 1,500 g. The negative pressure ventilator could also be used in a continuous negative pressure mode.

When using positive pressure ventilation, the conventional terminology is "positive end-expiratory pressure," but the principle of CPAP is exactly the same.

Alistair G. S. Philip, MD, FRCPE, FAAP
Editor-in-Chief, NeoReviews

Reference
1. Kattwinkel J, Fleming D, Chu CC, Fanaroff AA, Klaus MH. A device for administration of continuous positive airway pressure by the nasal route. *Pediatrics*. 1973;52:131–134.

Introduction

In the 1960s, hyaline membrane disease (HMD) was the major cause of neonatal death in the United States. Boston, Geller, and Smith (1) reported 100% mortality if neonates had Pao$_2$s of less than 100 mm Hg in the first 12 hours after birth, and Stahlman and associates (2) reported a 70% mortality if neonates were breathing 100% oxygen in the first 12 postnatal hours. Included among the deaths were infants who weighed more than 1,800 g at birth. Outcomes were similar in other centers. Available care often consisted of administering oxygen, intravenous fluids, and antibiotics and keeping patients warm. As a last ditch effort, some babies were mechanically ventilated.

Knowledge of the physiology of neonates and of their disease processes increased rapidly during this period. Smith (3) and Nelson and colleagues (4) demonstrated that neonates who had HMD had low lung compliance and a reduced functional residual capacity. Stahlman, (5) Rudolph and associates, (6) and many others demonstrated abnormalities in ventilation or the cardiovascular systems of affected neonates. John Clements isolated surfactant from the lung, (7) and Mary Ellen Avery and Jerry Mead (8) demonstrated a deficiency of surfactant in the lungs of neonates who died of HMD. Surfactant deficiency was associated with atelectasis. In detailed pulmonary and cardiovascular studies of neonates who had HMD, Chu and associates (9) demonstrated that a significant portion of the problem with this disease was due to mismatching of ventilation and perfusion and that grunting was an effort to counteract atelectasis (Figure).

Neonatal Intensive Care Units

The development of neonatal intensive care units (NICUs) in the early 1960s, such as that created by Dr. Mildred Stahlman at Vanderbilt University, provided an environment in which sick neonates could be cared for, questions could be asked and answered, and physiologic measurements (such as those used by Stanley James at Columbia University for research) (10)(11) could be made and used to treat patients. NICUs were an outgrowth of adult ICUs. In the late 1950s, surgeons and anesthesiologists in Sweden began to care for term postsurgical neonates in special areas of the adult ICU. (12)

Because HMD was the major cause of death in neonates, especially those born preterm, treatment of neonates who had HMD became the major focus of many developing NICUs. Bill Tooley organized the NICU at the University of California, San Francisco (UCSF) in 1963. From the studies of Chu and colleagues (9) and the attempts by Rod Phibbs and Ernie Guy at San Francisco General Hospital and by Bill Tooley at the UCSF to mechanically ventilate neonates who had HMD in the winter of 1960, it became clear that for this form of therapy to be effective, well-trained nurses were required. Fortunately Teresa Poirier, RN, an outstanding nurse and organizer who had the wonderful ability to get people to do the right thing and make them think it was their idea, was the head nurse in the nursery. She was very important in the development of this unit. Dr. Julius Comroe's understanding of the importance of NICUs for patient care and for research led him to provide a wide variety of help. John Clements offered the necessary constant questioning of what we were doing and unstinting help in research. John Severinghaus (the inventor of the carbon dioxide electrode) built a blood gas machine and placed it in the NICU to allow quick and frequent measurement of blood gases and pH. By the mid-1960s, we took this device to the delivery room to measure blood gases and pH in sick neonates immediately after birth.

I was given the opportunity to work in the NICU at UCSF through a series of events. I had lived in student housing near Rod Phibbs, where we became friends. Bill Hamilton became the new chair of anesthesia at UCSF in 1967. He and Bill Tooley had worked together in the Cardiovascular Research Institute at UCSF some years before and were good friends. Hamilton had been interested in HMD and its treatment while he was at the University of Iowa. The three of them decided that I might have something to contribute to the NICU because I had worked in the adult ICU and mechanically ventilated patients during my residency. I also had spent a considerable amount of time in the NICU during my residency and was interested in applying what I had learned from adults to neonates. Bill Hamilton gave me the opportunity to

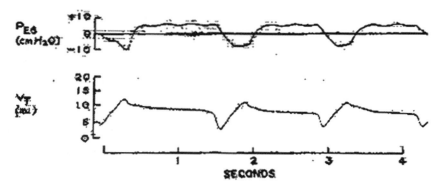

Figure. Tracing of esophageal pressure and tidal volume during grunting. Note rapid inspiration and prolonged expiration, with relatively positive intraesophageal pressure. Reprinted with permission from Chu et al. *Pediatrics.* 1967;40 (supp):709–782.

work full-time in the NICU with Bill Tooley, Rod Phibbs, and Joe Kitterman. I met Joe Kitterman during my residency while resuscitating a baby. Joe, more than anyone, taught me to question things and accept nothing as fact. He also taught me much of what I learned about neonatology in the early days. Because of my experience with mechanical ventilation in adults, I was given responsibility for pulmonary care in the NICU.

Early Mechanical Ventilation

Most mechanical ventilators available at the time were built to ventilate the lungs of adults, not those of sick pre-term neonates. Many of the machines were piston-driven and delivered a "constant" tidal volume. However, the compression volume of these piston-driven early machines often approached 1,000 mL. As a consequence, it was necessary to ventilate the lungs of neonates by setting the machine to deliver this 1,000 mL plus whatever tidal volume was estimated to be appropriate for the neonate (usually 10 mL/kg or 10 to 30 mL/ breath). Obviously, this was dangerous because the volume delivered to the neonate could vary significantly, depending on lung compliance and airway resistance. The Baby Bird and Puritan Bennett ventilators were subsequently developed for neonates, but they were often difficult to use, and it was difficult to wean patients who did improve from these devices. To do so required removing the patient from mechanical ventilation for progressively longer periods of time. Because the lung quickly collapsed when mechanical ventilation was discontinued,

weaning was long, arduous, and usually unsuccessful. In the end, many infants died because they could not be weaned from mechanical ventilation. Early experience at the University of Pennsylvania by Jack Downes, (13) at the Hospital for Sick Children in Toronto by Paul Swyer, (14) and at Stanford University by Penelope Cave-Smith and colleagues (15) demonstrated that some mechanically ventilated neonates (especially those requiring short-term mechanical ventilation) survived. However, many of the survivors had severe chronic lung disease (16) that persisted into adulthood. (17) It was obvious that we needed a better way to ventilate these neonates.

We noticed, while measuring pulmonary function in sick neonates in the delivery room, that increasing the ventilation rate during manual ventilation often resulted in an inadvertent positive end-expiratory pressure (PEEP) and improved blood gases. At the time, there was no simple, safe method of maintaining PEEP during mechanical ventilation or during weaning. Reducing the rate of ventilation led to atelectasis and hypoxemia. Gas trapping within the lung was considered a problem to be avoided by most physicians, based on work with normal lungs. Because the available mechanical ventilators frequently were ineffective, we and others sometimes ventilated neonates who had HMD by hand for 48 to 72 hours, using the Jackson-Reese system that commonly was employed to anesthetize infants and children. We learned early not to extubate the tracheas of these patients as soon as their blood gases improved

because more than 80% required reintubation. Following reintubation, they often were worse off than if tracheal extubation was delayed until we could slowly reduce the rate of ventilation while maintaining adequate oxygenation and carbon dioxide partial pressures. Much of the hand ventilation was performed by the nurses.

CPAP

At this point, several things came together that favored the development of CPAP. We had an ICU with sufficient well-trained nurses. We could make measurements and act immediately on the data. We understood the pathophysiology of HMD. It was clear that surfactant deficiency was the problem. We knew from the studies of Chu and associates (9) that grunting respiration maintained a positive pressure in the lungs of neonates who had HMD. Our previous experience with inadvertent gas trapping and PEEP suggested that applying a positive pressure to the oral end of the endotracheal tube during expiration would decrease atelectasis and improve oxygenation. Others also probably had been applying PEEP inadvertently during mechanical or hand ventilation. Because we frequently measured airway pressures during ventilation, we knew when we were applying PEEP and could correlate the presence of PEEP with blood gas findings.

The finding that really triggered the idea for CPAP in my mind was a paper by Harrison and associates from South Africa. (18) These authors demonstrated that when an endotracheal tube was inserted into the tracheas of neonates who had grunting respiration, Pao_2 and pH_a decreased and $Paco_2$ increased. Removing the endotracheal tube and allowing the neonate to resume grunting respiration improved all of these variables. The respiratory tracings presented in their article clearly documented positive pressure in the airway during grunting respiration (except during the very short period of inspiration). The same evening that I read this article, a 1-day-old newborn was sent to us who had respiratory distress and a Pao_2 of 28 mm Hg while breathing 100% oxygen. Initially he was believed to have cyanotic congenital heart disease and underwent cardiac catheterization. The heart was structurally and functionally normal. Based on our experience and that of others, this neonate had essentially a 100% chance of dying from his lung disease. We inserted an endotracheal tube and immediately attached a Jackson-Reese system to the endotracheal tube to generate a positive pressure during the expiratory phase of each breath while he breathed spontaneously. Within 5 minutes, his Pao_2 had risen to approximately 78 mm Hg. In less than 1 hour, the inspired oxygen had been reduced from 100% to 58% while the Pao_2 remained at 50 to 70 mm Hg. This was very unusual for an infant who had such serious HMD. Knowing that neonates who have HMD made and secreted surface-active material after 3 to 4 days of their disease, we maintained the applied end-expiratory pressure for 3 days before beginning to reduce the pressure. We subsequently weaned the neonate from CPAP in 5 days, and he made a complete recovery. He now runs a computer-related company in Japan.

Based on the response of this infant, we subsequently confirmed that applying a positive pressure during expiration to the lungs of neonates who had HMD improved oxygenation, functional residual capacity, and airway resistance and had variable effects on lung compliance. The 20 infants reported in our initial paper on CPAP (19) had Pao_2s of less than 50 mm Hg while breathing 100% oxygen, and many had apnea, cyanosis, and bradycardia before the initiation of CPAP.

Based on our own data and the data of others, the mortality of these patients should have been nearly 100%. In contrast, 80% of these first 20 patients survived, including seven who weighed less than 1,500 g at birth. During this same time, Llewellyn and Swyer in Toronto (20) demonstrated that applying PEEP during the exhalation phase of mechanical ventilation improved oxygenation of sick neonates, and Ashbaugh and colleagues (21) reported similar changes in mechanically ventilated adults. Based on our results, Dr. Robert Kirby built the Baby Bird ventilator out of existing parts, a device that allowed time-cycled flow ventilation, a continuous flow of gas during expiration, and the maintenance of PEEP. This was a major advance in neonatal mechanical ventilation.

Our original paper on CPAP was submitted to the New England Journal of Medicine, in great part to demonstrate the physiologic effects of CPAP. It was accepted for publication providing we placed the pulmonary function data in the archives. Ours was not a controlled trial; each patient served as her or his own control for physiologic measurements. We were still in the development stages of CPAP and continuing to refine it. One of the refinements was to add an underwater pop-off valve to the system to reduce the likelihood of causing a pneumothorax, which was done at the suggestion of John Clements. Until we had the system worked out, it was not possible to perform a controlled trial because once a trial started, the

system could not be changed until the trial was complete. The tone of the paper changed when the pulmonary function data were eliminated; it had a more clinical than a physiologic bent.

Conclusion

Looking back, one wonders why others did not develop CPAP earlier. All of the clues were there and in hindsight were obvious. I think the answer is related to the need for several factors to be in place: 1) an effective NICU where we could make measurements and act on them, 2) adequate numbers of nurses to provide needed care and make measurements frequently, and 3) an inquisitive environment where everything was questioned and there was no status quo. These were in place at UCSF, and I was given the privilege of working in this environment.

George A. Gregory, MD
Professor Emeritus Anesthesia and
Pediatrics
University of California School of
Medicine
San Francisco, CA

[To read the original article on treatment of HMD with CPAP written by Gregory and colleagues in 1971, which was reprinted with permission from New England Journal of Medicine, copyright © 1971, Massachusetts Medical Society, please go to: http://neoreviews.aappublications.org/cgi/content/full/5/1/e1/DC1]

References

1. Boston RW, Geller F, Smith CA. Arterial blood gas tensions and acid-base balance in the management of the respiratory distress syndrome. J Pediatr. 1966;68:74–89

2. Stahlman MT, Battersby EJ, Shepard FM, Blankenship WJ. Prognosis in hyalinemembrane disease: use of a linear discriminant. N Engl J Med. 1967;276:303–309

3. Smith CA. The Physiology of the Newborn Infant. Springfield, Ill: Chas. C. Thomas; 1959

4. Nelson NM, Prod'hom LS, Cherry RB, Lipsitz PJ, Smith CA. Pulmonary function in the newborn infant: the alveolar-arterial oxygen gradient. J Appl Physiol. 1963;18:534–538

5. Stahlman M. Treatment of cardiovascular disorders in newborns. Pediatr Clin North Am. 1964;11:363–400

6. Rudolph AM, Drorbaugh JE, Auld PA, et al. Studies of the circulation in the neonatal period. The circulation in the respiratory distress syndrome. Pediatrics. 1961;27:551–566

7. Clements JA. Surface tension of lung extracts. Proc Soc Exp Biol Med. 1957;95:170–172

8. Avery ME, Mead J. Surface properties in relation to atelectasis and hyaline membrane disease. Am J Dis Child. 1959;97:517–523

9. Chu J, Clements JA, Cotton EK, Klaus MH, Sweet AY, Tooley WH. Neonatal pulmonary ischemia: I. Clinical and physiological studies. Pediatrics. 1967;40(suppl):709–782

10. James LS, Weisbrot IM, Prince CE, Holiday DA, Apgar V. The acid-base status of human infants in relation to birth asphyxia and the onset of respiration. J Pediatr. 1958;52:379–394

11. James LS, Weisbrot IM, Prince CE, Holiday DA, Apgar V. Acid-base homeostasis of the newborn infant during the first 24 hours of life. *J Pediatr.* 1958;52: 395–403

12. Benson F, Celander O. Respirator treatment of pulmonary insufficiency in the newborn. *Acta Paediatr Scand.* 1959;118(suppl):49–50

13. Downes JJ. Mechanical ventilation of the newborn. *Anesthesiology.* 1971; 34:116–118

14. Swyer PR. Results of artificial ventilation. Experience at the Hospital for Sick Children, Toronto. *Biol Neonate.* 1970;16:148–54

15. Smith PC, Daily WJR, Fletcher G, Meyer HB, Taylor G. Mechanical ventilation of newborn infants. I. The effects of rate and pressure on arterial oxygenation of infants with respiratory distress syndrome. *Pediatr Res.* 1969; 3:244–254

16. Northway WH Jr, Rosan RC, Porter DY. Pulmonary disease following respirator therapy of hyaline membrane disease. *N Engl J Med.* 1967;276:357–36

17. Northway WH Jr. Bronchopulmonary dysplasia: thirty-three years later. *Pediatr Pulmonol.* 2001;23(suppl):5–7

18. Harrison VC, Heese H de V, Klein M. The significance of grunting in hyaline membrane disease. *Pediatrics.* 1968;41:549–559

19. Gregory GA, Kitterman JA, Phibbs RH, Tooley WH, Hamilton WK. Treatment of the idiopathic respiratory distress syndrome with continuous positive airway pressure. *N Engl J Med.* 1971;284:1333–1340

20. Llewellyn MA, Swyer PR. Positive expiratory pressure during mechanical ventilation in the newborn [abstract]. *Pediatr Res Program.* 1970:224

21. Ashbaugh DG, Petty TL, Bigelow DB, Harris TM. Continuous positive pressure breathing (CPPB) in adult respiratory distress syndrome. *J Thorac Cardiovasc Surg.* 1969;57:31–41

Historical Perspectives: Continuous Positive Airway Pressure (CPAP)

George A. Gregory

NeoReviews 2004;5;e1-e4

DOI: 10.1542/neo.5-1-e1

Antepartum Glucocorticoid Treatment

Introduction

The article chosen for this Historical Perspective was published in 1972 in *Pediatrics* (1) and emanated from New Zealand. We asked Dr. G.C. Liggins to provide perspective on how antepartum corticosteroids were introduced. As he notes, it took many years before this treatment gained acceptance. Dr. Liggins attributes this (in part) to resentment by neonatologists that obstetricians were intruding on their territory. In contrast, our perception is that the delay in acceptance was largely because obstetricians were unwilling to accept something that appeared in the pediatric literature. There was also concern about the long-term outcome in these infants, although follow-up of the original cohort showed no apparent differences. (2)

The consensus development conference on the "Effect of Corticosteroids for Fetal Maturation on Perinatal Outcomes" was held in early 1994 and published by the National Institutes of Health later that year. (3) This clearly documented advantages to antepartum corticosteroid administration not only with regard to respiratory distress syndrome, but also in reducing intraventricular hemorrhage and overall mortality in preterm infants.

Recent data from the Vermont Oxford Network, which reported on 118,448 very low-birthweight infants (501 to 1,500 g) from 362 centers, revealed an increase in the use of antenatal steroids in this population from approximately 25% in 1991 through 1992 to approximately 75% in 1997 through 1999. (4) The change was most noticeable around the time of the consensus development conference, with antenatal steroids administered to 33% in 1993, 49% in 1994, and 63% in 1995. (4)

Today, 30 years after the original report, antenatal corticosteroids have a well-deserved place in the perinatal therapeutic armamentarium.

Alistair G. S. Philip, MD, FRCPE, FAAP
Editor-in-Chief, NeoReviews

References

1. Liggins GC, Howie RN. A controlled trial of antepartum glucocorticoid treatment for prevention of the respiratory distress syndrome in premature infants. *Pediatrics.* 1972;50:515–525
2. MacArthur BA, Howie RN, Dezoete JA, Elkins J. School progress and cognitive development of 6 year old children whose mothers were treated antenatally with betamethasone. *Pediatrics.* 1982;70:99–105
3. *Report of the Consensus Development Conference on the Effect of Corticosteroids for Fetal Maturation on Perinatal Outcomes.* National Institute of Child Health and Human Development. NIH Publication No. 95–3784. November, 1994
4. Horbar JD, Badger GJ, Carpenter JH, et al for the members of the Vermont Oxford Network. Trends in mortality and morbidity for very low birth weight infants, 1991–1999. *Pediatrics.* 2002;110:143–151

Introducing Antepartum Corticosteroids

When I was appointed to an academic position in obstetrics/ gynecology at the University of Auckland in 1960, I looked for a research topic to pursue. My friend and colleague, Bill Liley, of fetal transfusion fame, suggested that I find a topic that was important and potentially solvable. Preterm labor was the obvious condition that I thought could be solved if the mechanism of term labor was discovered.

Circumstantial evidence pointed to a role for the fetal pituitary in initiating labor, which I decided to test experimentally. I developed a technique for destroying the pituitary in fetal sheep in New Zealand, then spent a sabbatical leave in the Veterinary School at the University of California, Davis. There my collaborator, the pathologist Peter Kennedy, and I found that sheep carrying hypophysectomized fetuses failed to start labor. I recall the mounting excitement as the first sheep reached term, then continued the pregnancy day by day until it was interrupted by cesarean section.

The next step was to find the mediator of the action of the pituitary, of which the adrenal seemed a likely candidate. Fetal adrenalectomy confirmed it. Back in New Zealand, we tested fetal cortisol as the next step in the chain by infusing it into the fetus, where it induced preterm labor. It seemed that we were well on our way to solving the problem of preterm labor. Unfortunately, although subsequent work confirmed the role of cortisol in many animal species, it was not true for human and other primate species.

However, serendipity stepped in at this point. Newborn lambs born preterm after fetal infusion of cortisol unexpectedly survived and had inappropriately mature lungs. The exciting possibility arose that the effect of corticosteroids on fetal sheep lungs might also apply to human fetal lungs. Corticosteroids administered to pregnant women crossed the placenta and depressed fetal adrenal function, as shown by the depressed excretion of estriol in maternal urine. Thus, the stage was set for a clinical trial in human pregnancy.

In collaboration with my neonatology colleague, Ross Howie, we designed and conducted a double-blind, controlled trial involving a large number of women in whom preterm labor threatened. Betamethasone was chosen as the treatment because the long-acting preparation we needed was a suspension, and a placebo ampule of identical appearance was difficult to prepare. The results, published in 1972, documented a drastic reduction in respiratory distress syndrome and neonatal mortality among treated infants. Nine controlled trials in various parts of the world confirmed our results.

Although this was one of the very few perinatal treatments shown to be effective in a controlled trial, its adoption in practice was remarkable slow. This was attributable primarily to unwillingness of professional organizations to support the treatment. It was nearly 20 years before the National Institutes of Health-sponsored Consensus Meeting and the British Royal College of Obstetricians and Gynecologists recommended antenatal administration of corticosteroids. Initially, there also were concerns about long-term adverse effects, and neonatologists tended to resent what they perceived as an intrusion of obstetricians into their territory.

Our more recent studies in fetal sheep showed that the effect of cortisol in accelerating lung maturation is enhanced by thyrotropin-releasing hormone (TRH). Because TRH crosses the human placenta, it could be administered to the mother. Unfortunately, controlled trials combining TRH with betamethasone showed no better outcome than betamethasone alone.

Professor G.C. (Mont) Liggins
University of Auckland
Auckland, New Zealand

[For the original article on antenatal corticosteroid administration, please go to: http://neoreviews.aappublications.org/cgi/data/3/11/e227/DC1 or http://pediatrics.aappublications.org/cgi/content/abstract/50/4/515]

Suggested Readings

Liggins GC. Premature parturition following infusion of corticotrophin or cortisol into fetal lambs. *J Endocrinol.* 1968;42:424–429

Liggins, Howie RN. A controlled trial of antepartum corticosteroid treatment for prevention of the respiratory distress syndrome in premature infants. *Pediatrics.* 1972;50:515–525

Liggins GC, Kennedy PC, Holm LW. Failure of initiation of parturition after electrocoagulation of the pituitary of the fetal lamb. *Am J Obstet Gynecol.* 1967; 98:1080–1086

Historical Perspectives: Antepartum Glucocorticoid Treatment
Alistair G. S. Philip and G. C. Liggins
NeoReviews 2002;3;227
DOI: 10.1542/neo.3-11-e227

Total Parenteral Nutrition

The difficulty in feeding very preterm infants is largely the result of their inability to adequately co-ordinate sucking and swallowing, posing the threat of aspiration. Because of this, withholding adequate nutrition was standard practice in many centers in the middle of the 20th century. Well-respected leaders, on both sides of the Atlantic Ocean, suggested that enteral feedings in premature infants be withheld for 2 to 3 days (see "Historical Perspectives: Immediate Feeding of Preterm Infants" by Dr Pamela Davies [1]).

Although intravenous administration of 10% dextrose was frequently attempted, there was the realization that glucose tolerance was limited and that daily caloric intake would usually not exceed 40 kcals/kg. At the same time, it was understood that an intake of 60 kcal/kg was needed to prevent tissue breakdown (catabolism).

In some centers, an aggressive approach was taken to feeding premature infants with breast milk (1), with some success. The importance of early extrauterine nutrition in subsequent brain development was emphasized in the late 1960s (2,3) and high-caloric peripheral intravenous alimentation in premature infants was described in 1971 (4).

Following the pioneering work of pediatric surgeons delivering total parenteral nutrition (TPN) to infants postoperatively (5), TPN was described in premature infants in 1972 and is amplified in this 2003 Historical Perspective by Drs. W.C. Heird and J.M. Driscoll. Today, TPN is one of the most important features of neonatal intensive care, allowing infants to receive nutritional support for weeks or even months. Recent improvements in neurodevelopmental outcome are certainly attributable in large measure to TPN delivered by central venous catheters.

Alistair G. S. Philip, MD, FRCPE, FAAP
Editor-in-Chief, NeoReviews

References

1. Davies P, Philip AGS. Historical Perspectives: Immediate Feeding of Preterm Infants. *NeoReviews.* 2004;2:29–32
2. Winick M, Rosso R. The effect of severe early malnutrition on cellular growth of human brain. *Pediatr Res.* 1969;3:181–184
3. Dobbing J. Undernutrition and the developing brain: the relevance of animal models to the human problem. *Am J Dis Child.* 1970;120:411–415
4. Benda G, Babson SG. Peripheral intravenous alimentation of the small premature infant. *J Pediatr.* 1971;79:494–498
5. Wilmore DW, Dudrick SJ. Growth and development in an infant receiving all nutrients exclusively by vein. *JAMA.* 1968;203:860–864

The report chosen for this Historical Perspectives (1) describes a study of the feasibility of total parenteral nutrition in low-birthweight (LBW) infants. This report was to have been followed by a randomized, controlled trial of total parenteral nutrition versus conventional nutrition management of LBW infants, which at that time was intravenous infusion of glucose with introduction of enteral feedings when tolerated. However, this planned trial was never completed. Despite a masked (then called "blinded") randomization scheme that would meet today's rigid standards, only one of the first 12 infants enrolled was assigned to the parenteral nutrition regimen!

This ill-fated trial was conceived by the two of us when we were enthusiastic, idealistic, and perhaps naïve young postdoctoral fellows at Babies Hospital and the College of Physicians and Surgeons of Columbia University. We were encouraged by our mentors, William Silverman, Stanley James, Jack Sinclair, and Bob Winters. Influenced by the findings of Myron Winick, who had just become Director of the Institute of Human Nutrition at Columbia, we reasoned that better early nutrition during the critical period of cellular growth of the brain of the preterm infant should, as observed in rats, prevent the irreversible effects of poor nutrition on brain growth and perhaps reduce the long-

term neurodevelopmental deficits of these infants. Unfortunately, such a trial has not been reported and, although still needed, is unlikely to be done.

The technique of parenteral nutrition that both we and Peden and Karpel (whose experience was published in the same issue of the *Journal of Pediatrics* (2)) evaluated was central vein delivery originally described by Wilmore and Dudrick (3) and subsequently used in term surgical infants by Filler and associates. (4) We and Peden and Karpel showed that the technique was feasible in infants weighing as little as 1,000 g at birth. However, it was far from risk-free. Thus, soon after publication of these reports in 1972, central vein delivery was virtually abandoned in favor of peripheral vein delivery. However, concern that the approximately 60 kcal/kg per day that could be delivered conveniently by peripheral vein was not sufficient to support utilization of a reasonable amino acid intake limited the use of parenteral nutrition in LBW infants.

Then, in the late 1970s, Tom Anderson, another young, enthusiastic postdoctoral fellow at Babies Hospital, conducted a small but important controlled clinical trial that demonstrated the efficacy of a peripheral vein parenteral nutrition regimen in providing approximately 60 kcal/kg per day as glucose plus 2.5 g/kg per day of amino acids. (5) The control group that received only an isocaloric intake of glucose was in negative nitrogen balance, but the group that received amino acids was in positive balance and showed other evidence of being anabolic. Moreover, there were only minor differences in plasma amino acid concentrations, blood acid-base status, or blood urea nitrogen concentrations between the groups. These findings have been confirmed over the past decade by a number of investigators. (6)(7)(8)(9)(10)(11) Currently, it is clear that infants who receive no amino acids lose up to 1% of their endogenous protein stores daily and that even very small infants who receive amino acids plus as few as 30 to 40 kcal/kg per day retain nitrogen, with the magnitude of retention being proportional to amino acid intake.

The availability of an acceptable parenteral lipid emulsion in the early 1980s helped overcome the problem of limited parenteral energy intake and prevented essential fatty acid deficiency. Today, despite a number of still unanswered questions, most infants who weigh less than 1,200 g at birth receive parenteral nutrition (although not necessarily exclusively) for a mean duration of nearly 3 weeks. (12) Many larger infants also are nourished parenterally, but usually for a shorter period. The most commonly used regimens provide an amino acid intake of 2.5 to 3.5 g/kg per day, an energy intake of 75 to 90 kcal/kg per day, and necessary vitamins and minerals. Central venous delivery, as originally described and as used in our feasibility study, rarely is employed today. When central vein delivery is required, the catheter usually is inserted percutaneously. Many of the problems encountered during the early days of parenteral nutrition remain (eg, infection, cholestasis), but many others have been resolved or circumvented (eg, acidosis, hyperammonemia, abnormal plasma amino acid concentrations). Thus, the technique that is practiced today appears to be reasonably safe and efficacious with respect to preserving lean body mass and promoting growth. However, we probably never will know if our initial assumption that it also would improve long-term neurodevelopmental outcome was correct.

Many other improvements in early nutrition management of LBW infants have been introduced since the early 1970s. Special nutrient-enriched preterm infant formulas are now available, as are supplements for human milk. Moreover, mothers of LBW infants are actively encouraged to provide human milk for feeding their infants. In addition, the technique of minimal enteral feeding, which is used widely, appears to have advantages. (13) Yet, most infants who weigh less than 1,200 g at birth are discharged weighing less than the 10th percentile of intrauterine standards. (14) Moreover, developmental deficits at school age and beyond persist. (15) Perhaps these are unrelated to early nutrition management, but a large body of data suggests otherwise. Certainly, poor nutrition management should be one of the easiest problems to remedy, although to date we have not done so, and until we do, we will not know the true impact of early nutrition, regardless of route of delivery, on subsequent outcome of the increasing number of surviving LBW infants.

William C. Heird, MD
Department of Pediatrics
Children's Nutrition Research Center
Baylor College of Medicine
Houston, TX

John M. Driscoll, Jr, MD
Department of Pediatrics
Columbia University
College of Physicians and Surgeons
Babies Hospital Columbia-Presbyterian
Medical Center
New York, NY

[For the original article by Driscoll, Heird, and associates regarding total intravenous alimentation in low-birthweight infants, which was reprinted with permission of the *Journal of Pediatrics*, please go to: http://neoreviews.aap publications.org/cgi/content/full/4/6/e137/DC1]

References

1. Driscoll JM Jr, Heird WC, Schullinger JN, Gongaware RD, Winters RW. Total intravenous alimentation in low-birth-weight infants: a preliminary report. *J Pediatr.* 1972;81:145–153

2. Peden VH, Karpel JT. Total parenteral nutrition in premature infants. *J Pediatr.* 1972;81:137–144

3. Wilmore DW, Dudrick SJ. Growth and development of an infant receiving all nutrients exclusively by vein. *JAMA.* 1968;203:860–864

4. Filler RM, Eraklis AJ, Rubin VG, Das JB. Long-term total parenteral nutrition in infants. *N Engl J Med.* 1969;281:589–594

5. Anderson TL, Muttart CR, Bieber MA, Nicholson JF, Heird WC. A controlled trial of glucose versus glucose and amino acids in premature infants. *J Pediatr.* 1979;94:947–951

6. Saini J, MacMahon P, Morgan JB, Kovar IZ. Early parenteral feeding of amino acids. *Arch Dis Child.* 1989;64:1362–1366

7. Van Lingen RA, van Goudoever JB, Luijendijk IHT, Wattimena JLD, Sauer PJJ. Effects of early amino acid administration during total parenteral nutrition on protein metabolism in pre-term infants. *Clin Sci.* 1992;82:199–203

8. Mitton SG, Garlick PJ. Changes in protein turnover after the introduction of parenteral nutrition in premature infants: comparison of breast milk and egg protein-based amino acid solutions. *Pediatr Res.* 1992;32:447–454

9. Rivera A, Bell EF, Bier DM. Effect of intravenous amino acids on protein metabolism of preterm infants during the first three days of life. *Pediatr Res.* 1993;33:106–111

10. Van Goudoever JB, Colen T, Wattimena JLD, Huijmans JGM, Carnielli VP, Sauer PJJ. Immediate commencement of amino acid supplementation in preterm infants: effect on serum amino acid concentrations and protein kinetics on the first day of life. *J Pediatr.* 1995;127:458–465

11. Kashyap S, Heird WC. Protein requirements of low birthweight, very low birthweight and small for gestational age infants. In: Raiha SM, Niels CR, eds. *Protein Metabolism During Infancy.* New York, NY: Raven Press; 1994:133–146

12. Lemons JA, Bauer CR, Oh W, et al. Very low birth weight outcomes of the National Institute of Child Health and Human Development Neonatal Research Network, January 1995 through December 1996. *Pediatrics.* 2001;107:e1. Available at: www.pediatrics.org/cgi/content/full/107/1/e1

13. Heird WC, Gomez MR. Total parenteral nutrition in necrotizing enterocolitis. *Clin Perinatol.* 1994:21:389–409

14. Ehrenkranz RA, Younes N, Lemons JA, et al. Longitudinal growth of hospitalized very low birth weight infants. *Pediatrics.* 1999;104:280–289

15. Hack M, Flannery DJ, Schluchter M, Cartar L, Borawski E, Klein N. Outcomes in young adulthood for very-low-birth-weight infants. *N Engl J Med.* 2002;346:149–157

Historical Perspectives: Total Parenteral Nutrition
William C. Heird and John M. Driscoll, Jr
NeoReviews 2003;4;137
DOI: 10.1542/neo.4-6-e137

The Introduction of Ultrasonography in Neonatal Cardiac Diagnosis

Alaina Kipps, MD* and Norman H. Silverman, MD, DSc (Med)†

Neonatal Echocardiography

The use of ultrasonography to detect cardiac abnormalities began in adults before being applied to pediatrics. It is not certain when the first application of this technique to a neonate occurred, but there was at least one report of the technique by 1972 (1). Dr Norman Silverman was certainly one of the first pediatric cardiologists to apply the technique to the fetus and neonate and for many years assisted his colleagues at the University of California in San Francisco. More recently he joined the faculty at Stanford University, where he provides stimulating discussions at many of the perinatal conferences. In this piece, written with Dr Alaina Kipps, he provides a detailed overview of the development of the technique and where things stand today.

Perhaps the most important aspect of this striking advance is that many disorders can be detected in the fetus prenatally, so that delivery can be scheduled at a center where cardiac surgery is readily available.

Alistair G. S. Philip, MD, FRCPE, FAAP
Editor-in-Chief, NeoReviews

Reference

1. Winsburg F : Echocardiography of the fetal and newborn heart. *Invest Radiol.* 1972;7:152–158.

Introduction

Before the advent of cardiac ultrasonography, diagnosis of cardiac disease in the neonate and preterm infant often was difficult. (1)(2) Frequently, neonatologists and cardiologists were pitted against each other, insisting on the accuracy of their clinical perspective of whether a patent ductus arteriosus was present and contributing to the respiratory complication, necrotizing enterocolitis, or apnea. From the cardiac perspective, such conflicts frequently could be solved only by cardiac catheterization, which entailed some risk, including transportation of the baby to the catheterization suite, invasion of the infant's vascular structure, and potential for bleeding and infection. At the end of the procedure, one group usually gloated at their clinical superiority, and the other group departed to nurse their egos.

The Development of Cardiac Ultrasonography

In the last few years of the 19th century, Pierre Curie, who along with his wife Marie Curie and Henri Bacquerell won the Nobel Prize for the discovery of radiographs in 1903, made the first contribution to the development of ultrasonography by discovering the piezoelectric phenomenon. (3) These two discoveries spawned the applied engineering of radiograph equipment and ultrasonography for medical usage. The piezoelectric phenomenon defines that when certain crystalloid substances are compressed, they emit electrical currents. The converse is also true, that is, when an electrical current is introduced into a crystalloid structure such as barium titanate, the crystal vibrates, setting up sound or ultrasonography waves. The vibrations are in the frequency of sound above the audible frequency of 35,000 Hz and termed ultrasound.

This conversion of mechanical to electrical energy is the phenomenon whereby the old phonographic recorder produced sound. The undulation of a needle in a groove of the record induced a vibration in a needle that, when amplified, led to the production of sound.

The first application of ultrasonography technology occurred in ships that had sonar where a crystal was excited electrically and produced an ultrasound wave that traveled through water at a known velocity. When it struck the hull of another ship, some of the waves bounced back to the sonar transmitter, now acting as a receiver. The time and size of the returning wave indicated the position and size of the other metal body. These sonar devices were installed in many ships and U boats.

At the end of the second World War, Inge Edler, working with Hertz, the son of the 1925 winner of the Nobel Prize in Physics, obtained an old sonar unit, modified it, and determined that the ultrasonography signal arose from the mitral valve (Fig. 1). The science of ultrasonography was so born. (4)(5) The transducer on the earliest clinical systems was a single crystal, which produced a reflective ultrasonography as if a small parallel beam of light (or sound) was directed through the heart. The amplitude of the signal was converted to a dot of brightness proportional to the amplitude of the signal, with the brightest signals arising from the highest amplitudes. This was called the brightness or B-mode of ultrasonography and is the standard method used for imaging today.

M-mode Echocardiography

Working with a single beam of ultrasonography, B-mode signals were difficult to interpret and, thus, were converted to a graphic of motion called M-mode. This technique is similar to the positive and negative deflections of an electrocardiogram that, before the paper moves, has the stylus riding up and down on a single line, but when the paper moves at a

---

*Resident in Pediatrics.
†Professor of Pediatrics, Director of the Pediatric and Fetal Echocardiographic Laboratories, Lucile Packard Children's Hospital and Stanford University, Palo Alto, Calif.

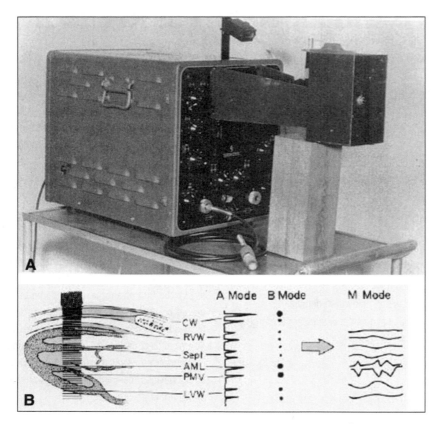

Figure 1. A. The first echocardiogram instrument of Edler and Hertz. A Polaroid® camera is mounted over an oscilloscope. B. The so-called icepick view of the heart passing through the chest wall (CW), right ventricular wall (RVW), ventricular septum (Sept), anterior mitral valvar leaflet (AML), posterior mitral valve (PMV), and left ventricular posterior wall (LVW). These are represented as a series of amplitude spikes, the height of which is proportional to the intensity of the reflective tissue. These are converted into a series of bright dots, where the intensity is proportional to their amplitude. When run over an oscilloscope or a paper, they create a motion image of depth to time, similar to an electrocardiogram. Because the motion was with respect to time, the procedure was termed M-mode echocardiography. Reprinted with permission from Elder I. Use of ultrasound as a diagnosis aid: effects on biologic tissues. *Acta Med Scan Suppl.*1961;370:39.

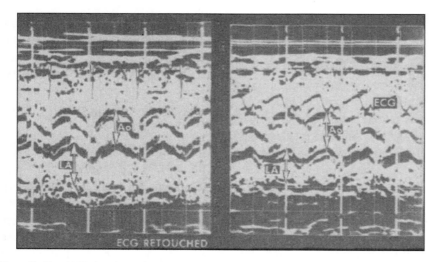

Figure 2. Two M-Mode echocardiograms passing through the right ventricular outflow tract and the aortic root (Ao) and the left atrium (LA). On the left is a preterm infant who has a patent ductus and on the right an infant who does not have a patent ductus. Note that the LA on the left is enlarged whereas on the right it is much smaller. These dimensions are related to the aortic root to yield the LA:Ao ratio.

calibrated rate, identifies the well-known features of the characteristic electrocardiogram. It is not surprising, therefore, that the electrocardiographic signal has become a standard accompaniment of all echocardiograms, providing an indication of the timing of a particular structure or event within the cardiac cycle. Initially, M-mode echocardiography was observed as a sweep of an oscilloscope, subsequently on paper, and finally on a television screen or monitor. The recognition of pericardial effusions by Harvey Feigenbaum (6) made it possible to define enlargement of the left atria with an early and primitive ultrasonographic instrument in preterm infants who had various forms of respiratory distress. (7) Because there were no standards established for the size of the left atrium, Rudolph suggested construction of a ratio of the size of the left atrium to a fairly rigid structure, the aortic root, which ran just in front of the atrium (Fig. 2) (Fig. 3).

The next major advance was made by Feigenbaum, who entered the field of echocardiography serendipitously when he borrowed an echoencephalograph from a neurologist. The technique of echoencephalography used amplitude modulation (A-mode) to determine midline shifts of the falx cerebri. Feigenbaum reaffirmed Edler's observations of a pericardial effusion in humans, findings subsequently confirmed in the animal laboratory. He derived the term "echocardiography" from echoencephalography. His early work culminated in his writing the first textbook on echocardiography. (8) He became a mentor

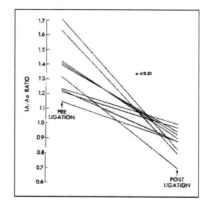

Figure 3. Left atrium-to-aortic root ratios before and after surgery in 10 pre-term infants who required ductus arteriosus ligation. The ratio diminished from an average of 1.3 to 0.67:1.

to many of the current leaders of echocardiography and participated in their training.

A spate of articles from investigators around the world identified means of evaluating cardiac function and anomalies. In the pediatric area, these observations were spurred by Richard Meyer in Cincinnati and Stanley Goldberg and his colleagues Hugh Allen and David Sahn and led to the first textbooks on the use of M-mode echocardiography in children and neonates. (9)(10) Higher-quality M-mode recordings in the pediatric age range became possible with the introduction of high-frequency 3.5- and 5-MHz transducers, which resolved the smaller and more superficial heart structures of infants.

In addition, the use of light-sensitive ultra-violet strip-chart recorders revolutionized the recording of studies from oscilloscope tracings by providing an opportunity for continuous recording of the structures that passed through the transducer beam (Fig. 4). Sophisticated studies, such as those by Solinger and colleagues in Louisville, as well as by Meyer, produced a rational approach to the complex problems of situs and malposition. (11)

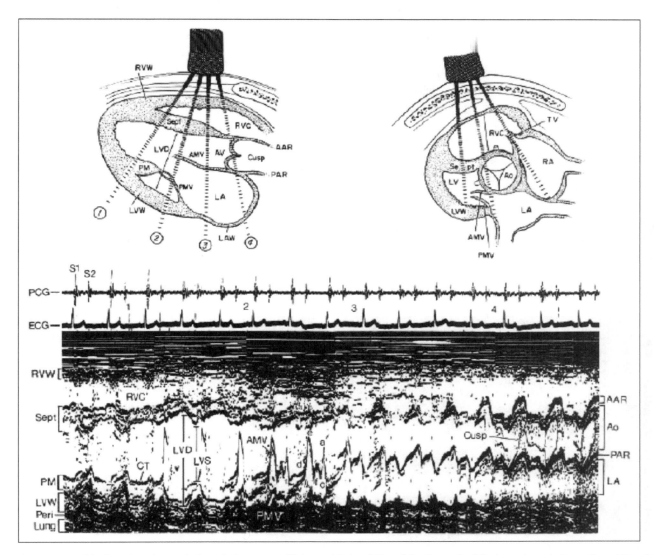

Figure 4. Diagrams of the heart in its long axis through the aorta and left ventricle (top left) and the short axis of the heart through the aortic root (top right). The position of the sound wave is depicted as arising from one of four positions as designated on the electrocardiogram (ECG) below. M-mode echocardiogram with phonocardiogram showing the first and second heart sounds (S1 and S2), the ECG, and the M-mode with the transducer swept from the apical to the basilar area of the heart are shown in the lower half of the illustration. Position 1 shows the right ventricular wall (RVW), the right ventricular cavity (RVC), interventricular septum (Sept), left ventricular cavity, papillary muscles, left ventricular wall (LVW), pericardium (Peri), and the lung. In position 2, as the transducer is swept cranially, the chordae tendineae (CT) are seen, and slightly above is the area when the maximal left ventricular dimensions are measured. The left ventricular dimensions in diastole (LVD) and systole (LVS) are seen. The mitral valve anterior and posterior leaflets (AMV and PMV) are seen further cranially. In position 3, the further cranial sweep shows the posterior leaflet developing into the left atrial wall and the anterior mitral valvar leaflet into the posterior aortic root (PAR). In position 4, the septum continues as the anterior aortic root (AAR). These areas define the dimensions of the aorta (AO) and the left atrium (LA). Reprinted from *Advances in Pediatrics*, vol 23, Silverman NH, pages 357–400, Copyright Elsevier (1976).

Contrast Echocardiography

The physiologic advantages of contrast echocardiography became evident with the work of Raymond Gramiak and colleagues in Rochester, New York. (12) These physicians noted that a cloud of echoes passed through the heart when indocyanine green dye was injected during dye dilution assessment of cardiac output. The remarkable phenomenon of strong echoes from the micro-bubbles in the cardiac chambers that were trapped in capillary circulations permitted validation of the site where they were injected. Soon it became evident that the passage of contrast dye from the right to the left heart could be detected through atrial, ventricular, or vascular shunts and that appropriate injections could identify shunting in the diagnosis of congenital heart diseases (Fig. 5). The Mayo Clinic group initially popularized this work in congenital heart disease, and such procedures became widely accepted for diagnosing congenital heart disease in children. (13)(14)(15) These techniques were greatly expanded by the development of two-dimensional (cross-sectional) echocardiography.

Two-dimensional Echocardiography

Although substantial numbers of articles were published on the use of M-mode echocardiography in congenital heart disease, the real breakthrough came with the introduction of two-dimensional or, as some prefer it, cross-sectional echocardiography. Development of a more graphic imaging modality had tremendous appeal. A number of approaches were used to refine the early systems, such as the rotating transducer and parabolic mirror, but the system was rather slow at only seven frames per second.

In 1968, Somer, a Dutch engineer, was instructed to develop a brain scanner for a large Dutch electronics conglomerate. His phased-array sector scanner system (Fig. 6) failed to impress executives of this company, who were not convinced that the instrument would have any practical value. Somer subsequently published papers on the instrument's design and characteristics. (16) His system was similar to that subsequently designed by Olaf Von Ramm and Frederick Thurston at Duke University. (17)

Of the many different techniques used for developing two-dimensional images (Fig. 7),

only the phased-array electronic system survives because of subsequent electronic developments in the ultrasonography armamentarium, which have incorporated color and other Doppler ultrasonography techniques directly from individual transducers.

The advent of cross-sectional techniques in the late 1970s allowed ultrasonographers to define tomographic images of the heart in real time that permitted "anatomic dissections" of the heart from the apex to the base. New techniques and positioning of the transducer led to the discovery of different and heretofore exquisite opportunities to image the heart. These views, available at http://neoreviews.aap publications.org/cgi/content/full/6/7/e315/DC1, included apical (Fig. 8) (Movie 1), suprasternal (Fig. 9) (Movie 2), and subcostal (Fig. 10) (Movie 3) views. (18)(19)(20)(21)(22) Now not only structural diseases could be identified, but functional assessment of the myocardium, its capacity for contraction, and the mass of the ventricles could be defined. (23)(24)

It was now possible to diagnose many cardiac conditions and to define complex cardiac defects, even in the human fetus. Working in Britain, Lindsay Allan marshaled the largest collection of fetal patients and, with her team, described a remarkable variety of fetal diseases, tracing their evolution in utero. (25)(26)(27)

The early 1980s saw a great number of publications about congenital heart disease. Although some lesions could be identified, their severity could not be assessed by morphologic methods and had to await further development of ultrasonography modalities.

Continuous-wave Doppler Ultrasonography

The next milestone was the introduction of continuous-wave Doppler ultrasonography by Holen, Hatle, and Angelsen, who developed the modified Bernoulli equation, which has become one of the most widely used (and misused) formulas in everyday pediatric echocardiography. (28)(29) Using a simplification of the Bernoulli equation:

$$(\text{Pressure Drop} = 4 \times \{\text{highest distal velocity}\}^2)$$

it became possible to define pressure differences across stenotic and regurgitant

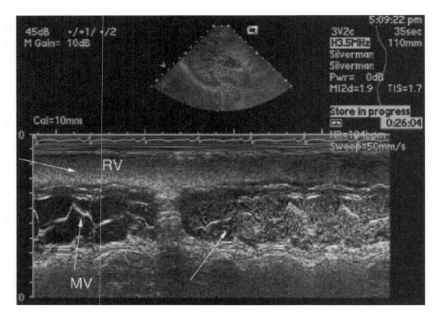

Figure 5. Contrast echocardiogram in a patient who has Rendu-Osler-Weber syndrome and pulmonary arteriovenous malformations. The venous injection of agitated saline shows the contrast effect in the right ventricle (RV) followed within three beats by the appearance of contrast in the left atrium behind the mitral valve (MV). Saline microcavitations of 100 to 200 microns in diameter are trapped in the pulmonary capillaries unless an arteriovenous malformation is present.

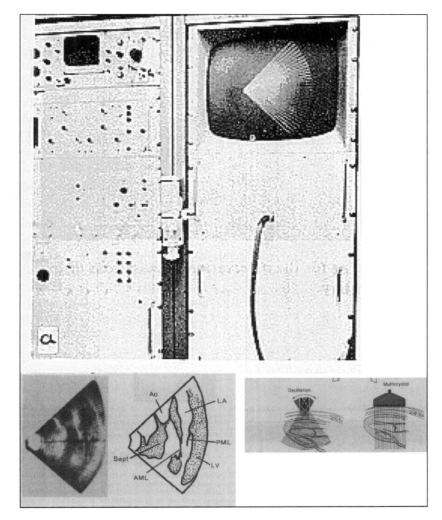

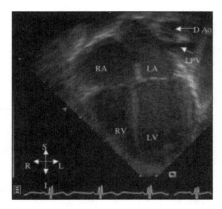

Figure 8. An apical four-chamber view of the heart obtained by placing the transducer over the cardiac apex and directing the plane through the heart. The right atrium (RA) is separated from the right ventricle (RV) by the tricuspid valve, the left atrium (LA) is separated from the left ventricle (LV) by the mitral valve, and the left pulmonary vein (LPV) enters the left atrium lateral to the descending aorta (D Ao). Orientation: I=inferior, L=left, R=right, S=superior.

valves, bands, aortopulmonary shunts, and patent ductus arteriosi (Fig. 11).

The application of this modality to pediatrics is perhaps the most quantitative advance since the development of two-dimensional echocardiography. The work of Holen and Hatle, who used Doppler ultrasonography with this equation, led to the accurate quantitation of pressure drops in aortic

Figure 6. Somer's first phased-array ultrasonography system, the size of two refrigerators (top). Diagrams of transducer array images from an electrically steered phased-array system and a large linear-array system that has not survived in modern ultrasonography (bottom right). An early ultrasonographic image and the diagram necessary to show what this poor image defined (bottom left). Reprinted from *Ultrasonics*, vol 6, J.C. Somer, "Electronic Sector Scanning for Ultrasonic Diagnosis," 153–159, (1968) with permission from Elsevier.

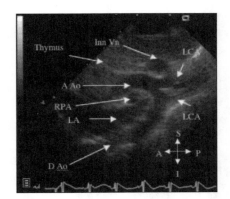

Figure 9. An image of the aorta and great arteries taken with the transducer placed in the suprasternal notch and directed in the plane of the aortic arch from the left scapula to the right midclavicular line. The innominate vein (Inn Vn) crosses the aortic arch. The ascending aorta (A Ao) continues into the aortic arch, giving rise to the left carotid (LCA) and left subclavian (LCA) arteries, and arches over the right pulmonary artery (RPA) and left atrium (LA) to become the descending thoracic aorta. (D Ao). Orientation: I = inferior, L = left, R = right, S = superior.

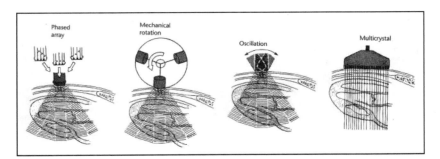

Figure 7. Diagrams of various techniques for making a two-dimensional image, including a phased-array system, a mechanical system involving rotation of several transducers, a mechanical oscillation system, and a multicrystal nonsteered system. Reprinted from Silverman NH. Newer noninvasive methods in pediatric cardiology: echocardiography, isotope angiography. *Adv Pediatr*. 1976;23:357–400, copyright 1976, with permission from Elsevier.

stenosis, pulmonary stenosis, and mitral stenosis. (28) (29) This technique also was applied to congenital heart diseases such as ventricular septal defects, measurement of pulmonary artery pressure from tricuspid regurgitation and pulmonary regurgitation, aortopulmonary shunts, and patent ductus arteriosus.

These observations were extended further to the fetus. The modality was valuable not only for systolic gradients, but also for valvar insufficiencies. (30)(31)(32)(33)(34)(35)(36)(37)

Doppler techniques also permitted evaluation of the flow characteristics across valves as well as the quantitation of flow and cardiac ouput. (38)(39)(40)

Perhaps the most valuable development of the pulsed Doppler technique was the emergence of the Doppler color flow technique. Fish described a system in 1975, (41) and Brandestini introduced a system using a multigate Doppler superimposed on M-mode tracings in 1979. (42) However, it was a development by Japanese engineers that led to the incorporation of the multigate Doppler color system into a cross-sectional format. The work of Omoto did much to bring this technique to the attention of the rest of the world. His experiences led to the publication of the first book on Doppler color flow. The first article to appear on the subject of Doppler color flow in congenital heart disease was by Kyo and colleagues. (43) Sahn's group was the first to explore the potential of the color flow method fully in pediatric cardiology. (44)(45) Ludomirski and colleagues (46) published an article about the efficacy of the Doppler color flow method for detection of muscular ventricular septal defects.

Early Doppler color flow systems were large and cumbersome to use, the images were of poor quality, and the color spectral output was insensitive. Modern equipment developed in the United States took Doppler color flow to a new plane of quality that now provides the opportunity to examine congenital heart

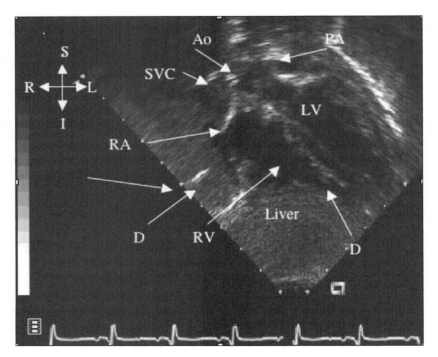

Figure 10. Subcostal echocardiogram in a healthy patient obtained by placing the transducer in the subxiphoid space and angling the plane toward the heart. As originally described by Bierman, moving the plane from posterior to anterior, the two atria connect to their respective ventricles posteriorly and the two ventricles to their respective great arteries anteriorly. Orientation: I = inferior, L = left, R = right, S = superior.

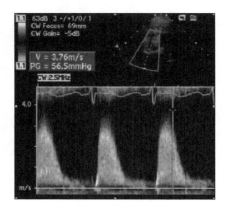

Figure 11. A continuous wave Doppler frame passed into the ascending aorta in a patient who has aortic stenosis. The dotted line in the reference image is placed in the ascending aorta and the resultant Doppler signal obtained. Using the modified Bernoulli equation (see text), the pressure difference was predicted to be 56.5 mm Hg.

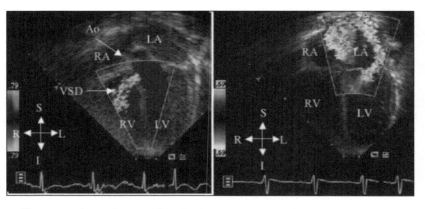

Figure 12. Images taken in the apical four-chamber plane show the advantage of Doppler color flow for defining lesions. The left frame shows a perimembranous ventricular septal defect (VSD), with a Doppler color jet shunting into the right ventricle (RV) across the defect. The right frame shows mitral regurgitation, with the color jet shunting from the left ventricle (LV) across the mitral valve and into the left atrium (LA). Ao = aorta, RA = right atrium, RV = right ventricle. Orientation: I = inferior, L = left, R = right, S = superior.

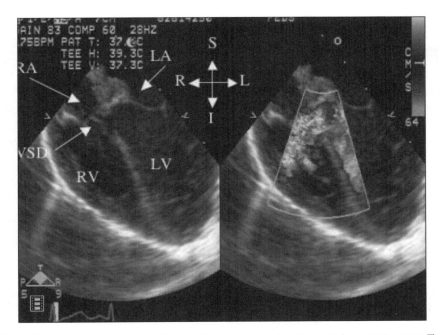

Figure 13. Transesophageal echocardiogram taken prior to surgical closure in the operating room. The ventricular septal defect (VSD) is confirmed to be perimembranous. The image at left is a raw image; the image at right has simultaneous superimposition of Doppler color flow information, showing the shunt crossing the defect from the left to the right ventricle. LA = left atrium, LV = left ventricle, RA = right atrium, RV = right ventricle. Orientation: I = inferior, L = left, R = right, S = superior.

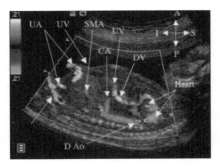

Figure 15. A fetal echocardiogram demonstrating the value of the Doppler color flow imaging of the vascular system. The fetus is imaged in its long axis. The descending aorta (D Ao) can be traced into the iliac artery (IA) and thence into the umbilical artery (UA). The umbilical vein (UV) drains through the ductus venosus (V) and thence to the heart. The major branches of the descending aorta—the celiac artery (CA), the superior mesenteric artery (SMA), and the IA— can be seen. In the raw image, the heart can be seen in a sagittal body plane. Orientation: A = anterior, I = inferior, P = posterior, S = superior.

disease by mapping shunts, stenosis, and abnormal flow (Fig. 12) (Movies 4 and 5).

Transesophageal echocardiography, created for passage in adult-size patients, was miniaturized by Japanese entrepreneurs (Fig. 13) (Movie 6). The technique also has been applied successfully to fetal cardiac diagnosis to define flow within the vascular system and the heart (Figs. 14, 15, 16) (Movies 7, 8, 9).

Conclusion

These ultrasonography techniques have provided an armamentarium for anatomic, physiologic, and developmental capabilities

that can make surgery possible in many instances without cardiac catheterization. (47) The diagnosis and management of most neonatal cardiac diseases can be managed with ultrasonographic cardiac diagnosis alone. The diagnosis and follow-up of patent ductus treatment has become standard with ultrasonography, whether managed with surgical or medical therapy.

Among the many other developments in cardiac ultrasonography are Doppler methods for assessing systolic and diastolic function, wall stress, and strain. New three- and four-dimensional methods for examining cardiac

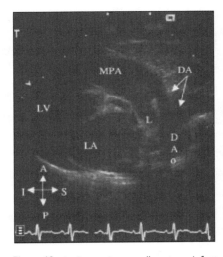

Figure 16. An image in a small preterm infant taken from the precordium in a view termed the ductus cut, which is a sagittal view parallel to the spine and passing through the pulmonary artery (PA), the ductus arteriosus (DA), and the descending aorta (D Ao). MPA = main pulmonary artery, L = left pulmonary artery, LV = left ventricle, LA = left atrium. Orientation: A = anterior, I = inferior, P = posterior, S = superior.

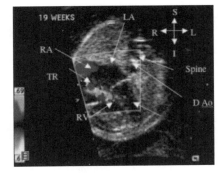

Figure 14. A fetal echocardiogram taken in an infant who has Ebstein malformation at 19 weeks' gestation. The features are shown in the still frame, but the movie shows the displaced tricuspid valve and enlarged right atrium. LA = left atrium, LV = left ventricle, RA = right atrium, RV = right ventricle. Orientation: I = inferior, L = left, R = right, S = superior.

structure use one-beat acquisition of an entire volume of cardiac information. This information can be sliced and viewed from many different perspectives. These modalities, now on the forefront of cardiac ultrasonography, no doubt will be the subject of a future review as a description of previous developments in the evolution of ultrasonographic technology.

References

1. Rudolph AM, Auld PAM, Golinko RJ, Paul MH. Pulmonary vascular adjustments in the neonatal period. *Pediatrics*. 1961;28:28–34

2. Rudolph AM, Scarpelli EM, Golinko RJ, Gootman N. Hemodynamic basis for clinical manifestations of patent ductus arteriosus. *Am Heart J*. 1964;68: 447–458

3. Silverman NH. Pediatric cardiac imaging: a historical perspective and future challenges. *Isr J Med Sci*. 1996;32:892–903

4. Edler I. Early echocardiography. *Ultrasound Med Biol*. 1991;17:425–431

5. Edler I, Gustafson A, Kerelefors T, Christensson B. Ultrasound cardiology. *Acta Med Scand Suppl*. 1961;370:5–123

6. Feigenbaum H, Waldhausen JA, Hyde LP. Ultrasound diagnosis of pericardial effusion. *JAMA*. 1965;191:711–714

7. Silverman NH, Lewis AB, Heymann MA, Rudolph AM. Echocardiographic assessment of ductus arteriosus shunt in premature infants. *Circulation*. 1974;50:821–825

8. Feigenbaum H. *Echocardiography*. Philadelphia, Pa: Lea & Febiger; 1972

9. Meyer RA. *Pediatric Echocardiography*. Philadelphia, Pa: Lea & Febiger, 1977

10. Goldberg SJ, Allen HD, Sahn DJ. *Pediatric and Adolescent Echocardiography: A Handbook*. Chicago, Ill: Year Book Medical Publishers; 1975

11. Solinger R, Elbl F, Minhas K. Deductive echocardiographic analysis in infants with congenital heart disease. *Circulation*. 1974;50:1072–1096

12. Gramiak R, Shah PM, Kramer DH. Ultrasound cardiography: contrast studies in anatomy and function. *Radiology*. 1969;92:939–948

13. Seward JB, Tajik AJ, Spangler JG, Ritter DG. Echocardiographic contrast studies: initial experience. *Mayo Clin Proc*. 1975;50:163–192

14. Seward JB, Tajik AJ, Hagler DJ, Ritter DG. Peripheral venous contrast echocardiography. *Am J Cardiol*. 1977;39:202–212

15. Seward JB, Tajik AJ, Hagler DJ, Ritter DG. Contrast echocardiography in single or common ventricle. *Circulation*. 1977;55:513–519

16. Somer JC. Electronic sector scanning for ultrasonic diagnosis. *Ultrasonics*. 1968;6:153–159

17. von Ramm OT, Thurstone FL. Cardiac imaging using a phased array ultrasound system. I. System design. *Circulation*. 1976;53:258–262

18. Silverman NH, Schiller NB. Apex echocardiography: a two-dimensional technique for evaluating congenital heart disease. *Circulation*. 1978;57:503

19. Snider AR, Silverman NH. Suprasternal notch echocardiography: a two-dimensional technique for evaluating congenital heart disease. *Circulation*. 1981;63:165–173

20. Bierman FZ, Fellows K, Williams RG. Prospective identification of ventricular septal defects in infancy using subxyphoid two-dimensional echocardiography. *Circulation*. 1980;62:807–817

21. Bierman FZ, Williams RG. Subxyphoid two-dimensional imaging of the interatrial septum in infants and neonates with congenital heart disease. *Circulation*. 1979;60:80–90

22. Bierman FZ, Williams RG. Prospective diagnosis of d-transposition of the great arteries in neonates by subxyphoid two dimensional echocardiography. *Circulation*. 1979;60:1496–1502

23. Schiller NB, Acquatella H, Ports TA, et al. Left ventricular volume from paired biplane two-dimensional echocardiographs. *Circulation*. 1979;60:547

24. Silverman NH, Ports TA, Snider AR, Schiller NB, Carlsson E, Heilbron DC. Determination of left ventricular volume in children: echocardiographic and angiographic comparisons. *Circulation*. 1980;62:548

25. Allan LD, Tynan MJ, Campbell S, Wilkinson JL, Anderson RH. Echocardiographic and anatomical correlates in the fetus. *Br Heart J*. 1980;44:444–451

26. Allan LD, Tynan MJ, Campbell S, Anderson RH. Identification of cardiac malformations by echocardiography in the midtrimester fetus. *Br Heart J*. 1981;46:358–362

27. Allan LD, Little D, Campbell MJ, Whitehead M. Fetal ascites associated with congenital heart disease. *Br J Obstet Gynaecol*. 1981;88:453–455

28. Holen J, Aaslid R, Landmark K, Simonsen S. Determination of pressure gradient in mitral stenosis with a non-invasive ultrasound Doppler technique. *Acta Med Scand*. 1976;199:455–460

29. Hatle L, Angelsen BA, Tromsdal A.Non-invasive assessment of aortic stenosisby Doppler ultrasound. *Br Heart J*. 1980;43:284–292

30. Kosturakis D, Allen HD, Goldberg SJ,Sahn DJ, Valdes-Cruz LM. Noninvasivequantification of stenotic semilunar valveareas by Doppler echocardiography. *J Am Coll Cardiol*. 1984;3:1256–1262

31. Frantz EG, Silverman NH. Doppler ultrasound evaluation of valvar pulmonary stenosis from multiple transducer positions in children requiring pulmonary valvuloplasty. *Am J Cardiol*. 1988;61:844–849

32. Murphy DJ Jr, Ludomirsky A, Huhta JC. Continuous-wave Doppler in children with ventricular septal defect: noninvasive estimation of interventricular pressure gradient. *Am J Cardiol*. 1986;57:428–432

33. Musewe NN, Smallhorn JF, Benson LN, Burrows PE, Freedom RM. Validation of Doppler-derived pulmonary arterial pressure in patients with ductus arteriosus under different hemodynamic states. *Circulation*. 1987;76: 1081–1091

34. Fyfe DA, Currie PJ, Seward JB, et al. Continuous-wave Doppler determination of the pressure gradient across pulmonary artery bands: hemodynamic correlation in 20 patients. *Mayo Clin Proc*. 1984;59:744–750

35. Kosturakis D, Goldberg SJ, Allen HD, Loeber C. Doppler echocardiographic prediction of pulmonary arterial hypertension in congenital heart disease. *Am J Cardiol*. 1984;53:1110–1115

36. Marx GR, Allen HD, Goldberg SJ. Doppler echocardiographic estimation of systolic pulmonary artery pressure in pediatric patients with interventricular communications. *J Am Coll Cardiol*. 1985;6:1132–1137

37. Marx GR, Allen HD. Accuracy and pitfalls of Doppler evaluation of the pressure gradient in aortic coarctation. *J Am Coll Cardiol*. 1986;7:1379–1385

38. Sanders SP, Yeager S, Williams RG. Measurement of systemic and pulmonary blood flow and Qp/Qs ratio using Doppler and two-dimensional echocardiography. *Am J Cardiol*. 1983;51:952–956

39. Goldberg SJ, Sahn DJ, Allen HD, Valdes-Cruz LM, Hoenecke H, Carnahan Y. Evaluation of pulmonary and systemic blood flow by 2-dimensional Doppler echo-cardiography using fast Fourier transform spectral analysis. *Am J Cardiol*. 1982;50:1394–400

40. Cloez JL, Schmidt KG, Birk E, Silver-man NH. Determination of pulmonary to systemic blood flow ratio in children by a simplified Doppler echocardiographic method. *J Am Coll Cardiol*. 1988;11:825–830

41. Fish PJ. Multichannel direction resolving Doppler angiography. In: Kazner E, ed. *Second European Congress on Ultrasonics in Medicine, Munich, 1975*. Amsterdam, The Netherlands: Excerpta Medica; 1975:72

42. Brandestini MA, Eyer MK, Stevenson JG. M/Q mode echocardiography. The synthesis of conventional echo with multi-gate Doppler. In: Lancée CT, ed. *Echocardiography*. The Hague/Boston, Mass: Maartinus Nijhoff; 1979:441–446

43. Kyo S, Takamoti S, Ueada K, et al. Clinical significance of newly developed real-time two-dimensional echocardiogra-phy in congenital heart disease with special reference to the assessment of intracardiac shunts. *Proceedings of the 43rd Meeting of the Japanese Society of Ultrasonics in Medicine*. 1983;43:465–466

44. Sahn DJ. Real-time two-dimensional Doppler echocardiographic flow mapping. *Circulation*. 1985;71:849–853

45. Swensson RE, Sahn DJ, Valdez-Cruz LM. Color flow mapping in congenital heart disease. *Echocardiography*. 1985;2:545–549

46. Ludomirsky A, Huhta JC, Vick GW III, Murphy DJ, Danford DA, Morrow WR. Color Doppler detection of multiple ventricular septal defects. *Circulation*. 1986; 74:1317–1322.

47. Tworetzky W, McElhinney D, Brook MM, Reddy VM, Hanley FL, Silverman NH. Echocardiographic diagnosis alone for the complete repair of major congenital heart defects. *J Am Coll Cardiol*. 1999;33:228–233

Historical Perspectives: The Introduction of Ultrasonography in Neonatal Cardiac Diagnosis

Alaina Kipps and Norman H. Silverman

NeoReviews 2005;6;e315-e325
DOI: 10.1542/neo.6-7-e315

Use of Methylxanthines in the Management of Apneic Attacks in the Newborn

For many years, treatment of apnea was initiated with either aminophylline or theophylline, given intravenously or orally. Treatment was continued with theophylline or caffeine. With both agents, it was standard practice to measure blood levels to be sure that therapeutic levels had been achieved or to avoid toxicity. More recently, caffeine has emerged as the more reliable treatment (1, 2, 3). Uptake seems to be reliable and toxic levels are rare with standard dosing. Some consider it unnecessary to measure caffeine levels, because it frequently takes several days for results to return from the laboratory.

In a large randomized controlled trial (of more than 2,000 very-low-birthweight infants) using caffeine, not only was the number of episodes of apnea decreased, but also a beneficial effect was noted on the development of bronchopulmonary dysplasia (1).

Alistair G. S. Philip, MD, FRCPE, FAAP
Editor-in-Chief, NeoReviews

References
1. Schmidt B, Roberts RS, Davis P et al. Caffeine therapy for apnea of prematurity. *N Engl J Med*. 2006;354:2112–2121
2. Natarajan G, Lulic-Botica M, Aranda JV. Clinical pharmacology of caffeine in the newborn. *NeoReviews*. 2007;8:e214–e221
3. Charles BG, Townsend SR, Steer PA, Flenady VJ, Gray PH, Shearman A. Caffeine citrate treatment for extremely premature infants with apnea : population pharmacokinetics, absolute bioavailablity, and implications for therapeutic drug monitoring. *Ther Drug Monit*. 2008;30:709–716

The Background

I trained in pediatric respiratory medicine and cardiology in Oxford and Liverpool. When I was appointed a Consultant Pediatrician, I continued to research and expand my interest in these specialties further. At the time (1968 to 1970), we studied the treatment of asthma in toddlers by using aminophylline suppositories. With the use of 10 to 20 mg/kg per day of aminophylline, suppositories resulted in beneficial clinical responses and serum levels of 10 to 20 mcg/mL. More importantly, no serious adverse effects were observed. During these years, the duties of a Consultant Pediatrician in the United Kingdom included the care of the newborn and supervision of the special care baby unit at the local maternity hospital. The total number of babies born in my local hospital was about 3,000 per year.

The First Steps

During 1969, a preterm baby in the special care unit developed numerous apneic attacks that lasted 30 seconds or longer and were associated with periods of bradycardia and hypoxia. Although ventilatory support was useful in managing each severe episode, the attacks resumed as soon as the ventilatory support was withdrawn. Other means, such as external stimulation or increasing the ambient oxygen concentrations, were unsuccessful in prevented subsequent apnea. Sadly, the baby, whose birthweight was 1,205 g, died 18 days after birth. At the postmortem examination, a small intraventricular hemorrhage was found in addition to some evidence of hypoxic damage to parts of the gut. The baby had not been treated with aminophylline.

A search of the medical literature for any other management strategies was unfruitful. In fact, the literature on apnea in the newborn and its management in 1969 and 1970 was limited to a few papers that described the incidence of the attacks, which were poorly defined as lasting 15, 20, or more than 30 seconds. There was, however, agreement that prolonged and frequent attacks would lead to hypoxic brain damage and, in the absence of respiratory flow, most likely were due to a lack of respiratory effort (ie, central apnea). Also, it was recognized that such episodes differed from periodic breathing (apnea of 2 to 3 seconds' duration alternating with regular breathing patterns).

Because I had a good working knowledge of the actions of aminophylline, I wondered whether the drug could be useful in the management and prevention of prolonged apnea in the preterm baby, especially because aminophylline was known to act on the respiratory center. Following discussions with various colleagues, we agreed to address the subject further at our next Regional Pediatric Meeting, usually attended by 20 to 30 pediatricians who had different pediatric interests and specialties.

The Regional Meeting, 1970

There was a fair amount of interest in the subject of apnea management with aminophylline that was mixed with a fair amount of skepticism. It was suggested, however, that if any pediatrician wished to use aminophylline for the management of apnea, he or she should discuss the issue fully with the parents or other local colleagues. Further, if such an approach was used, accurate records and observations should be kept and the results reported to subsequent meetings. The dose of aminophylline was agreed upon by meeting participants (see below). During subsequent months, aminophylline suppositories were used by colleagues elsewhere in three babies, and the reported results were encouraging. One of the babies was treated by Dr. Douglas Gairdner in Cambridge, who was then the editor of the *Archives of Diseases in Childhood*. He suggested to me that there was sufficient positive evidence to embark on a formal study of 10 consecutive babies.

The Dose

A pharmaceutical company formulated aminophylline suppositories for our study of asthmatic attacks in toddlers. The chemists were willing to scale the formulation of the suppository to any lower level that we desired. Following discussions, we extrapolated that a 5-mcg suppository administered every 6 hours for three doses initially would be clinically safe. The subsequent use of suppositories would depend on the clinical situation and patient response. We also agreed that technical problems would prevent us from studying dose responses of aminophylline in these very small babies. Hence, the dose used remained empiric. Aminophylline is well absorbed when administered rectally (excellent blood supply), provided the suppository is inserted properly and the infant is supervised by experienced medical and nursing staff.

The Study

The Regional Research Committee approved the study and allowed funding for the purchase of additional equipment and support of a research Fellow. During the next 2 years, 10 babies were studied, and the results were discussed at a number of meetings. The results were submitted for publication and accepted under the heading of "Short Reports." (1)

Feedback

In Europe and the United Kingdom, pediatricians reported positive responses to the use of methylxanthines, but no formal studies were published until three articles in the United States confirmed the efficacy of methylxanthines in the management of apnea in preterm babies. (2) Subsequently, studies from around the world testified to the value of these agents in the management of apnea. Other studies explored the use of caffeine (3) and other stimulants such as doxapram. (4) The Cochrane Database of Systemic Reviews showed that caffeine was as effective as theophylline in providing short-term reductions in the incidence of apnea in preterm babies and was better tolerated and easier to administer. (5) The review concluded that intravenous doxapram and intravenous methylxanthines were similar in their short-term effects, but the trials were too small to exclude any important difference between the therapies. Double-blind studies of methylxanthines for the treatment of apnea of prematurity (6) demonstrated that the administration of 2.5 mg/kg per day caffeine base (ie, equivalent of 5 mg/kg per day caffeine citrate) intravenously or orally for approximately 10 days was effective and safe.

Recent Observations

During the past few years, methylxanthines have been shown to reduce the frequency of postoperative apnea and the use of assisted ventilation in the preterm baby. (5) In addition, methylxanthines have been beneficial in the management of apnea in respiratory syncytial virus-associated infections in the neonate and infant. (7)(8) The long-term effects, if any, of methylxanthine use in the preterm infant are unknown. It has been suggested that because methylxanthines are antagonists of adenosine A1 and A2a receptors and adenosine is neuroprotective, methylxanthine use may lead to neurologic impairment. (9) However, results of cohort studies of the long-term outcome of babies treated with methylxanthines are reassuring. (10)(11) It is possible that some of the undesirable effects of methylxanthines may be related to the doses (eg, too high a dose (12) or erroneous formulation of the dose (13)). Nonetheless, it is only right and proper to conduct controlled, long-term studies of methylxanthines in the management of apnea in the pre-term infant.

Jan A. Kuzemko, MD, FRCP (Ed. and Lond.)
Paediatrician (ret.)

[For the original article by Kuzemko and Paala on aminophylline treatment of apnea in the newborn, which is reprinted with permission from the *Archives of Disease in Childhood* and the British Medical Association, please go to: http://neoreviews.aappublications.org/cgi/content/full/4/3/e62/DC1]

References

1. Kuzemko JA, Paala J. Apneic attacks in the newborn treated with aminophylline. *Arch Dis Child.* 1973;48:404–406

2. Aranda JV, Gorman W, Bergsteinsson H, Gunn T. Efficacy of caffeine in treatment of apnea in the low-birth-weight infant. *J Pediatr.* 1977;90:467–472

3. Bairam A, Boutroy MJ, Badonnel Y, Vert P. Theophylline versus caffeine: comparative effects in treatment of idiopathic apnea in the preterm infant. *J Pediatr.* 1987;110:636–639

4. Barrington KJ, Finer NN, Peters KL, Barton J. Physiologic effects of doxapram in idiopathic apnea of prematurity. *J Pediatr.* 1986;108:124–129

5. Henderson-Smart DJ, Steer PA. Methylxanthine treatment for apnea in preterm infants. *Cochrane Database Syst Rev.* 2001;(3):CD000140

6. Erenberg A, Leff RD, Haack DG, et al. Caffeine citrate for the treatment of apnea of prematurity: a double-blind placebo-controlled study. *Pharmacotherapy.* 2000;20:644–652

7. Bruhn FW, Mokrohisky ST, McIntosh K. Apnea associated with respiratory syncytial virus infection in young infants. *J Pediatr.* 1977;90:382–386

8. Johnston DM, Kuzemko JA. Virus-induced apnea and theophylline. *Lancet.* 1992;340:1352

9. Fredholm BB. Astra Award Lecture: adenosine, adenosine receptors and the actions of caffeine. *Pharmacol Toxicol.* 1995;76:93–101

10. Gunn TR, Metrakos K, Riley P, et al. Sequelae of caffeine treatment in preterm infants with apnea. *J Pediatr.* 1979;94:106–109

11. Ment LR, Scott DT, Ehrenkranz RA, Duncan CC. Early childhood developmental follow-up of infants with GMH/IVH: effect of methylxanthine. *Am J Perinatol.* 1985;2:223–227

12. Hoecker C, Nelle M, Poeschl J, et al. Caffeine impairs cerebral and intestinal blood flow velocity in preterm infants. *Pediatrics.* 2002;109:784–787

13. Narayanan M, Schlueter M, Clyman RI. Incidence and outcome of a 10-fold indomethacin overdose in premature infants. *J Pediatr.* 1999;135:105–107

Historical Perspectives: Use of Methylxanthines in the Management of Apneic Attacks in the Newborn
Jan A. Kuzemko
NeoReviews 2003;4;62
DOI: 10.1542/neo.4-3-e62

Transcutaneous Blood Gas Measurement

Introduction

This 2003 Historical Perspective draws attention to the remarkable feat achieved by Renate and Albert Huch in the early 1970s, which seemed magical at the time. This was the development of an electrode that measured the partial pressure of oxygen at the skin surface ($tcPo_2$), which reflected the oxygen tension in arterial blood. (1) Subsequently, continuous transcutaneous measurement demonstrated that intermittent arterial blood gas measurements provided only a glimpse of the dynamic variations that occur with different procedures in the neonatal intensive care unit (NICU). In addition, it was not long before the use of two electrodes demonstrated shunting through the ductus arteriosus. (2)

Later in the same decade, this same team produced a complementary electrode to measure the partial pressure of carbon dioxide ($tcPco_2$). (3) The measurement of both $tcPo_2$ and $tcPco_2$ allowed greatly improved management of assisted ventilation. There was one significant disadvantage of $tcPo_2$ monitoring, which was the need to move the electrode every few hours to prevent skin injury from the heating device. As a result, when pulse oximetry became available, monitoring of oxygen saturation became more popular. However, as the Huchs point out, most pulse oximeters have a problem with movement artefact (although this may have been resolved with some devices), and they cannot detect hyperoxemia. Consequently, transcutaneous blood gas monitoring (particularly $tcPco_2$) remains an important adjunct in the NICU, especially early in the course of respiratory disease.

Alistair G. S. Philip, MD, FRCPE, FAAP
Editor-in-Chief, NeoReviews

References

1. Huch R, Huch A, Lübbers DW. Transcutaneous measurement of blood PO_2 ($tcPO_2$): method and applications in perinatal medicine. *J Perinat Med.* 1973;1:183–191
2. Yamanouchi I, Igarashi I. Ductal shunt in premature infants observed by $tcPO_2$ measurements. In: Huch A, Huch R, Lucey JF, eds. *Transcutaneous Blood Gas Monitoring. Birth Defects: Original Article Series.* Vol. 15. New York, NY: AR Liss; 1979:323–340
3. Huch A, Huch R, Seiler D, Galster H, Meinzer K, Lübbers DW. Transcutaneous PCO_2 measurement with a miniaturized electrode. *Lancet.* 1977;i:982–983

Transcutaneous Po_2 in Newborns: An Electrode in the Family

Göttingen: We Meet

When we met in the German university city of Göttingen in 1959, Albert was a medical student and Renate was still in high school. After qualifying, Albert studied respiratory physiology at the Max Planck Institute for Experimental Medicine in Göttingen while Renate completed her medical studies. We married in 1964 and moved some miles south to Marburg, another medieval university city, in 1967 for Albert to join the Department of Obstetrics and Renate the Institute of Physiology, headed by Dietrich Lübbers, the oxygen physiologist. (1) Over the years, the Lübbers group had worked on oxygen measurement using spectrophotometry (oxygen saturation) and polarography (oxygen pressure). In particular, they had analyzed and refined the Clark Po_2 principle. (2)

Marburg: We Measure Oxygen Saturation and Make a False Start

At that time, Erich Saling's fetal blood analysis (FBA) had just entered obstetric medicine. (3) By enabling the detection of oxygen deficiency in blood samples from the fetal scalp in the birth canal, the FBA opened a major window on the "dark world of the fetus" during labor and delivery. However, the invasive, noncontinuous nature of this oxygen status information spurred us on to further research.

With the added stimulus of the Lübbers Institute setting, we began by measuring oxygen saturation. The Institute had developed a spectrophotometer that measured the reflection spectrum from the skin over a wide range of wavelengths in several microseconds. We reconstructed it with modifications that yielded spectra from newborns' heads in the visible spectral range. We were blessed with a ready-made volunteer in the person of our 4-month-old daughter, who had a precocious taste for clinical research (which she now exercises as an academic radiologist).

It was obvious to the naked eye that breathing pure oxygen made the two oxygen saturation peaks steeper, but quantifying these increases in saturation remained an insolvable problem. Many years later, of course, pulse oximetry cleverly overcame this problem with the aid of modern electronics and increased computer power. Back in 1967 and 1968, our computer was a DEC PDP-8, retailing at $18,000, that had a then "staggering" 4 KB of memory. This modern classic filled an entire room and generated an immense amount of heat. Because our spectrophotometer required a dark surround for measurement, we could only open the windows at night to get rid of the heat. Accordingly, we made all our baby skin measurements in the late evening.

Later in Zurich, at our 1984 symposium *The Roots of Today's Perinatal Medicine*, we grew nostalgic over those early days, listening to Lilly Dubowitz recount her own research in newborns—the only research subject possible, as she explained, for a physiologist who had three children younger than the age of 3 years. (4) The upshot of this period was that, despite many attempts and a compliant volunteer, we failed to obtain any quantitative information on oxygen saturation.

Marburg: We Measure Oxygen Partial Pressure Instead and Are on Our Way

Despite our early false start, we simply could not abandon our ambition of devising a method of continuous noninvasive monitoring of fetal oxygen status that would parallel, for example, the monitoring of fetal heart rate. In the absence of an accessible fetus, we continued with babies as our favored research subjects. We decided to switch from measuring oxygen saturation to measuring oxygen partial pressure.

At least three important contributions in this field created a platform for further research:

- *The development of the Clark Po_2 electrode and the success of the Lübbers group in miniaturizing the platinum/silver electrode system.* Among other advantages, miniaturization meant less oxygen consumption by the electrode itself, which was a critical prerequisite for accurate quantification, given the small amount of oxygen diffusing through intact skin.

- *The demonstration by Baumberger and Goodfried (5) and Rooth and coworkers (6) that oxygen in a heated liquid surrounding the skin equilibrates with the oxygen in the skin.* This finding enabled the measurement of Po_2 in the liquid with the aid of a given ratio. Rooth and coworkers showed that after a finger was immersed in heated potassium chloride solution, Po_2 in the liquid equilibrated with arterial Po_2 levels after 20 minutes.

- *The systematic skin Po_2 measurements reported in 1966 and 1967 by Evans and Naylor. (7)* These physiology and dermatology partners used a Po_2 electrode suspended on the skin in such a way that the electrode was virtually weightless, thereby preventing compression of the underlying capillaries. Hyperemia was achieved either by pharmacologic means or by infrared radiation. Although arterial levels were not measured on skin, and the whole

construction was too clumsy for clinical application, respiratory maneuvers and oxygen breathing could be monitored on skin. They did not continue their studies, despite being very close to resolving these problems, and when we met Evans in 1971, he was kind enough to say that he was glad we had been able to do so.

Marburg: Our Transcutaneous Electrode Takes Shape

We began our measurements with a catheter Po_2 electrode that was guided by a micrometer screw onto the skin. The cover was attached to the skin by vacuum. With this setup, we could demonstrate a relationship between the changes in Po_2 measured on the skin surface and those in arterial blood. The experience we gained with this electrode led us to develop a flat, buttonlike electrode that had three separate cathodes arranged in a triangle. Identical readings from all three cathodes indicated that the electrode was attached properly. Our use of a quick-setting plastic material greatly improved adhesion, decreased the risk of compressing the underlying capillaries, and enabled the infant to move freely (Figure).

When we tried to perform skin measurements under constant temperature conditions, we made what turned out to be a crucial observation. The electrode was affixed with the plastic to an adult's forearm, and the entire forearm was immersed in a thermostatically controlled water bath. Skin

Po_2 increased more than could be accounted for by the temperature of the electrode itself; the warm water clearly induced the local hyperemia. This prompted us to incorporate an electric heating system in the silver anode of the electrode. The hyperperfusion response to the local heat-induced vasodilation was so good that the weight of the electrode no longer compressed the capillaries. This made it possible simply to attach the electrode to a hairless part of the skin with a double-sided self-adhesive ring. Our first simultaneous intra-arterial and transcutaneous Po_2 recordings during various respiratory maneuvers were made in an adult population that had asthma and showed close agreement. (8) Long-term monitoring of arterial Po_2 finally was looking like a realistic prospect.

Marburg: The Swedish Connection

A knock on the laboratory door one day in 1972 introduced us to Gosta Rooth from Sweden, who was based in Lund at the time and was destined to become the first professor of perinatal medicine in Europe at Uppsala. He had been working on fetal acid-base status for almost 20 years. It was the beginning of a long collaboration in Sweden, Germany, and later Switzerland and of a wonderful friendship. Together we systematically evaluated tcPo_2 in various patient populations: adults, newborns, and fetuses. We plumbed the method's potential, mapped its boundaries, and in our joint publications reported a number of physiologic firsts and clinical applications, all achieved by continuous noninvasive recording. In particular, we devised the oxycardiorespirogram, which monitors postnatal cardiopulmonary adaptation by combining tcPo_2 with the beat-to-beat heart rate and respiratory waveform. (9)

Marburg: More Visitors to Our Door

Another notable friend and enthusiastic promoter of the neonatal application of tcPo_2 was Jerold Lucey, editor of *Pediatrics* and Professor of Pediatrics at the University of Vermont Medical Center in Burlington. He was fascinated by the possibility of monitoring small newborns and arranged to meet us in 1974 at an international congress in Europe. He promoted tcPo_2 in the United States by organizing a tour for us through

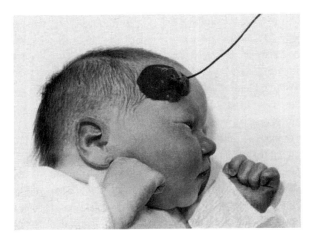

Figure 1. Transcutaneous electrode for measurement of Po^2.

major neonatal centers. His was one of the first departments, along with some in Europe, to receive our electrode systems virtually on a loan basis before industrial production by the German medical device manufacturers, Dräger in Lübeck and Hellige in Freiburg, got off the ground. *Pediatrics* published the first multicenter evaluation of $tcPo_2$ in neonatal intensive care in 1975. (10)

Marburg: Victory Over Industry

Eberhardt and coworkers were an industry-based group researching a similar device. The first good clinical data achieved with our system motivated the Roche Kontron group to bring their product onto the market a little rashly, before it had been evaluated fully. Their electrode had a high intrinsic oxygen consumption and was heated to only 43°C instead of our 45°C (a feature that they marketed as an advantage). Gabriel Duc, Professor and Chairman of Neonatology at the University Hospital in Zurich, told us of his disappointment over unsatisfactory results with the Roche electrode. He proposed bolstering the credibility of $tcPo_2$ by organizing a comparative trial of the rival systems in severely ill newborns in Zurich. The $tcPo_2$ values measured with our system largely agreed with the arterial values; the Roche Kontron values proved to be substantial underestimates. This led to a publication that advanced the cause of transcutaneous blood gas monitoring (11) and at the same time, in career terms, was the first step in our eventual move to Zurich.

Marburg: The Years of Consolidation

Visitors during our final years in Marburg were primarily neonatologists and anesthesiologists who needed to confirm with their own eyes that arterial Po_2 could be monitored reliably through intact skin. Many prolonged their stay, in some cases for a whole year, conducting systematic studies with us. These visitors included Jerold Lucey (Burlington), Hans Ueli Bucher (Zurich), Harald Schachinger (Berlin), and Joyce Peabody (Boston/Burlington). Subsequent publications brought more physiologic and clinical firsts, centered (in an obstetrics department) on the unborn child and specifically how labor,

maternal position, medication, and maternal oxygen breathing influenced fetal oxygenation; respiratory adaptation of the healthy newborn in the first postnatal week; and distinctive maternal breathing features during delivery.

These were the consolidation years in continuous noninvasive monitoring. We began working intensively with industry. Electrodes almost identical to our prototypes were brought onto the market. In 1978, we organized our first international symposium, attended by many of the world's leading figures in blood gas measurement. They included Leland Clark, the father of the Clark electrode, who surprised us with a then-popular lyric from the pop group, The Sweet:

Love is like oxygen
Love is like oxygen
You get too much, you get too high, too high
Not enough and you're gonna die

and pronounced $tcPo_2$ a "long-awaited breakthrough" in clinical medicine. Various awards began coming our way, and in late 1978, we were offered the posts in Zurich— Albert as Professor and Chairman of the Department of Obstetrics and Renate as Professor and Head of the Perinatal Research Unit—that we were to occupy for the next 25 years.

Zurich: Coming to Terms With Our Dream

Our motivation from the beginning was the dream of monitoring fetal oxygenation during the hours of greatest risk, ie, during delivery. The fetus was our target patient, with the newborn no more than a halfway stage that was privileged by its ease of access. Even though our $tcPo_2$ technique had yielded new and important physiologic and clinical data despite formidable constraints (application to the fetus was possible only after rupture of the membranes and with the cervix dilated at least 3 to 4 cm), we were forced to recognize that it fell irremediably short of the Holy Grail of routine monitoring during birth. Transcutaneous measurement requires maximal vasodilatation under the oxygen electrode, a type of peripheral arterialization. In newborns and preterm infants, this is possible even in very sick children, apparently because their capacity for

protective vasoconstriction is less developed than in later life or, as we found, than in the birth canal. Marked superficial vasoconstriction evidently occurs in the fetus in the presence of oxygen deficiency, which is "physiologic" to a certain degree during passage through the birth canal. As a result, a $tcPo_2$ value in the birth canal no longer relates closely to a central arterial value; rather, it reflects only the local situation. Under clinical conditions, it becomes difficult to differentiate with confidence between local vasoconstriction and true oxygen deficiency.

Zurich: A Final Look Back

In the 1980s, a rival system, pulse oximetry, swept through intensive care units across the world for monitoring oxygen saturation through intact skin. Thanks to the ingenious idea of basing measurement solely on pulsations that parallel the action of the heart and light absorbance changes caused only by volume changes, individual factors such as tissue volume, skin perfusion, and color became irrelevant. Compared with the technically and physiologically more complex $tcPo_2$, pulse oximetry was simple to perform, and the device could be attached easily to newborns with no individual calibration.

Which is best in newborns: Po_2 or So_2? Pulse oximetry in infants has two crucial disadvantages. One is technical, the problem of movement artefacts, and the other is inherent in the principle of saturation measurement, namely, that it cannot detect hyperoxemia. This can be circumvented only by measuring Po_2 in blood or transcutaneously, thus resolving the debate to the mutual advantage of each technique. Far from competing against one another, each complements the other in neonatal intensive care. The Huch family is happy to have added its tessera to the expanding mosaic of progress in neonatal medicine.

Renate and Albert Huch

[To read the original article on measurement of transcutaneous Po_2 in newborns published by the Huchs in 1973, which was reprinted with permission from *the Journal of Perinatal Medicine,* please go to: http://neoreviews.aappublications.org/cgi/content/full/4/9/e223/DC1]

References

1. Lübbers DW. Methods of measuring oxygen tensions of blood and organ surfaces. In: Payne JP, Hill DW, eds. *Oxygen Measurements in Blood and Tissues.* London, England: Churchill; 1966:103

2. Clark LC Jr. Monitor and control of blood and tissue oxygen tension. *Trans Am Soc Artif Intern Organs.* 1956;2:41

3. Saling E. *Das Kind im Bereich der Geburtshilfe.* Stuttgart, Germany: Georg Thieme Verlag; 1966

4. Dubowitz L, Dubowitz V. Gestational age of the newborn - evolution of the score. In: Rooth G, Saugstad OD, eds. *The Roots of Perinatal Medicine.* Stuttgart, Germany: Georg Thieme Verlag; 1985:31

5. Baumberger JP, Goodfried RB. Determination of arterial oxygen tension in man by equilibration through intact skin. *Fed Proc.* 1951;10:10

6. Rooth G, Sjostedt S, Caligara F. Bloodless determination of arterial oxygen tension by polarography. *Science Tools, The LKW Instrument J.* 1957;4:37

7. Evans NTS, Naylor PFD. The systemic oxygen supply to the surface of human skin. *Respir Physiol.* 1967;3:21–37

8. Huch A, Huch R, Arner B, Rooth G. Continuous transcutaneous oxygen measured with a heated electrode. *Scand J Clin Lab Invest.* 1973;31:269–275

9. Huch R, Huch A, Rooth G, Fallenstein F, Schachinger H. *An Atlas of Oxygen-Cardiorespirograms in Newborn Infants.* London, England: Wolfe Medical Publishing Ltd; 1983

10. Huch R, Huch A, Albani M, et al. Transcutaneous PO_2 monitoring in routine management of infants and children with cardiorespiratory problems. *Pediatrics.* 1976;57:681–690

11. Duc G, Bucher HU, Micheli JL. Is transcutaneous PO_2 reliable for arterial oxygen monitoring in newborn infants? *Pediatrics.* 1975;55:566–567

Historical Perspectives: Transcutaneous Blood Gas Measurement

Alistair G. S. Philip, Renate Huch and Albert Huch

NeoReviews 2003;4;223

DOI: 10.1542/neo.4-9-e223

Maternal Serum Alpha-fetoprotein and Fetal Abnormalities

Introduction

This 2004 Historical Perspective is in a slightly different format, but should be of considerable interest to readers of *NeoReviews*.

Professor Nicholas Wald is an epidemiologist who has evaluated and written about a variety of topics, but he is best known for his work on screening methods, particularly in the area of maternal serum alpha-fetoprotein (AFP) and fetal abnormalities. Because of his continuing heavy commitments and to minimize the disruption of his schedule, I posed a number of questions to him, to which he responded with detailed answers. Before moving to his responses, some background information seems in order.

Shortly before publication of the article highlighted here, evaluation of amniotic fluid in cases of open spina bifida and other neural tube defects had shown increased levels of AFP. (1) Somewhat later, it was shown that abdominal wall defects, as well as neural tube defects, could contribute to increased levels of amniotic fluid AFP. (2) In his responses, Professor Wald documents the sequence of events that followed, noting that Professor David Brock in Edinburgh described the association of increased levels of maternal serum alpha-fetoprotein (MSAFP) with fetal anencephaly, which triggered the idea that this also might be true of open spina bifida. Thus, MSAFP was used as a screening tool for the detection of neural tube and abdominal wall defects. Elevated MSAFP levels were noted in other "at-risk" pregnancies (3) and twin pregnancies. (4) To provide better standardization, Professor Wald introduced the concept of "multiples of the median" (MoM) at different gestational ages.

Approximately a decade passed before the association was made between low MoMs for AFP and chromosomal defects, particularly Down syndrome. Soon thereafter, several other serum markers for Down syndrome were described, and by linking them to maternal age, screening became increasingly valuable. In the early 1980s, Dr James Haddow of the Foundation for Blood Research (FBR) in Scarborough, Maine, spent a sabbatical in London with Professor Wald. The FBR had been established with the primary focus of evaluating proteins that might be valuable as diagnostic aids. Dr Haddow recognized the value of MSAFP (initially using high levels, but later incorporating low levels) and in collaboration with Professor Wald established MSAFP screening both regionally and later at a nationwide reference laboratory. (5)(6)

At present, linking these serum markers not only to maternal age, but also to findings of prenatal ultrasonography, has resulted in screening that produces a very high detection rate of both Down syndrome and trisomy 18, (7) with a reduction in the numbers of false-positive findings. This decreases the anxiety that can be created for many mothers and helps to minimize the difficulty in making decisions about continuing or terminating a pregnancy.

Alistair G. S. Philip, MD, FRCPE, FAAP
Editor-in-Chief, NeoReviews

References

1. Brock DJH, Sutcliffe RG. Alphafetoprotein in antenatal diagnosis of anencephaly and spina bifida. *Lancet.* 1972;ii:197
2. Clarke PC, Gordon YB, Kitau MJ, Chard T, McNeal AD. Alpha-fetoprotein levels in pregnancies complicated by gastrointestinal abnormalities of the fetus. *Br J Obstet Gynaecol.* 1977;84:285–289
3. Brock DJH, Barron L, Watt M, Scrimgeour JB, Keay AJ. Maternal plasma alphafetoprotein and low birth weight: a prospective study throughout pregnancy. *Br J Obstet Gynaecol.* 1982;89:348–351
4. Wald NJ, Barker S, Peto R, Brock DJH, Bonnar J. Maternal serum alpha-fetoprotein levels in multiple pregnancy. *Br Med J.* 1975;i:651–652
5. Haddow JE, Kloza EM, Smith DE, Knight GJ. Data from an alphafetoprotein pilot screening program in Maine. *Obstet Gynecol.* 1983;62:556–560
6. Haddow JE, Palomaki GE, Knight GJ, et al. Prenatal screening for Down's syndrome with the use of maternal serum markers. *N Engl J Med.* 1992;327:588–593
7. Palomaki GE, Neveux LM, Knight GJ, Haddow JE. Maternal serum-integrated screening for trisomy 18 using both first-and second-trimester markers. *Prenat Diag.* 2003;23:243–247

Questions and Answers

What were you doing in 1974 or shortly before then? Where were you based?

I was in the Department of the Regius Professor of Medicine, which was based in the Radcliffe Infirmary in Oxford, England. Sir Richard Doll (known for his work showing that cigarette smoking was an important cause of lung cancer) was the Regius Professor at the time. I held a junior academic medical position in the field of epidemiology.

How did you become interested in AFP?

This was prompted by a case report from David Brock and his colleagues in Edinburgh published in 1973. They reported an anencephalic pregnancy in which the AFP level in maternal serum was raised. (1) I had collected a bank of antenatal serum samples at the time with the intention of exploring the possible relationship between influenza infection in pregnancy and childhood leukemia. For various reasons, the prospects for the success of this project were slim, and I was looking for another scientific question to investigate using the antenatal serum samples I had collected. The observation that AFP was associated with anencephaly led me to suspect that maternal serum AFP might be associated with spina bifida as well.

With whom did you collaborate?

Collection of the antenatal serum samples required the cooperation of my obstetric colleagues at the maternity hospital in Oxford (the John Radcliffe), but other than that, there was little need for collaboration. I instituted a system in which remnant blood samples taken during antenatal care (the small amount left in a syringe that would otherwise be thrown away) was retained; the patient's identification label stuck onto the syringe; and the syringe sent to a small laboratory for centrifugation, separation, and storage. Separately, I collected details of all the births from the maternity hospital, so I could link the blood samples to these birth details.

Did you have previous contact with David Brock?

I had no contact with David Brock until after I had read his paper and contacted him with a view to collaborating. I suggested that I retrieve the antenatal serum samples from the pregnancies with open neural tube defects, match them each with two controls, and give them to him blind so he would not know which were cases and which were controls. He agreed, and within a few days, traveled from Edinburgh to Oxford to collect the sera, carry out the AFP measurements, and let me have the results. He did this within about a week, and the paper was published shortly afterwards in April 1974. (2)

Who else was influential in your thinking?

On this issue at this time, no one. I wanted to put the antenatal sera I had collected to good use. The AFP project came to me one Saturday morning when I had gone into the office with no one around. I contacted David Brock on the following Monday morning.

What provided the clue that maternal serum testing, rather than amniotic fluid testing, might be fruitful?

There was not much of a clue to this. The earlier study with amniotic fluid had shown increased AFP with both anencephaly and spina bifida. (3) Once I had contacted David Brock, he indicated that despite the evidence that anencephaly was associated with raised MSAFP, there was no evidence that this applied to open spina bifida. Of course, the possibility of screening was of much greater importance with respect to spina bifida than it was to fatal abnormalities such an anencephaly.

When was "triple testing" introduced?

This was introduced in 1988 at St. Bartholomew's Hospital following research that combined three advances into one: 1) reduced AFP levels in aneuploidies, (4) later shown to be reasonably specific for Down syndrome; (5) 2) increased concentrations of human chorionic gonadotropin (hCG) in Down

syndrome pregnancies; (6) and 3) reduced estriol concentrations in Down syndrome pregnancies. (7) We developed a simple method of combining these markers into a single test, (8) which became known as the triple test (to be followed later by the quadruple test). (9) It now probably is the primary method of screening for Down syndrome in economically developed parts of the world.

How important was the collaboration with the FBR and Jim Haddow? When was "multiples of the median" introduced?

The MoM was introduced early. It was a concept that emerged (again I think on a quiet weekend) that would enable AFP values to be standardized simply for both gestational age and screening laboratory. I presented the concept at a meeting in Paris organized by the geneticist Andre Boué, and the paper was published in the proceedings of INSERM (Institute National de la Sante et Recherche Medicale). (10) MoM subsequently was used in the United Kingdom Collaborative AFP study of Down syndrome screening and has been accepted widely. The link with Jim Haddow and FBR was an important complementary collaboration. FBR were instrumental in recognizing the value of screening and disseminating the principles of screening widely throughout the United States. Their annual course has been very valuable in this respect. They have collaborated in a number of areas, perhaps the most important of which was introducing me to Jack Canick and catalyzing the collaboration that led to the triple test that was published jointly in the *British Medical Journal* in 1988. (8)

How important was the finding of nuchal translucency in Down syndrome?

This finding was important. The initial observation was made by Szabo in Hungary, (11) following observations made by Benacerraf in Boston in the second trimester of pregnancies. (12) Subsequently, Nicolaides developed and promoted the measurement as a method of screening, initially on its own and then with maternal age. In 1997, the first trimester "combined test" was described in which nuchal translucency was combined with maternal age, pregnancy-associated plasma protein-A (PAPP-A), and free betahCG in the first

trimester (13) and later was adopted by Nicolaides and his colleagues. (14)

Where do we stand today?

Today we have a screening test for Down syndrome that is very effective, with a detection rate of about 90% and a false-positive rate of 2%. This is based on the "integrated test," which uses two first trimester markers (nuchal translucency and PAPP-A) and the quadruple test markers in the second trimester. All six markers are combined with maternal age to produce a single estimate of risk. The test was described in the *New England Journal of Medicine* in 1999, (15) and the screening performance of the test was corroborated in a multicenter study supported by the United Kingdom Government Health Technology Assessment Research and Development Research Programme (the SURUSS report). (16) Even though the integrated test is the most effective and safe method of screening, different screening tests still remain, and different groups have tended to become wedded to the test that they have adopted. So, in some places the triple test persists, some use the quadruple test, others promote the first-trimester combined test, and a few have started to introduce the integrated test.

Summation

A common thread running through this history is the recognition that the combination of different tests into a single evaluation can improve the discriminatory ability of a test significantly. I think it was the mathematical and statistical environment in which I was steeped in Oxford that gave me the statistical insights into doing this. My collaboration with Howard Cuckle helped in this respect, and the collaboration with the FBR was very helpful from the laboratory perspective. For example, they provided me with purified AFP that we labeled in the physics department of Reading University to set up our AFP radioimmunoassay. Another influence was my exposure to clinical pathology. As a junior doctor while a resident clinical pathologist, I had to get up in the middle of the night to perform bilirubin estimations for rhesus hemolytic disease of the newborn. There was no automated method. I felt that one could be developed. The Professor of

Clinical Pathology kindly set aside time for me to work on this, and eventually I managed to put bilirubin measurements on the Technicon Autoanalyser, making what was once a tricky manual assay into a simple automated one. This work led to my first publication, (17) and the experience, influenced as it was by an interest in epidemiology and public health, encouraged me to develop epidemiology linked to laboratory science, which has been a theme throughout my research career.

All this could not really have been successful without the support and good will of one's immediate colleagues, including, of course, all the heads of departments in which I worked as well as colleagues from different disciplines in different centers throughout the world. Many became friends who were interested in and willing to talk about new ideas in an open, relaxed, and inspiring way.

Nicholas J. Wald, DSc (Med), FRCP, FRS
Director, Wolfson Institute of Preventive
Medicine
Barts and The London Queen Mary's School
of Medicine and Dentistry
England

EDITOR'S NOTE: See also Welch KK, Malone FD. Advances in prenatal screening: nuchal translucency ultrasonography in the first trimester. NeoReviews. 2002;3:e202–e208. Available at: http://neoreviews.aappublications. org/cgi/content/full/3/10/e202

[To view Professor Wald's groundbreaking study on the relationship of spina bifida and anencephaly with MSAFP, which was reprinted with permission from Elsevier (*The Lancet*. 1974;i:765–767), please go to: http://neoreviews.aappublications.org/cgi/ content/full/5/12/e507/DC1]

References

1. Brock DJH, Bolton EA, Monaghan JM. Prenatal diagnosis of anencephaly through maternal serum alpha-fetoprotein measurement. *Lancet*. 1973;ii: 923–924

2. Wald NJ, Brock DJH, Bonnar J. Prenatal diagnosis of spina bifida and anencephaly by maternal serum AFP measurement: a controlled study. *Lancet*. 1974;i:765–767

3. Brock DJH, Sutcliffe RG. Alpha-fetoprotein in antenatal diagnosis of anencephaly and spina bifida. *Lancet*. 1972;ii:197

4. Merkatz IR, Nitowsky HM, Macri JN, Johnson WE. An association between low maternal serum alpha-fetoprotein and fetal chromosomal abnormalities. *Am J Obstet Gynecol*. 1984;148:886–894

5. Cuckle HS, Wald NJ. Screening for Down's syndrome using serum alpha-fetoprotein. *Br Med J (Clin Res Ed)*. 1985;291:349

6. Bogart MH, Pandian MR, Jones OW. Abnormal maternal serum chorionic gonadotropin levels in pregnancies with fetal chromosome abnormalities. *Prenat Diagn*. 1987;7:623–630

7. Canick JA, Knight GJ, Palomaki GE, Haddow JE, Cuckle HS, Wald NJ. Low second trimester maternal serum unconjugated oestriol in pregnancies with Down's syndrome. *Br J Obstet Gynaecol*. 1988;95:330–333

8. Wald NJ, Cuckle HS, Densem JW, et al. Maternal serum screening for Down's syndrome in early pregnancy. *Br Med J*. 1988;297:883–887

9. Wald NJ, Hackshaw AK, Huttly W, Kennard A. Empirical validation of risk screening for Down's syndrome. *J Med Screen*. 1996;3:185–187

10. Wald NJ. The detection of neural tube defects by screening maternal blood. In: Boué A, ed. *Prenatal Diagnosis. Les Colloques d'INSERM*. 1976;61:227–238

11. Szabo J, Gellan J, Szemere G. [Nuchal edema as an ultrasonic sign of trisomy 21 during the first trimester of pregnancy] *Orv Hetil*. 1992;133:3167–3168 (Hungarian)

12. Benacerraf BR, Gelman R, Frigoletto FD Jr. Sonographic identification of second trimester fetuses with Down's syndrome. *N Engl J Med*. 1987; 317:1371–1376

13. Wald NJ, Hackshaw AK. Combined ultrasound and biochemistry in first-trimester screening for Down's syndrome. *Prenat Diagn*. 1997;17:821–829

14. Bindra R, Heath V, Liao A, Spencer K, Nicolaides KH. One-stop clinic for assessment of risk for trisomy 21 at 11–14 weeks: a prospective study of 15, 030 pregnancies. *Ultrasound Obstet Gynecol*. 2002;20:219–225

15. Wald NJ, Watt HC, Hackshaw AK. Integrated screening for Down's syndrome on the basis of tests performed during the first and second trimesters. *N Engl J Med*. 1999;341:461–467

16. Wald NJ, Rodeck C, Hackshaw AK, Walters J, Chitty L, Mackinson AM. First and second trimester antenatal screening for Down's syndrome: the results of the Serum, Urine and Ultrasound Screening Study (SURUSS). *J Med Screen*. 2003;10: 56–104; and *Health Technol Assess*. 2003;7:1–77

17. Billing B, Haslam R, Wald N. Bilirubin standards and the determination of bilirubin by manual and Technicon Auto-Analyzer methods. *Ann Clin Biochem*. 1971;8:21–30

Historical Perspectives: Maternal Serum Alpha-fetoprotein and Fetal Abnormalities
Alistair G. S. Philip and Nicholas J. Wald
NeoReviews 2004;5;e507-e510
DOI: 10.1542/neo.5-12-e507

Neonatal Transillumination

Transillumination is a technique that had been used for many years to detect intracranial pathology. In particular, cases of hydranencephalus could be detected easily using a simple flashlight in a darkened room. A new and improved method of detection involved a high-intensity light source, which was called a "Chun gun" (after its inventor) and allowed norms to be established (1).

The significant advance that we highlight here occurred in the 1970s. This was the use of a fiberoptic high-intensity light source to detect air leaks, such as pneumothorax, pneumomediastinum, or pneumoperitoneum. The leader in this field was Dr Lawrence Kuhns, a radiologist in Ann Arbor, Michigan.

This 2005 Historical Perspective is contributed by Dr Steven Donn who was a resident in Vermont when I was a junior faculty member. We both came under the influence of Dr Jerry Lucey (see Historical Perspective on Phototherapy, page 60), who happened to know a thing or two about light and had installed a high-intensity fiberoptic light for use in the Vermont neonatal intensive care unit. As he notes, Dr Donn moved to Michigan to do his neonatal fellowship and came under the influence of Dr Kuhns. Together they wrote a monograph on pediatric transillumination, which included its use not only for air leaks, but also for various other situations (eg, using light to facilitate cannulation of arteries or veins and transilluminating masses such as hydronephrosis or encephaloceles etc).

Alistair G. S. Philip, MD, FRCPE, FAAP
Editor-in-Chief, NeoReviews

References
[See also Dr Donn's reference list]
1. Vyhmeister N, Schneider S, Cha C. Cranial transillumination norms of the premature infant. *J Pediatr.* 1977;91:980–982.

Introduction

As a fledgling intern in pediatrics at the University of Vermont in 1975 to 1976, my first experience with transilluminating the chest of a preterm newborn who had a pneumothorax was an unforgettable milestone in my training. I was amazed at how rapid, non-invasive, and inexpensive this technique was, and how it enabled immediate intervention without the inordinate delays usually involved in obtaining emergency radiography in the middle of the night. What surprised me even more was to learn that this was a relatively new neonatal diagnostic technique, with the first report from Lawrence Kuhns and cow-orkers at the University of Michigan having been published only a few months earlier. (1) Neonatal intensive care was a relatively new proposition in those days. Mechanical ventilation only recently had been introduced as a standard practice, and the incidence of pneumothorax and other thoracic air leaks in the presurfactant era was very high. Of course, every medical student was taught to transilluminate the skull of a newborn as part of the neonatal neurologic assessment, but this novel approach to using high-intensity visible light to diagnose a pneumothorax rapidly and accurately was exciting. Moreover, it was something even an intern could do.

By a quirk of fate, 2 years later I moved to Ann Arbor for a fellowship in neonatal-perinatal medicine. One of the first babies I encountered was a newborn in whom unilateral hydronephrosis was suspected. While I was standing at the bedside discussing possible diagnostic tests with the house staff, Larry Kuhns entered the neonatal intensive care unit (NICU) wheeling a high-intensity fiberoptic light. After darkening the room, Larry transilluminated the baby's flank, and the sight drew everyone to the bedside like moths to a flame. Afterwards, we introduced ourselves and had a brief discussion. I told Larry of my interests in intraventricular hemorrhage and noninvasive intracranial pressure monitoring, and he suggested that we might be able to collaborate on some clinical projects during my fellowship.

Expanding Use

Subsequently, I learned that Larry had been a fully trained pediatrician before subspecializing in pediatric radiology. He understood neonatology and had a real clinical inquisitiveness. He also had had a very positive influence on a number of my predecessors in the neonatology fellowship program, including Mike Wyman, Frank Bednarek, and Pat Wall, and they had contributed several landmark papers describing the use of transillumination in the NICU. (2)(3) I also was impressed by the expanded uses of transillumination I observed during those first few weeks of my fellowship, including detection of pneumoperitoneum and as an aid to venipuncture and peripheral arterial cannulation.

As the decade of the 1970s closed, a number of important clinical contributions on transillumination appeared in the literature. Cabatu and Brown described the use of transillumination to diagnose and treat pneumopericardium. (4) Buck and associates (5) reported the use of light to aid in the diagnosis of intra-abdominal pathology (this work also was directed by Larry Kuhns). Several reports documented improved success in achieving vascular access using transillumination. (6)(7)(8)(9) The portable transilluminator became a standard piece of equipment in neonatal intensive care.

Documentation

Larry also perfected the ability to photograph transillumination procedures (10) and assembled an impressive atlas of color slides depicting virtually every neonatal condition amenable to diagnosis by transillumination. It was a tremendous reference resource. Multiple users, including myself, often commented that Larry should publish it. His reply caught me off guard when he said, "Why don't *we* do it?" He and I had established a strong collaboration and had published a few papers together. I was at the midpoint of my fellowship and thought that this would be a worthwhile pursuit, so I allowed myself to be talked into doing it. After we sent a few inquiries to publishers, Year Book expressed an interest in producing the monograph, and the task began. Despite Larry's extensive atlas, I wondered whether there actually would be enough material to write the proposed 100-page monograph.

I learned much about the properties of light and transillumination during the preparation of the monograph. I suppose it finally made all of those undergraduate physics classes worthwhile. I also learned that although transillumination only recently had been described in neonatal circles, its use in medicine dated back to 1831, when Richard Bright first described his observation of candlelight shining visibly through the head of a macrocephalic adult, presumably with massive hydrocephalus. Numerous publications over the next 150 years described the use of visible light to distinguish solid structures from cystic and to use the optical properties of tissues to define anatomy.

The evolution of the monograph was an educational experience for me. I learned about the medical publishing industry, the process of dealing with multiple contributors, and the necessity of good organizational skills. I also learned that having a coauthor to motivate, support, and challenge is not a luxury; it is a necessity. *Pediatric Transillumination* (11) was released in 1983. Perhaps it was not the best timing because it was overshadowed by the newer, more glamorous imaging modalities, computed tomography and ultrasonography. Still, it is one of the only reference sources on diagnostic transillumination of the newborn.

Into the Future

The technologic advances of the 1990s have expanded the applications of light in medicine. Many devices now in use, such as pulse oximeters, use light to detect changes in physiologic states. Fiberoptic cables enable the use of light as a signal carrier, producing a "cleaner" signal. Therapeutic uses of light also have increased dramatically. In addition to phototherapy, lasers have been added to the treatment of several neonatal diseases, such as retinopathy of prematurity and arteriovenous malformations. Light beyond the visible spectrum also is used as a diagnostic source. In the immediate future, near-infrared spectroscopy, for example, may answer many questions about cerebral blood flow and metabolism.

Although ultrasonography and magnetic resonance imaging largely have replaced transillumination as the gold standards of neonatal diagnosis, there is still a place for the transilluminator in the NICU. Thoracic air leaks and abdominal perforations still occur and require immediate diagnosis and treatment. Babies still require vascular access, and "seeing is believing." Today, when I see young house officers transilluminating a newborn's chest, it seems so matter of fact. I often wonder if they have any concept of how it all started. Maybe I need to show them the light.

Steven M. Donn, MD, FAAP
Professor of Pediatrics
Director, Division of Neonatal-Perinatal Medicine
C.S. Mott Children's Hospital
University of Michigan Health System
Ann Arbor, Mich.

[To read the original article on the use of transillumination for diagnosing pneumothorax, published in 1975, please go to: http://neoreviews.aappublications.org/cgi/content/full/6/3/e112/DC1 or http://pediatrics.aappublications.org/cgi/content/abstract/5/6/3/355]

References

1. Kuhns LR, Bednarek FJ, Wyman ML, et al. Diagnosis of pneumothorax or pneumomediastinum in the neonate by transillumination. *Pediatrics.* 1975; 56:355–360

2. Uy J, Kuhns LR, Wall PM, et al. Light filtration during transillumination of the neonate: a method to reduce heat buildup in the skin. *Pediatrics.* 1976;60: 308–312

3. Wyman ML, Kuhns LR. Accuracy of transillumination in the recognition of pneumothorax and pneumomediastinum in the neonate. *Clin Pediatr.* 1977; 16:323–324

4. Cabatu EE, Brown EG. Thoracic trans-illumination: aid in the diagnosis and treatment of pneumopericardium. *Pediatrics.* 1979;64:958–960

5. Buck JR, Weintraub WW, Coran AG, et al. Fiberoptic transillumination: a new tool for the pediatric surgeon. *J Pediatr Surg.* 1997;12:451–463

6. Wall PM, Kuhns LR. Percutaneous arterial sampling using transillumination. *Pediatrics.* 1977;59(suppl):1032–1035

7. Pearse RG. Percutaneous catheterisation of the radial artery in newborn babies using transillumination. *Arch Dis Child.* 1978;53:549–554

8. Cole FS, Todres ID, Shannon DC. Technique for percutaneous cannulation of the radial artery in the newborn infant. *J Pediatr.* 1978;92:105–107

9. Feldman BH. Arterial cannulation in the newborn infant. *J Pediatr.* 1978; 93:161–162

10. Martin AJ, Kuhns LR, Gutowski D, et al. Production of a permanent radiographic record of transillumination of the neonate. *Radiology.* 1977;122: 540–541

11. Donn SM, Kuhns LR. *Pediatric Transillumination.* Chicago, Ill: Year Book Medical Publishers, Inc; 1983

Historical Perspectives: Neonatal Transillumination
Steven M. Donn
NeoReviews 2005;6;e112-e114
DOI: 10.1542/neo.6-3-e112

A Look Back: The Clinical Initiation of Pharmacologic Closure of Patent Ductus Arteriosus in the Preterm Infant

Pharmacologic Closure of Patent Ductus Arteriosus

Manipulation of the ductus arteriosus with pharmacologic agents has played an important role in neonatology during the past 30 years or so. Not only was closure considered to be important, primarily in substantially preterm infants, but maintaining patency of the ductus arteriosus with prostaglandin E has been a life-saving strategy for certain forms of congenital heart diseases (1).

One of the most interesting (to me) facts about the introduction of pharmacologic closure of patent ductus arteriousus (PDA) is that there was a 10-fold difference in the dose of indomethacin described in the two studies published in 1976, which are described by Dr Friedman. It is rather remarkable that more side effects were not observed by Friedman and colleagues using the higher dose. As smaller and smaller infants have been treated, the potential for side effects has appreciated increasingly.

At the present time, caution is advised when trying to close the ductus arteriosus in very preterm infants (2). It is suggested that a large number of PDAs will close spontaneously. Indomethacin is not without toxicity, primarily due to decreased renal blood flow and urine output, but also decreased blood flow to the gut. On the other hand, evidence supports the use of low-dose indomethacin to minimize severe intraventricular hemorrhage and reduce the incidence of PDA in very-low-birthweight infants.

Alistair G. S. Philip, MD, FRCPE, FAAP
Editor-in-Chief, NeoReviews

References

1. Elliot RA, Starling MB, Neutze JM. Medical manipulation of the ductus arteriosus. *Lancet.* 1975,i:140–142
2. Gien J. Contoversies in the management of patent ductus arteriosus. *NeoReviews.* 2008,9:e477–e482

Introduction

When pharmacologic closure of patent ductus arteriosus (PDA) using indomethacin in the preterm infant was introduced in 1976, there was a paucity of knowledge about the factors controlling the caliber of the ductus arteriosus both before and after birth. Additionally, mortality and morbidity of prematurity (associated with what was then usually referred to as hyaline membrane disease) was remarkably high in the early 1970s.

As early as the 1950s, some neonatologists recognized PDA as a complication of what later became designated as "respiratory distress syndrome" (RDS), although it was not until the advent of intermittent mandatory ventilation (IMV) and continuous positive airway pressure (CPAP) that the concept gained prominence. Patency of the ductus appeared to be a major complication, especially in the smallest of preterm babies (at that time, < 1,350 g]) and usually carried a terminal prognosis. The advent of IMV and CPAP kept these small babies alive for a sufficient period of time for the patent ductus to become recognized progressively as a distinct clinical entity and an important early complication of preterm birth. Observant neonatologists noted that babies who had RDS often improved up to a point, beyond which they worsened. The usual story was that the baby experienced ventilatory failure, was treated with mechanical ventilation, and began to improve, with lower inspired oxygen requirements. After a few days, when discussions ensued about taking the baby off the ventilator, the infant's improvement would cease. The radiographic picture changed from a clearing of the initial ground glass appearance coupled with a relatively small heart to an enlarging heart and the pulmonary edema of congestive heart failure due to a left-to-right shunt across the PDA.

Operative Closure

Beginning in the mid-1960s, aggressive surgeons advocated operative closure of the PDA in these small preterm infants, but multiple centers consistently reported unacceptably high postoperative morbidity and mortality rates. In more than a dozen series from 1974 to 1977, the mortality rates after surgical ligation varied from 21% to 70%; significant morbidity was seen in the surviving infants. In the early 1970s, it was not unusual for neonatal intensive care units to report a mortality of 70% for infants weighing less than 1,000 g, whether or not the ductus was ligated or medical management was attempted with fluid restriction, maintenance of hematocrit, diuretics, and digitalis. Infants weighing 1,001 to 1,350 g fared little better. More aggressive approaches to ventilatory intervention reduced this mortality, although these infants still required prolonged ventilatory management. However, a relationship between bronchopulmonary dysplasia and positive pressure ventilation with high inspired oxygen concentrations was recognized at that time.

Pathophysiology of PDA

Also in the 1970s, laboratory efforts to understand the pathophysiology and clinical approaches to detect patency of the ductus more accurately were underway. The latter employed sequential assessment of pulmonary surfactant maturity, pulmonary vascular resistance as reflected by echocardiographically derived right ventricular systolic time intervals, left atrial-to-aortic root dimension ratios, and serial chest radiographs in seeking to establish the dynamic relationships between the pulmonary and systemic vascular circuits and differentiate the contribution to RDS of surfactant deficiency from that of pulmonary hyperperfusion. All of these efforts sought to define the relative contributions of the altered hemodynamics due to a PDA, in addition to surfactant deficiency or developmental immaturity, on the clinical condition of these infants.

Until the 1970s, it was assumed that the ductus arteriosus was a passively open channel during fetal life and that it constricted postnatally by undefined molecular mechanisms in response to the abrupt rise in arterial Po_2 that accompanies the first breath after birth. Many decades earlier, classic guinea pig experiments showed the initial and reversible stimulus of increased arterial oxygen concentration to smooth muscle contraction and resultant closure of the PDA. (1) The greatly increased incidence of PDA in human neonates born at high altitudes also supported the concept that oxygen played a role in determining the caliber of the ductus arteriosus. Rudolph and associates showed that responsiveness of the ductus arteriosus to increased oxygen increases with gestational age. Studies of isolated PDA strips demonstrated that the oxygen response was not affected by blocking the actions of acetylcholine or norepinephrine, the neurotransmitters of the parasympathetic and sympathetic nervous systems, respectively. Results of subsequent experiments focusing on the role of the autonomic nervous system in modulating normal closure of the PDA were inconclusive or contradictory. (2) Other studies showed that the response of the PDA to oxygen was modified or eliminated by altering cyclic nucleotides and intracellular calcium levels.

The first suggestion that prostaglandins (PGs) played a role in ductus physiology was made in 1972 when Starling and Elliott showed in puppies and calves that exogenous PGF_2-alpha caused closure of the ductus arteriosus. (3) In these experiments, high arterial oxygen saturation was required to maintain the PGF_2-alpha response. PGE_2 dilated the ductus arteriosus, and inhibitors of prostaglandin synthesis reduced the PGF_2-alpha responses in a high-oxygen environment. Later, whole animal freezing experiments on fetal rodents and rabbits demonstrated that PG synthesis inhibition resulted in PDA constriction. (4) When I heard a presentation of

these latter findings at a national meeting, I immediately considered the possibility of employing a pharmacologic approach to closure of the PDA in preterm infants. First, however, I took the idea to my basic science laboratories.

Fetal Lamb Studies

Beginning in the mid-1960s, my laboratory had a major investment in studying the physiologic, pharmacologic, biochemical, and ultrastructural properties of the developing heart. Our studies on cardiac muscle and whole heart isolated from the fetal and newborn lamb and adult sheep had revealed striking age-dependent differences in cardiac mechanics, the compliance characteristics of both ventricles, myocardial energetics, and the development of myocardial autonomic control as well as major ultrastructural alterations as the heart developed from fetal to adult life. (5) After I moved in 1968 from the National Heart Institute in Bethesda, Maryland, to help start the new medical school at the University of California, San Diego, Dr Abraham Rudolph at the University of California, San Francisco, a pioneer and leader in the field of fetal physiology, graciously accepted my request to teach me the techniques necessary to instrument the fetal lamb chronically.

After days as a house guest of the Rudolphs and taking copious notes watching Abe insert a variety of catheters and flow meters in the intact fetal lamb in his laboratory, I returned to San Diego. We then developed methods for examining left ventricular function in the chronically instrumented fetal lamb. (6) Thus, we could continuously monitor internal left ventricular dimensions and pressures in the fully recovered, intact, undisturbed fetus in utero without the need for anesthesia. Previous studies of cardiac performance in the fetus would have been derived from acute exteriorized fetal lamb experiments. Our approach avoided the multiple problems associated with anesthesia, acute experimentation, and their confounding effects on the fragile fetus. The sonocardiometry methods we employed in these studies placed tiny piezoelectric crystals opposite one another on the endocardial surface of the left ventricle, which were excited

with a burst of energy. The time required for each ultrasonic burst to pass from one transducer to the other was converted to a voltage, and because sound velocity in blood is known, the voltage readings could be converted into a distance, allowing continuous assessment of ventricular dimensions. Placing these crystals across the PDA of the sheep fetus was a much simpler task than inserting them onto the endocardial surface of the left ventricle, and in some preliminary experiments in which ductus dimensions thereby were monitored continuously, we administered dissolved 100-mg capsules of indomethacin by suppositories to the pregnant ewes. Rapid major constriction of the fetal ductus arteriosus was obvious. My colleagues and I subsequently published many articles using the chronically instrumented fetal lamb ductus approach as well as studies of the PG biochemistry of homogenates of the fetal ductus arteriosus, lung, and other vessels in an effort to understand the mechanisms of vasodilatation and vasoconstriction of the ductus arteriosus. (7)(8)

Clinical Studies

Armed with evidence that inhibition of PG synthesis by indomethacin was a powerful constrictor of the fetal ductus arteriosus, we formulated a compelling request to the University's Institutional Review Board to attempt medical closure of the PDA in small, at-risk preterm infants who had RDS. We received permission to administer indomethacin orally or via suppository in such infants who otherwise would have undergone surgical ligation. However, we had to overcome a major turf issue. Louis Gluck, the remarkable neonatologist who pioneered the concept and development of neonatal intensive care units, objected to anyone but his division's faculty participating in direct management of "his" nursery patients, except as consultants. Fortunately, we enjoyed mutual respect as faculty colleagues, but it still took my threat to accuse him of interfering with academic freedom before the first baby was given indomethacin. The details of this initial clinical trial can be found in our article in the *New England Journal of Medicine*. (9) In six consecutive infants, we observed dramatic clinical improvement within 24 hours of indomethacin administration, extubation was achieved without difficulty, and all physical findings attributed to PDA and heart failure promptly disappeared. We had used high doses of indomethacin in this first group of infants, two of whom experienced transient renal dysfunction.

We were convinced that the findings strongly suggested the need for further studies of inhibition of the synthesis of PGs to close the PDAs of preterm infants; the extremely high morbidity and mortality seen in infants who had RDS and PDA provided abundant justification to pursue nonsurgical methods to alter the course of this common complication of preterm birth. In our later studies of more than 150 infants in whom indomethacin was employed for ductal closure, we reported detailed analyses of the organ system effects of this form of treatment as well as clinical outcomes; comparisons of indomethacin treatment with ligation; and the longitudinal assessment of psychomotor development, postnatal growth, and vision and hearing. (10)(11) We also worked successfully with Merck, Sharpe and Dome and the United States Food and Drug Administration to justify and make available an intravenous preparation of indomethacin that would allow precise dosing in preterm babies, and we participated in the national collaborative controlled trial funded by the National Institutes of Health, which further validated the pharmacologic approach to PDA closure in preterm infants. (12)

An Aside

There is an interesting side story to our publication in the *New England Journal of Medicine* of the first clinical application of pharmacologic closure. Immediately after our success with the first six infants in the UC San Diego nurseries, I wrote the article that was submitted. After a relatively short review period, the *Journal* accepted the article for publication without the necessity for changes in the manuscript. When I received this notification, I called Dr Abraham Rudolph at UC, San Francisco, who earlier had so willingly taught me chronic instrumentation techniques to access the fetal circulation, and who had a long and abiding interest in the physiology of the ductus arteriosus. I told him that we had a paper accepted by the *New England Journal* on using indomethacin to close the PDA in "preemies" who had RDS and asked if he had thought of attempting a similar approach. He told me that he and his associate, Dr Michael Heymann, had been applying this same treatment to babies in their nurseries. I asked him how long it would take them to prepare a manuscript of their experience, and he replied that they could rapidly put their findings into manuscript form. I then called Dr Arnold Relman, then editor of the *New England Journal of Medicine*, and asked if he would defer publication of my article until receiving the manuscript from Drs Rudolph and Heymann. I asked only that if the San Francisco manuscript was judged suitable for publication in the *Journal* that my article appear first and theirs second, and he was agreeable to this arrangement. I called Abe Rudolph back and gave him this news. He and Mike Heymann promptly wrote and submitted their manuscript and, indeed, the San Diego and San Francisco (13) manuscripts soon appeared back-to-back in the same issue of the *New England Journal of Medicine*. Drs Rudolph, Heymann, and I then collaborated on an article for the *Journal of Pediatrics* (14) in which we updated our experience and reported additional preliminary experimental data. We also proposed a dosage regimen using the smaller doses initially employed by the San Francisco group. They continue to be used to this day and avoid the problems of serious renal dysfunction.

Conclusion

In retrospect, it appears fair to say that permission to pursue human experimentation was less difficult to accomplish almost 30 years ago than it is today, but the upshot of our going forward to administer indomethacin to these preterm babies resulted in an explosion of both basic and clinical investigations in laboratories and nurseries around the world. Further, countless young infants have been spared the necessity of a surgical approach to a cardiovascular problem. It is also true that an untold number of these little patients are alive today as a result of this and subsequent advances to the field, particularly the introduction of surfactant therapy. What I am not a sufficiently facile writer to indicate in this brief reminiscence is the great excitement and fun it was to participate in the many subsequent basic science and clinical studies that suggested themselves after this introduction of a new and novel clinical approach to improving the outlook for the most fragile of pediatric patients.

William F. Friedman, MD
J.H. Nicholson Professor of Pediatrics
(Cardiology)
Chairman Emeritus
Department of Pediatrics
Senior Associate Dean for Academic Affairs
David Geffen School of Medicine at UCLA
Los Angeles, CA

EDITOR'S NOTE: For current thoughts on pharmacologic closure of PDA, see the August, 2003 issue of *NeoReviews*.

[To read the original article on pharmacologic closure of PDA written by Dr Friedman and colleagues in 1976, which was reprinted with permission from the New England Journal of Medicine and copyrighted by the Massachusetts Medical Society, please go to: http://neoreviews.aappublications.org/cgi/content/full/4/10/e259/DC1]

References

1. Kennedy JA, Clark SL. Observations on the ductus arteriosus of the guinea pig in relation to its method of closure. *Anat Rec.* 1941;79:349

2. Heymann MA, Rudolph AM. Control of the ductus arteriosus. *Physiol Rev.* 1975;55:62–78

3. Starling MB, Elliot RB. The effects of prostaglandins, prostaglandin inhibitors and oxygen on the closure of the ductus arteriosus, pulmonary arteries, and umbilical vessels in vitro. *Prostaglandins.* 1974;8:187–203

4. Sharpe GL, Larsson KS, ThalmeB.Studies on closure of the ductus arteriosus. XII. In utero effects of indomethacin and sodium salicylate in rats and rabbits. *Prostaglandins.* 1975;9:585–596

5. Friedman WF. The intrinsic physiologic properties of the developing heart. *Progr Cardiovasc Dis.* 1972;15:87–111

6. Kirkpatrick SE, Covell JW, Friedman WF. A new technique for the continuous assessment of fetal and neonatal cardiac performance. *Am J Obstet Gynecol.* 1973;116:963–972

7. Friedman WF, Printz MP, Kirkpatrick SE, Hoskins EJ. The vasoactivity of the fetal lamb ductus arteriosus studied in utero. *Pediatr Res.* 1983;17:331–337

8. Skidgel RA, Friedman WF, Printz MP. Prostaglandin biosynthetic activities of the fetal lamb ductus arteriosus, other blood vessels and lung tissue. *Pediatr Res.* 1984;18:12–18

9. Friedman WF, Hirschklau MJ, Printz MP, Pitlick PT, Kirkpatrick SE. Pharmacological closure of patent ductus arteriosus in the premature infant. *N Engl J Med.* 1976;295:526–529

10. Merritt TA, DiSessa TG, Feldman BH, Kirkpatrick SE, Gluck I, Friedman WF. Closure of the patent ductus arteriosus with ligation and indomethacin: a consecutive experience. *J Pediatr.* 1978;93:639–646

11. Merritt TA, White CL, Coen RW, Friedman WF, Gluck L, Rosenberg M. Preschool assessment of infants with a patent ductus arteriosus: comparison of ligation and indomethacin therapy. *Am J Dis Child.* 1982;136:507–512

12. Gersony WM, Peckham GJ, Ellison RC, Miettinen OS, Nadas AS. Effects of indomethacin in premature infants with patent ductus arteriosus: results of a national collaborative study. *J Pediatr.* 1983;102:895–906

13. Heymann MA, Rudolph AM, Silverman NH. Closure of the ductus arteriosus in premature infants by inhibition of prostaglandin synthesis. *N Engl J Med.* 1976;295:530–533

14. Friedman WF, Heymann MA, Rudolph AM. Commentary: new thoughts on an old problem–patent ductus arteriosus in the premature infant. *J Pediatr.* 1977;90:338–340

Historical Perspectives: A Look Back: The Clinical Initiation of Pharmacologic Closure of Patent Ductus Arteriosus in the Preterm Infant

William F. Friedman

NeoReviews 2003;4;259

DOI: 10.1542/neo.4-10-e259

Fetal Blood Sampling

Several dramatic advances in maternal-fetal medicine were seen in the 1970s, and not all were immediately accepted in the United States or elsewhere. Antepartum glucocorticoid treatment to prevent respiratory distress syndrome (see Liggins 1972, p. 93–94); prevention of Rhesus incompatibility (see Bowman 1978, p. 124–127); assessment of fetal lung maturity (see Spellacy 1971, p. 86–88); and fetal blood sampling all emerged in this decade. Suddenly, the fetus became "accessible" and the handful of obstetricians who specialized in maternal-fetal medicine spawned a whole new generation of obstetricians interested in the fetus. The American Society for Maternal-Fetal Medicine was founded in 1977.

In actuality, there were two different kinds of fetal blood sampling. The first was used to evaluate the fetus during pregnancy, initially to follow cases of Rhesus incompatibility and to detect hemoglobinopathies, and later to detect or assess the status of the fetus in other suspected disorders, such as chromosomal abnormalities and intrauterine growth restriction. Blood sampling was from the umbilical cord close to its insertion into the placenta. In the United Kingdom (and Europe), it was generally referred to as "cordocentesis," while in the United States, it was usually referred to as "percutaneous umbilical blood sampling" or "PUBS."

The second kind of fetal blood sampling was performed during labor in the form of fetal scalp blood sampling, to evaluate for asphyxia, and was pioneered by Professor Erich Saling in Berlin, Germany, with results published as early as 1962. This latter technique never gained strong support in the United States, but it was used successfully in some centers. Currently, fetal scalp pH measurement seems to have been replaced by lactate measurements in parts of Europe. The literature on fetal scalp blood sampling has been comparatively sparse in the last decade. As noted in this 2004 Historical Perspective by Professor Charles Rodeck, the use of cordocentesis (or PUBS) has also declined in recent years because of other recent technical advances.

Alistair G. S. Philip, MD, FRCPE, FAAP
Editor-in-Chief, NeoReviews

Reference

1. Saling E. Fetal scalp blood sampling. *Am J Obstet Gynecol.* 2006;194:896–899

Introduction

In 1975, I was a clinical lecturer at King's College Hospital Medical School, trying to organize a major study on fetal monitoring without much success. The following year, Stuart Campbell moved to King's as head of department and asked what were my interests. Here was an opportunity to drop the fetal monitoring project! I said I was interested in more direct access to the fetus, such as fetoscopy, and asked if he thought it had a future. His friend John Hobbins at Yale was doing some work in that area, and he suggested that I visit and look into it. I had a very enjoyable 2 weeks there in September 1976, observed two cases, and returned to England with a Dyonics Needlescope in my luggage.

Early Approaches

Dyonics was a small company in Woburn near New Haven, Connecticut, and the Needlescope was a 1.7-mm diameter modified arthroscope. It made fetoscopy a clinical possibility because it could be introduced percutaneously under local anesthesia and on an outpatient basis. Previous attempts at fetoscopy by Valenti, (1) Scrimgeour, (2) and others used larger diameter endoscopes and required a laparotomy—an approach that never entered clinical practice. The Needlescope was used by several groups in North America, including Hobbins at Yale, Benzie in Toronto, and Perry in Montreal. Hobbins and Mahoney (3) reported a technique for obtaining fetal blood in 1974, but it had some drawbacks. It could be used only if the placenta was posterior because the risks of perforating an anterior placenta (eg, fetal bleeding and placental separation) were deemed to be too high. Also, the samples obtained usually consisted of a mixture of fetal red cells, amniotic fluid, and sometimes maternal blood. They were taken by passing a 27-gauge needle down the side channel of the cannula, puncturing a fetal vessel on the chorionic plate of the posterior placenta under direct vision, and aspirating while pulling the tip back into the amniotic fluid. Such mixed samples usually were adequate for prenatal diagnosis of hemoglobinopathies because the diagnosis was based on globin chain production by the fetal reticulocytes.

Placentacentesis was another method of obtaining fetal red cells for prenatal diagnosis of hemoglobinopathies that was being used by the San Francisco group (4) and a collaboration of teams from Boston and University College London. The aim was to introduce a needle into the placenta, usually "blindly" (ie, without ultrasonographic guidance), and to perforate fetal vessels on the chorionic plate. This procedure made the anterior placenta amenable to sampling, but the aspirates usually were less suitable for diagnosis than those obtained by the Hobbins and Mahoney technique. In approximately 15% of cases, the number of fetal red cells was inadequate and the procedure had to be repeated. Furthermore, there was a 10% fetal mortality rate due to exsanguination. As fetoscopy became more widespread, most centers abandoned placentacentesis.

Ultrasonographically Guided Fetoscopy

At King's, we decided to focus on fetoscopy and to make it an ultrasonographically guided procedure, using the recent advances in real-time ultrasonography. One of our motivations was prenatal diagnosis of the hemoglobinopathies because the immigrant population in South London provided the highest concentration of the sickle cell gene in Europe. In addition, we had a hemophilia center and were interested in diagnosing severe hemophilia prenatally. To do this, we had to obtain uncontaminated fetal plasma in which coagulation had not been initiated. The samples obtained with the then current techniques would not suffice.

Thus, we had two goals: 1) to use fetoscopy whether the placenta was anterior or posterior and 2) to obtain pure fetal blood every time. We began with patients who were having second-trimester termination of pregnancy; they received intra-amniotic prostaglandins after the fetoscopy, which initially was performed under general anesthesia. Every week I carried an ADR realtime scanner to nearby Dulwich Hospital, which was the location of our gynecology department. The anesthetist cynically observed that the fetoscope was another gadget doomed to be discarded on the surgical scrap heap!

Breaking the Rules

To achieve our two goals we had to break two cardinal rules. The first was "Keep to the midline," which was based on the possibility of the trocar in a lateral approach damaging bowel or major uterine vessels. However, to avoid perforating an extensive anterior placenta, an extremely lateral entry into the uterus frequently had to be used. In my experience of some 2,000 fetoscopies, there never were any maternal complications. The puncture site was selected with great care using ultrasonography. By 18 weeks' gestation, the uterus had pushed bowel aside, and the major vessels were too deep in the pelvis. Readiness to adopt a lateral approach combined with careful ultrasonographic planning and selection of the entry point enabled the safe use of the fetoscope whatever the placental site.

The second rule that we broke was "Don't touch the cord." It was believed that this was dangerous because of the likelihood of bleeding or umbilical vessel spasm. The first time I broke this taboo and punctured a vessel at the base of the cord, the choice was either to touch the cord or not to obtain a sample, thereby failing to make a diagnosis for the patient. The problem had been that puncturing chorionic plate vessels (the Hobbins/

Mahoney technique) was difficult when the placenta was anterior and the fetoscope entry was lateral. The view was across the surface of the chorionic plate, and the vessels could not be seen readily; conversely, the cord insertion stood out like a beacon. The vessels had acquired a white covering, the Wharton's jelly, so that they lost some of their color, but they were, of course, larger, and it still was possible to distinguish umbilical arteries from vein. It was with some trepidation that I plunged the tip of the 27-gauge needle into a vessel at the base of the cord. There was no hint of spasm! Furthermore, pure fetal blood was aspirated into the 1-mL syringe far more easily and quickly than from chorionic plate vessels, and after withdrawal of the needle, there was much less bleeding into the amniotic fluid. The Wharton's jelly closed the puncture hole and acted as a hemostat.

New Diagnostic Possibilities

It rapidly became clear that this was a reliable and safe technique. (5)(6) The ease of aspiration of fetal blood meant that coagulation was not initiated during the process. Further, Reuben Mibashan, director of our Haemophilia Centre, could perform accurate coagulant assays for factors VIII and IX (7) as well as other factors on 100-mcL aliquots. It also was clear that 4 to 5 mL of blood could be taken from a fetus at 20 weeks' gestation without causing any harm.

It was not long before six to eight patients a week were coming for prenatal diagnosis of hemoglobinopathies and hemophilia A and B from all over Europe and further afield. Other diagnostic possibilities became possible using fetal red cells, white cells, platelets, and plasma. Normal physiologic ranges could be studied and differences between umbilical artery and vein blood documented. New diagnostic procedures, such as fetal skin and liver biopsy, were performed fetoscopically, as were the first successful percutaneous intravascular fetal transfusions. The latter transformed the prognosis for fetuses that had early severe hydropic hemolytic disease. We felt the age of fetal medicine had dawned! (8)(9)

Further Changes

Change has been rapid, largely due to improvements in ultrasonographic technology. Fetoscopy was an ultrasonographically guided procedure, but the final placement of the needle was performed under direct endoscopic vision. In the early 1980s, ultrasonographic equipment enabled the needle to be guided solely by ultrasonography. (10)(11) By the mid-1980s, all centers were taking fetal blood by ultrasonographic guidance. It was easier to perform, less invasive than fetoscopy, and led to a further increase in the number of physicians capable of performing the procedure, the indications for the procedure, and the number of patients undergoing it.

Since the heyday of fetal blood sampling in the 1990s, there has been a steep decline in its use. The reasons for this include better noninvasive assessment of fetal anemia and intrauterine growth restriction (by Doppler ultrasonography); molecular techniques for the prenatal diagnosis of genetic diseases (by chorionic villus sampling), fetal rhesus genotyping, and fetal infection; and above all, polymerase chain reaction for chromosome analysis on amniotic fluid. In most fetal medicine units, fetal blood sampling has become sufficiently infrequent to make it impossible to give all trainees a practical experience and even to maintain the skills of experts. It is vital not to lose this expertise entirely because therapeutic interventions such as fetal gene or stem cell therapy in the future may require access to the fetal vascular compartment. (12)

Professor Charles H. Rodeck
Department of Obstetrics and Gynaecology
Royal Free and University College Medical School
University College London
London, England

[To read the original article describing fetal blood sampling by fetoscopy written by Rodeck and Campbell in 1978 and reprinted with permission from the *British Medical Journal*, please go to: http://neoreviews.aap publications.org/cgi/content/full/5/6/e229/DC1]

References

1. Valenti C. Endoamnioscopy and fetal biopsy: a new technique. *Am J Obstet Gynecol.* 1972;114:561–564

2. Scrimgeour JB. Other techniques for antenatal diagnosis. In: Emery AEH, ed. *Antenatal Diagnosis of Genetic Disease.* New York, NY: Churchill Livingstone; 1973:41–57

3. Hobbins JC, Mahoney MJ. In utero diagnosis of hemoglobinopathies: technic for obtaining fetal blood. *N Engl J Med.* 1974;290:1065–1067

4. Kan YW, Valenti C, Guidotti R, Carnazza V, Reider RF. Fetal blood sampling in utero. *Lancet.* 1974;i:79–80

5. Rodeck CH, Campbell S. Sampling pure fetal blood by fetoscopy in second trimester of pregnancy. *Br Med J.* 1978;2:728–730

6. Rodeck CH, Campbell S. Umbilical cord insertion as source of pure fetal blood for prenatal diagnosis. *Lancet.* 1979;i:1244–1245

7. Mibashan RS, Rodeck CH, Thumpston JK, et al. Plasma assay of fetal factors VIII C and IX for prenatal diagnosis of haemophilia. *Lancet.* 1979;i:1309–1311

8. Rodeck CH, Nicolaides KH. Fetoscopy and fetal tissue sampling. *Br Med Bull.* 1983;39:332–337

9. Rodeck CH. An intrauterine odyssey. *Yearbook Obstet Gynaecol.* 2002; 10:26–41

10. Bang J, Bock JE, Trolle D. Ultrasound guided fetal intravenous transfusion for severe rhesus haemolytic disease. *Br Med J.* 1982;284:373–374

11. Daffos F, Capella-Pavlovsky M, Forestier F. Fetal blood sampling via the umbilical cord using a needle guided by ultrasound. Report of 66 cases. *Prenat Diagn.* 1983;3:271–277

12. David AL, Themis M, Waddington SN, et al. The current status and future direction of fetal gene therapy. *Gene Ther Molec Biol.* 2003;7:181–209

Historical Perspectives: Fetal Blood Sampling

Charles H. Rodeck

NeoReviews 2004;5;e229-e231

DOI: 10.1542/neo.5-6-e229

Prevention of Rh Hemolytic Disease of the Newborn

Introduction

The accompanying 2002 article by Dr. John Bowman was contributed in response to a request to place his important paper (1) into context. Dr. Bowman is the former Medical Director of the Winnipeg Rh Laboratory and a Distinguished Professor Emeritus at the University of Manitoba. Although not the first to describe the use of Rh immune globulin, the clinicians in Winnipeg were leaders in the use of antenatal prophylaxis. At present, Rh isoimmunization is extremely rare, in large measure because of the pioneers described by Dr. Bowman. Antenatal administration of anti-D immune globulin now is "standard operating procedure," but this was not always the case. It is important to understand how the problem of Rh isoimmunization has been virtually eliminated from neonatal practice.

Alistair G. S. Philip, MD, FRCPE, FAAP
Editor-in-Chief, NeoReviews

Reference

1. Bowman JM, Chown B, Lewis M, Pollock JM. Rh isoimmunization during pregnancy: antenatal prophylaxis. *Can Med Assoc J.* 1978;118:623–627

Addressing Rh Hemolytic Disease of the Newborn

Rh hemolytic disease was reported initially by a French midwife in 1609. She described the birth of twins: the first, who was pale and bloated with fluid (hydrops fetalis), died within minutes of birth; the second, in much better condition, became deeply jaundiced in the first 3 days after birth, developed rigidity, lay in a position of opisthotonus (kernicterus), and died on the fourth day after birth.

Hydrops fetalis and kernicterus were not linked again until 323 years later. In 1932, Diamond and associates determined that they were simply different aspects of a spectrum representing the same disorder. The more severe, hydrops, was characterized by hemolysis of fetal red blood cells that produced severe anemia, followed by hepatosplenomegaly, extramedullary erythropoiesis, and the outpouring of immature nucleated fetal red cells, from which Diamond coined the diagnostic term "erythroblastosis fetalis."

Uncovering the cause of the fetal red blood cell hemolysis had to await the discovery of the Rh blood group system by Landsteiner and Wiener in 1940 and the subsequent determination in 1941 by Levine that the cause of hemolytic disease was the exposure of an Rh(D)-negative woman to fetal Rh(D)-positive red cells. Her body developed an immunoglobulin (Ig)G Rh(D) antibody that traversed the placenta from mother to fetus, causing subsequent fetal red blood cell hemolysis that set in motion the mechanism leading to hydrops or kernicterus.

Before 1945, the mortality rate from hemolytic disease of the newborn was 50%, evenly divided between kernicterus and hydrops. In the Province of Manitoba (population 1 million), there were 90 to 100 deaths from Rh hemolytic disease each year (10% of all perinatal deaths). Extrapolating to the United States, in the same era, Rh hemolytic disease caused approximately 15,000 perinatal deaths annually.

With the introduction of exchange transfusion by Wallerstein in 1945, perinatal mortality was halved. Following the introduction of induced early delivery by Chown in 1951, perinatal mortality was further reduced to 16%. Additional management measures, including amniotic fluid spectrophotometry (Liley, 1961), intraperitoneal blood transfusion (Liley, 1963), periumbilical blood sampling (Daffos, 1981), and intravascular fetal transfusion (Rodeck, 1981; Beck, 1982), reduced perinatal mortality to about 3% in highly skilled perinatal management units.

Further reductions in perinatal mortality from Rh hemolytic disease required the development of a means of preventing maternal Rh immunization.

The Scientific Basis of Rh Immunization Prevention

In 1900, Von Dungern (1) conducted what certainly had to be considered, at the time, a most completely nonapplied basic scientific experiment. He injected ox red blood cells into a group of rabbits. The rabbits obligingly produced ox red blood cell antibodies. He then injected a second group of rabbits with the same ox red blood cells (antigen), followed by an injection of serum from the first group of rabbits (antibody). The second group of rabbits did not develop ox red blood cell antibodies. Thus, Von Dungern proved the axiom that the presence of passive antibodies to an antigen prevents active immunization to the antigen. There are two provisos to this axiom: passive antibody must be present before active immunization has begun, and an adequate amount of passive antibody must be present.

One might have thought that Landsteiner, a contemporary of Von Dungern and surely familiar with the German literature, would have realized, following Levine's application of his and Wiener's discovery of the Rh system, that Rh immunization was preventable. In fact, almost 25 years elapsed before Von Dungern's experiment was put to practical use.

Rh Immunization Prevention Trials

Almost simultaneously, Freda, Gorman, and Pollack (2) in New York and New Jersey and Clarke and colleagues (3) in Liverpool, England, began work on Rh prevention. Clarke initially used high-titer Rh plasma; the United States researchers always used a gamma globulin produced from plasma with a very high Rh(D) antibody content (anti-DIgG). In the United States, anti-DIgG was licensed for Rh prophylaxis on July 1, 1968.

The Western Canada Clinical Trial

Very shortly after the work began in New York and Liverpool, Zipursky and Chown began similar experiments in Winnipeg, Canada. Initially, Rh(D)-negative male volunteers were injected with Rh(D)-positive red blood cells, followed by Rh(D) antibody in the form of Rh immune globulin (anti-DIgG). This experiment, which documented protection against Rh immunization, was followed by a clinical trial, coordinated by Chown, in Rh(D)-negative women in Western Canada. (4) In the trial, women delivering Rh(D)-positive babies who had no evidence of Rh immunization were given anti-DIgG in doses varying from 145 to 435 mcg within 3 days after delivery. Among the 1,216 women treated in this manner, none had evidence of Rh immunization 6 months after delivery. Of 500 exactly similar women not given anti-DIgG, 36 (7.2%) showed evidence of Rh immunization within 6 months after delivery.

On the basis of this clinical trial, Rh immune globulin for Rh prophylaxis in Canada was licensed in December 1968. Again, it is almost certain that anti-DIgG always will prevent Rh immunization if it is administered in adequate doses before active Rh immunization has begun. Because a 300-mcg dose was selected in the United States, this dose was set as the standard in Canada. In many other countries, 100 to 125 mcg is the standard postpartum dose, and it appears to be almost equally effective.

Rh Immunization During Pregnancy

In the Winnipeg part of the Western Canada Clinical Trial, we were surprised to discover that 5 of 210 Rh(D)-negative primiparas given anti-DIgG already were Rh immunized at the time of delivery and were not protected by anti-DIgG administered after delivery. This observation was contrary to the belief that Rh immunization always occurred after delivery. We decided to study this phenomenon further and, if necessary, to embark on a clinical trial of antenatal Rh prophylaxis. (5) Of 3,533 Rh(D)-negative women who began their pregnancies with no evidence of Rh immunization and delivered Rh(D)-positive babies, 62 (1.8%) had evidence of Rh immunization by the time of delivery (5 women [0.14%] before 28 weeks' gestation).

The Antenatal Rh Prophylaxis Trial

In parallel with the previous study, a clinical trial of antenatal Rh prophylaxis was initiated. (5) Exactly similar Rh(D)-negative women due to deliver in two selected Winnipeg hospitals were given 300 mcg of anti-DIgG at 28 weeks and 34 weeks of gestation and after delivery if they delivered Rh(D)-positive babies. Of 1,358 women treated in this manner and delivering Rh(D)-positive babies, one had evidence of Rh immunization at 28 weeks of gestation (a logistic failure rate of 0.07% versus the anticipated rate of 1.8%). The remaining 1,357 women had no evidence of Rh immunization 6 months after delivery, a protection against Rh immunization during pregnancy rate of 96%. On the basis of this study, anti-DIgG was licensed for antenatal administration in Canada on July 1, 1975.

The Antenatal Rh Prophylaxis Service Program

Because of calculations (based on the IgG half-life of about 28 days) that 20 to 30 mcg of anti-DIgG would be present in the maternal circulation 12 weeks after injection of 300 mcg, it was decided that the antenatal Rh prophylaxis service program would consist of only one injection of 300 mcg of anti-DIgG (at 28 weeks' gestation), followed by another injection of 300 mcg 12 weeks later either before or after delivery. (6) Of 1,086 women in this program who delivered Rh(D)-positive babies, two (0.2%) had evidence of Rh immunization at 28 weeks' gestation (the time of injection of anti-DigG) and were considered logistic failures. The remaining 1,084 had no evidence of Rh immunization at 6 months after delivery, with a protection rate of 90% (comparing actual failures with the anticipated rate) and the only failures being logistic failures.

The Grandmother Theory

It has been postulated that the appearance of Rh immunization during pregnancy is due to immunization of the Rh(D)-negative mother in infancy due to the reverse passage of Rh(D)-positive maternal red blood cells into her circulation at the time of her birth. Although there is one well-documented instance of reverse maternal fetal transfusion, (7) reverse maternal fetal hemorrhage plays little or no role in Rh immunization because antenatal Rh prophylaxis is so successful.

Rh Immunization After Abortion

There is a well-documented 2% incidence of Rh immunization following spontaneous abortion, which increases to 4% to 5% after induced abortion. For this reason, all Rh(D)-negative women who abort should be given Rh prophylaxis. If a 50-mcg mini-dose is available, this will provide sufficient protection in the first trimester. An Rh(D)-negative woman who threatens to abort should be given 300 mcg of anti-DigG and the dose repeated every 12 weeks if her pregnancy continues.

Rh Prophylaxis After Amniocentesis

There is a risk for a placenta that is implanted on the anterior uterine wall to be traumatized at amniocentesis, with subsequent fetomaternal hemorrhage. (8) An Rh(D)-negative unimmunized woman undergoing amniocentesis for genetic reasons or to determine fetal pulmonary maturity, therefore, is at risk of fetomaternal hemorrhage and Rh immunization. Although ultrasonographic placental localization reduces the risk, it does not remove it entirely. Such women should receive 300 mcg of anti-DIgG at the time of amniocentesis, with the dose repeated every 12 weeks until delivery.

Massive Fetomaternal Transplacental Hemorrhage

The protective effect of anti-DIgG is dose-dependent. It can prevent Rh immunization

Table 1. Current Rh Prophylaxis Recommendations

1) An Rh(D)-negative unimmunized woman should receive 300 mcg of anti-DIgG intramuscularly (120 mcg intravenously) after delivery of an Rh(D)-positive baby.

2) A similar woman should be given Rh prophylaxis after abortion or threatened abortion unless the father of her conceptus is known to be Rh(D)-negative. If her pregnancy continues, prophylaxis should be repeated every 12 weeks.

3) A similar woman should receive 300 mcg of anti-DIgG after amniocentesis unless the father of her conceptus is known to be Rh(D)-negative. Prophylaxis should be repeated every 12 weeks until delivery.

4) 300 mcg of anti-DIgG should be given at 28 weeks of gestation to every Rh(D)-negative unimmunized woman and repeated in 12 weeks if she has not delivered.

5) If a fetomaternal hemorrhage is greater than 25 mL, 300 mcg of anti-DIgG should be administered for each 25 mL or part thereof in the maternal circulation. If intravenous anti-DIgG is given, the dose is 300 mcg for every 45 mL or part thereof in the maternal circulation.

6) An Rh(D)-negative woman who is Rh immunized, no matter how weak her Rh(D) antibody, will NOT benefit from receipt of anti-DIgG.

7) Anti-DIgG should NOT be given to Rh(D)-negative babies born of Rh(D)-positive mothers.

completely up to an Rh antigen exposure of 1 mL of Rh(D)-positive blood for every 10 mcg of anti-DIgG administered intramuscularly. Thus, the standard dose of 300 mcg protects up to an exposure of 30 mL of Rh(D)-positive blood (15 mL of red blood cells). Experimentally, when 300 mcg of anti-DIgG was administered to Rh(D)-negative male volunteers following injection of 30 to 450 mL of Rh(D)-positive blood, 35% of subjects became Rh immunized. (9) If a fetomaternal hemorrhage exceeds 30 mL of Rh(D)-positive red blood cells, multiple doses of anti-DIgG should be given (Table). If possible, all Rh(D)-negative women should be screened for massive fetomaternal hemorrhage after delivery. However, if this is not possible, it should be noted that only 0.2% of women have a fetomaternal hemorrhage in excess of 30 mL of fetal blood, and only 35% (if Rh(D)-negative and delivering Rh(D)-positive babies) become Rh immunized following a single injection of 300 mcg of anti-DIgG, a failure of protection rate of 0.07% (1 in 1,400).

Attempts to Suppress Rh Immunization

Attempts have been made to suppress weak active Rh immunization by the administration of anti-DIgG during pregnancy. (10) Such attempts have been uniformly unsuccessful, demonstrating that anti-DIgG prevents Rh immunization but will not suppress it once it is present, no matter how weak in amount.

Intravenous Rh Immune Globulin

Most Rh immune globulin is prepared by the Cohn cold ethanol precipitation method. IgG prepared by this method is effective and has a good safety record. However, the efficiency of yield from starting plasma is low, and cold ethanol precipitation produces an anti-complementary IgG that obviates intravenous administration. Small amounts of residual IgA are present. There is one report of an anaphylactic reaction in a woman who had anti-IgA and received cold ethanol anti-DIgG intramuscularly. (11)

Hoppe et al (12) have prepared an anti-DIgG by ion exchange column chromatography. The IgG is very pure and can be administered safely intravenously. The ion exchange column preparation method has been adapted for use in North America. An intravenous anti-DIgG is now licensed for use in the United States and Canada. (13) Solvent detergent viral destruction and viral filtration steps make this product as safe from viral contamination as possible. When administered intravenously, anti-DIgG is twice as effective microgram-for-microgram as intramuscularly administered product because anti-D levels in the maternal circulation are immediate and twice as high. Because its half-life when administered intravenously is no greater, the antenatal prophylaxis dose is the same (300 mcg) as the intramuscular dose. In Canada, the postdelivery intravenous dose is 120 mcg.

Clinical trials and service programs (13) in which thousands of doses of anti-DIgG have been given intravenously show that this agent is as effective as intramuscular IgG. Its advantages are: greater purity and less likelihood of producing a reaction, greater efficiency of yield from anti-D plasma, lower dose, and less discomfort when administered intravenously.

John M. Bowman, OC, MD, FRSC
Distinguished Professor Emeritus
Department of Paediatrics and Child Health
Faculty of Medicine
University of Manitoba
Winnipeg, Canada

[For the original article on Rh prophylaxis, please go to: http://neoreviews.aappublications.org/cgi/content/full/3/11/e223/DC1]

References

1. Von Dungern F. Beitrage zur Immunitatslehr. *Munch Med.* 1900;47:677

2. Freda VJ, Gorman JG, Pollack W. Successful prevention of experimental Rh sensitization in man with an anti-Rh gamma 2 globulin antibody preparation: a preliminary report. *Transfusion.* 1964;4:26

3. Clarke CA, Donohue WTA, McConnell RB, et al. Further experimental studies in the prevention of Rh haemolytic disease. *Br Med J.* 1963;1:979

4. Chown B, Duff AM, James J, et al. Prevention of primary Rh immunization: first report of the Western Canadian Trial. *Can Med Assoc J.* 1969;100:121

5. Bowman JM, Chown B, Lewis M, Pollock JM. Rh isoimmunization during pregnancy: antenatal prophylaxis. *Can Med Assoc J.* 1978;118:623

6. Bowman JM, Pollock JM. Antenatal prophylaxis of Rh isoimmunization: 28 weeks' gestation service program. *Can Med Assoc J.* 1978;118:627

7. Bowman JM, Lewis M, DeSa DJ. Hydrops fetalis caused by massive materno-fetal transplacental hemorrhage. *JPediatr.* 1984;104:769

8. Bowman JM, Pollock JM. Transplacental fetal hemorrhage after amniocentesis. *Obstet Gynecol.* 1985;66:749

9. Pollack W, Ascari WQ, Kochesky RJ, et al. Studies on Rh prophylaxis. 1. Relationship between doses of anti-Rh and size of antigenic stimulus. *Transfusion.* 1971;11:333

10. Bowman JM, Pollock JM. Reversal of Rh alloimmunization: fact or fancy? *Vox Sang.* 1984;47:209

11. Rvat L, Parent M, Rvat C. Accident survenu apres injection de gammaglobulines anti-Rh dû à la présence d'anticorps anti-gamma A. *Presse Med.* 1970;7:2072

12. Hoppe HH, Mester T, Hennig W, et al. Prevention of Rh immunization. Modified production of IgG anti-Rh for intravenous application by ion exchange chromatography (IEC). *Vox Sang.* 1973;25:308

13. Bowman JM, Friesen AD, Pollock JM, Taylor WE. Win Rho: Rh immunoglobulin prepared by ion exchange for intravenous use. *Can Med Assoc J.* 1980;123:1121

Historical Perspectives: Prevention of Rh Hemolytic Disease of the Newborn

Alistair G. S. Philip and John M. Bowman

NeoReviews 2002;3;223

DOI: 10.1542/neo.3-11-e223

Intensive Care and Cranial Ultrasonography at UCH in London

Introduction

This 2003 Historical Perspective is written by Osmund Reynolds. When I requested a personal reminiscence of how his research and article on detection of brain damage in preterm infants via cranial ultrasonography originated, I asked that he include the setting in which this advance occurred. His entertaining response provides a perspective on the evolution of neonatal care at University College Hospital (UCH), London. This recollection of the introduction of neonatal care at UCH is included in Part 1; part 2 focuses on the more specific introduction of cranial ultrasound imaging.

It should be mentioned that the pace of development of neonatal intensive care in the United Kingdom generally was much slower than in the United States and some other countries. Indeed, in 1980, there were only 12 neonatal consultant posts for the entire UK. It is generally recognized that UCH was one of the leaders in this arena not only for the UK, but also for the world. For a more detailed discussion of the development of intensive care in the UK, the reader is referred to one in a series of "Witness Seminars" developed by the Wellcome Institute for the History of Medicine, for which Professor Reynolds was the major consultant. (1)

Alistair G. S. Philip, MD, FRCPE, FAAP
Editor-in-Chief, NeoReviews

Reference

1. Origins of neonatal intensive care in the UK. In: Christie DA, Tansey EM, eds. *Wellcome Witnesses to Twentieth Century Medicine*. Vol. 9. London, United Kingdom: Wellcome Trust; 2001:1–75

Part 1: Background and Intensive Care

Introduction

I first became interested in perinatal medicine in 1955 while undertaking a physiology BSc degree at St. Thomas' Hospital Medical School in London. The head of the department was Professor Henry Barcroft (son of Sir Joseph), and Maureen Young was a lecturer. She taught me to measure blood gases using the Roughton-Scholander syringe; duplicate samples took about three quarters of an hour. After qualifying in medicine, I became a house physician on Professor Peter Sharpey-Shafer's adult medical unit, which was an extremely stimulating environment with a very strong group of physiologically orientated investigators. Steve Semple taught me how to mechanically ventilate adults with chronic bronchitis and take arterial samples for blood gas analysis. When the houseman got mumps, I was drafted to do a pediatric job and became hooked. By chance, I was faced with an epidemic of bronchiolitis, so it seemed obvious to measure the arterial blood gases. (1)

Around that time, I remember Herbert Barrie using Ian Donald's "puffer" ventilator on some very preterm infants. Maureen Young had worked with Donald in the 1950s on his negative pressure ventilator.

On the strength of the bronchiolitis studies, I obtained a fellowship at Harvard, working at Children's Hospital in Dav Cook's laboratory, where Marcello Orzalesi was one of the luminaries. I became involved in developing a model of hyaline membrane disease (later called respiratory distress syndrome [RDS]) in the pre-term lamb (2) and began to gain some insight on how one might ventilate surfactant-deficient lungs.

In 1964, I went back to London, where Sharpey-Shafer had intended that I should start an academic pediatric department at St. Thomas'. Unfortunately, he died while I was in Boston. Luckily, Leonard Strang wanted someone who knew how to operate on sheep, so I joined him in his newly established academic department at University College Hospital (UCH) Medical School. Leonard had

spent a year in Dav Cook's laboratory, just before I went there, doing his very important work on changes in the pulmonary circulation at birth. For several years I helped Leonard with a series of related investigations, including studies of lung permeability and of the mechanisms of fetal lung liquid secretion and its absorption at birth. It was during this period that the idea dawned that "massive pulmonary hemorrhage" in the newborn was usually hemorrhagic pulmonary edema. (3)

Leonard, like Sharpey-Shafer, established a strong physiologically based department at UCH. The staff included, among others, Colin Normand and Jean Smellie (who were at UCH before Leonard), Richard Olver, Robert Boyd, Dafydd Walters, Jonathan Shaw, Rodney Rivers, and Bernadette Model. Bit by bit, I infiltrated the neonatal unit, where Colin Normand and Jean Smellie were working, together with Leonard, and over the next few years, I gradually took over the running of it. Intensive care for preterm and ill babies was introduced at UCH in the mid-1960s.

Changing the Care of Preterm Infants

At that time, there was deep suspicion about the wisdom of applying new techniques such as mechanical ventilation to fragile infants, especially very preterm ones.* The anxiety arose because a number of studies, particularly by Cecil Drillien in Edinburgh, had shown that about two thirds of very low-birthweight (VLBW) (<1,500 g) survivors born in the 1940s and 1950s were handicapped at school age. The general view was that these infants had been damaged before birth, so any attempts to help them live would inevitably lead to an unacceptable increase in handicap in the community.

However, in those days very little was known about the physiology of preterm

---

*The suspicion continued in some quarters...in 1981 Margaret Thatcher said to me, "You're one of those people who give babies oxygen to breathe and make them blind."

infants. It was customary to deprive them of fluid and food for many days after birth (because of the risk of aspiration), and some did not regain their birthweight for several weeks. Little was known about temperature control, and methods for supporting breathing were only very rarely available. It seemed inevitable that many of the survivors had suffered from potentially brain-damaging insults, such as hypoxemia, acidemia, hypotension, hypoglycemia, hyperbilirubinemia, and undernutrition. Possibly avoidance of these and other adverse influences, arising largely because of immaturity of organ systems and iatrogenesis, might improve the outcome. Accordingly, a program of care was introduced at UCH that included closely involved obstetricians, swift resuscitation by pediatricians using endotracheal intubation, strict asepsis, careful temperature control, monitoring of vital signs, early feeding by fine nasogastric catheter, measurement of arterial blood gases and pH, avoidance of biochemical insults, attention to hemostasis, and mechanical ventilation if required. Because very few (sometimes no) housestaff were quickly available, nurses were taught to intubate and initiate ventilation.

Early on, only about 30% of ventilated infants (of all birthweights) survived, (4) but later there were rapid improvements after discovering that Pao_2 and $Paco_2$ could be varied independently of one another by suitable manipulations of the ventilator settings and that oxygenation was related to mean airway pressure in infants who had hyaline membrane disease. (5) Initially, celebratory corks popped when a potentially healthy baby was weaned off the ventilator, in contrast to the gloom that tends to supervene today if an infant is not weaned. In 1969, a small ventilator was attached to a portable incubator so apneic infants could be transported successfully from outlying hospitals. (6) Total parenteral nutrition via percutaneous long silastic catheters was introduced by Jonathan Shaw in 1970 (7), and continuous positive airway pressure in 1971. Surfactant replacement and antenatal steroids came along much later.

Follow-up of Infants

Because we were very worried about the outcome for survivors, in case our hypothesis

was wrong, we started a follow-up study on January 1, 1966, that has been going on ever since, with Ann Stewart, until very recently, in charge. The first results were published in 1971. (8) Of 72 surviving VLBW infants born from 1966 through 1969, 59 (87%) were believed to be progressing normally at a mean corrected age of 2 years 3 months (9 mo through 4 y, 3 mo). Not long after, results from 95 survivors at a mean age of 5 years 2 months confirmed earlier findings. This report caused something of a storm and was widely disbelieved. However, Cecil Drillien sat in at the follow-up clinic (wearing battle dress) and became convinced.

We knew that because the children were still very young, some would show more signs of trouble later on, and so it was proved, although almost all were attending normal school. (9) Nevertheless we felt obliged to publish our early results because they seemed so strikingly different from those of Drillien and several other authors in the 1950s and 1960s. It appeared important to make at least a preliminary statement countering the policy of benign neglect that previous poor results had encouraged. Our findings formed part of the basis for the introduction of regional services for ill babies and their mothers in the UK. We were, however, criticized on a number of grounds, most particularly because our study was from a single center and was not a population study. Our response was that when starting an innovative program of intensive care that was associated with a sudden drop in mortality to well below the national average for VLBW infants, the most important question was: "Are they mostly OK or are they mostly frightful?" If the latter finding was true, we would have shut up shop. Population studies were for later.

The Long View

Many other groups' experiences were broadly similar to ours, with sharply increasing survival rates for the larger VLBW infants and, more recently, extremely low-birthweight (ELBW) (<1,000 g) babies. In 1981, we attempted to ascertain overall outcome for VLBW infants by surveying the world literature. (10) We concluded that the 1960s and

1970s had witnessed a steady increase in survival rate and that the proportion of survivors who had major handicaps (abnormalities that in the long term were likely to affect, in an important way, the individual's ability to lead a normal life or obtain satisfactory employment) had remained constant at 6% to 8% of live births. There was insufficient evidence to form any opinion about the prevalence of lesser problems. This study was widely interpreted as showing that "intensive care does not reduce handicap." When asked to explain, particularly to managers and politicians, I found it helpful to tell them that the mother of a VLBW infant had a much better chance than previously of taking home a healthy infant and a much lower chance of having to bury a dead one, but in between there was a comparatively small population of infants who would have problems and whose size was not changing much. Some studies showed a reduction; others an increase. In later years, justified anxiety developed over the size of this subpopulation among ELBW infants, particularly the smallest ones, as their chances of survival continued to increase.

Osmund Reynolds, CBE, MD, FRS
Emeritus Professor of Neonatal Paediatrics
University College London
London, United Kingdom

References

1. Reynolds EOR. The effect of breathing 40% oxygen on the arterial blood gas tensions of babies with bronchiolitis. *J Pediatr.* 1963;63: 1135–1139

2. Reynolds EOR, Jacobson HN, Motoyama EK, et al. The effect of immaturity and prenatal asphyxia on the lungs and pulmonary function of newborn lambs. The experimental production of respiratory distress. *Pediatrics.* 1965;35:382–392

3. Cole VA, Normand ICS, Reynolds EOR, Rivers RPA. Pathogenesis of hemorrhagic pulmonary edema and massive pulmonary hemorrhage in the newborn. *Pediatrics.* 1973;51:175–187

4. Adamson TM, Collins LM, Dehan M, Hawker JM, Reynolds EOR, Strang LB. Mechanical ventilation in newborn infants with respiratory failure. *Lancet.* 1968;ii: 227–231

5. Herman S, Reynolds EOR. Methods for improving arterial oxygen tension in infants mechanically ventilated for severe hyaline membrane disease. *Arch Dis Child.* 1973;48: 612–617

6. Blake AM, Collins LM, Langham J, Reynolds EOR. Portable ventilator-incubator for newborn infants with respiratory failure. *Lancet.* 1970;ii:25

7. Shaw JCL. Parenteral nutrition in the management of sick low birthweight infants. *Pediat Clin North Am.* 1973;20:338–358

8. Rawlings G, Reynolds EOR, Stewart A, Strang LB. Changing prognosis for infants of very low birthweight. *Lancet.* 1971;i: 516–519

9. Stewart A, Turcan D, Rawlings G, Hart S, Gregory S. Outcome for infants at high risk of major handicap. In: *Major Mental Handicap: Costs and Methods of Prevention.* Ciba Foundation Symposium 59 (new series). Amsterdam, The Netherlands: Elsevier; 1978:151–171

10. Stewart AL, Reynolds EOR, Lipscomb AP. Outcome for infants of very low birth-weight: survey of world literature. *Lancet.* 1981;i:1038–1041

Part 2: Introduction of Ultrasonography
Establishing Professional Collaborations

University College Hospital (UCH) is the hospital attached to the large multifaculty college, University College London, that forms a major part of the University of London. The neonatal unit, therefore, can call on a wide range of local expertise to solve problems. Close ties were established early on with many departments, including obstetrics, physiology, anatomy, and most particularly, medical physics.

In the 1960s, physicists and clinicians rarely interacted, primarily because the clinicians were too haughty, and the physicists did not know how to approach them with their bright ideas for useful innovations. However, contact eventually was made, partly because the neonatal unit and medical physics department were geographically very close and especially because there was much willingness and interest on both sides. It soon became clear that mutually exciting projects could be undertaken. The first was the development and introduction by Dawood Parker, Linda Soutter, and Dave Delpy in the early 1970s of an umbilical artery catheter-tip oxygen electrode. (1) The first version had been miniaturized from a large device for measuring the Po_2 of Lake Windermere. The electrode was especially useful because Pao_2 had been found to vary substantially with changes in ventilator settings, making

intermittent sampling wholly inadequate. It was tested in sheep before being used in babies. It was also used (in a series of exceedingly tedious studies) to test the accuracy in vivo of the newly introduced transcutaneous Po_2 electrodes for estimating Pao_2. Later, Parker and Delpy devised a transcutaneous electrode for estimating Pao_2 and $Paco_2$ simultaneously.

Focusing on the Brain

Major attention in the neonatal unit shifted from the lungs to the brain in the mid-1970s because autopsy studies showed that cerebral pathology, particularly intraventricular hemorrhage or periventricular hemorrhage (PVH), was very common in VLBW infants. Also, it was clear from follow-up studies that some of VLBW survivors continued to suffer from neurodevelopmental problems, particularly cerebral palsy. There was an obvious need for noninvasive methods of investigating the brain. In 1978, Papile and her colleagues published their important study using computed tomography (CT), which showed that an unexpectedly large proportion of surviving VLBW infants had PVH. (2) However, to use CT, infants had to be transported to the machine, and there was concern about radiation. Something simpler was required.

The obstetrician Ian Donald moved from St. Thomas' Hospital to Hammersmith Hospital and was then appointed Regius Professor of Midwifery at the University of Glasgow, where he arrived in 1954. Previously, his main interest had been in mechanical ventilation in the newborn (see Part 1), but shortly after his arrival in Glasgow he, together with the engineer Tom Brown, invented obstetric ultrasonography. He delighted in tinkering with machinery left lying about after the war. For example, he used an altimeter to measure ventilator pressure, and a United States Air Force flying mask placed upside down on the baby's face to apply mask ventilation. His first (A-scan) ultrasonography studies were performed in 1955 with a Henry Hughes Supersonic Flaw Detector for the nondestructive testing of metals. He soon linked up with Tom Brown to introduce the first two-dimensional (B-scan) scanner, which evolved into the first

commercial machine, the Diasonograph, in the early 1960s. (3)

Roland Blackwell arrived in the UCH Medical Physics Department in 1966. He was and is a major authority on obstetric ultrasonography. In the 1970s, great strides were made in the technological aspects of ultrasonography scanners, particularly by the Advanced Diagnostic Research Corporation (ADR), of Tempe, Arizona, which marketed the first commercial linear-array real-time scanner in 1974, and the ADR 2130, which was a big advance, in 1976. Blackwell acquired one of these machines in 1977, and he soon was obtaining remarkably good images of the fetal brain in utero. This happened at precisely the same time as we had realized that we needed brain imaging in the neonatal unit, and Roland was keen to try it because it would help him interpret his fetal images. Ultrasonography had, in fact, previously been used to scan various organs in newborns, but few attempts had been made to image the brain (although some information was acquired using articulated-arm static scanners). (4) A major problem was the difficulty of obtaining good contact between the rather bulky linear-array probe and the infant's curved head. Also, as in many other areas, techniques used in infants were often scaled down from those used in adults. Ultrasonic waves do not penetrate the adult skull, and it seems to have been assumed that the same would be true of neonates.*

Ultrasonographic Imaging of the Brain

Our first attempts to image the brain were made early in 1978. (5) The ADR 2130 machine was small and portable, and it proved easy to scan babies in their incubators. A 5-mHz probe was used (and later a 7-mHz one was added). The primary initial problem was acoustic contact. A rubber glove filled with water and a small tank with a thin polythene base were tried, but both were

---

*In 1978, a Select Committee of the House of Commons that was investigating perinatal mortality in the UK (and which I was advising) visited the UCH neonatal unit and saw cranial scanning in progress. The Labour chairman, Renee Short, asked us to scan the brain of one of the Conservative members. No image appeared. "I always knew it," said she.

unpopular because of the perceived risk of drowning the baby. Karen Pape joined us at this time as a visiting fellow from the Hospital for Sick Children, Toronto. She had spent the previous year with Jonathan Wigglesworth at Hammersmith Hospital, where they wrote their famous book on perinatal brain damage. (6) Karen was in the right place at precisely the right time. We had lined up three potential areas of investigation from which she could choose: transcephalic impedance, intracranial Doppler, or cranial ultrasonography. She unhesitatingly took up ultrasonography and, together with Roland Blackwell and his colleague Geoff Cusick, made it her own.

The contact problem was swiftly solved by applying copious quantities of contact gel to the baby's head. (The nurses made it very plain that cleaning up was totally the responsibility of the ultrasonographers.) The images seemed pretty good, so a formal study was undertaken between September 1978 and January 1979. The brains were repeatedly scanned for 31 of the 34 infants born at fewer than 33 weeks of gestation who were admitted to the neonatal unit. Horizontal and coronal scans were obtained (Fig. 1). A freeze-frame attachment allowed detailed examination and measurement of ventricular dimensions. Records were kept as Polaroid® photographs and on videotape. All the equipment was mounted on a small trolley, and no logistical problems were encountered. Comparisons were made with CT and autopsy in the seven infants who died. The normal appearance of the brain was described, and we concluded that we could identify hemorrhage into the germinal layer and ventricles, hydrocephalus, cerebral edema, and loss of brain tissue in the periventricular region (later recognized as periventricular leukomalacia [PVL]) and the cortex. These findings were published in the *Lancet* in June 1979 (7), and Karen Pape presented them to the Society for Pediatric Research.

It was not until this study was completed that we discovered the anterior fontanelle (which shows how slow on the uptake one can be). One Sunday morning we were doing a ward round, and Tony Lipscomb placed the probe over the fontanelle (Fig. 2). We had,

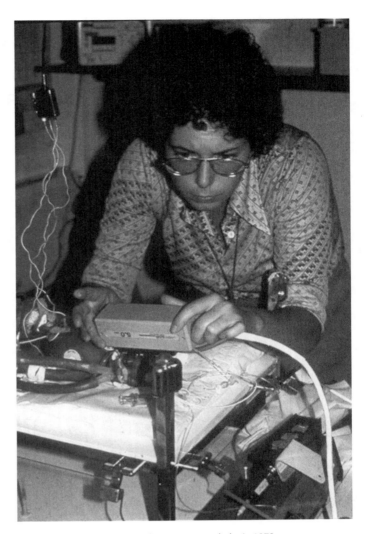

Figure 1. Karen Pape scanning the brain of a very preterm baby in 1978.

by chance, chosen the right baby and were astonished by what we saw. He had ventricular dilatation, and the ventricular system and cerebral anatomy were well displayed. Fontanelle scanning then became part of the routine and provided satisfactory images, provided the fontanelle was not very small. A letter was dispatched to the *Lancet* and published in July 1979 that included the first published image of a fontanelle scan (Fig. 3) of the infant described previously. (8). In the same issue, a letter appeared from Richard Cooke stating that he was performing fontanelle scanning in Rotterdam (which we did not know at the time) and that a sector scanner gave better images than the linear-array. Karen Pape went back to Canada soon thereafter.

Ros Thorburn presented our results to a conference in Oxford in September 1979,

where Richard Cooke showed fontanelle scans obtained with his Advanced Technology Labs (ATL) 850A sector scanner. (9) In December 1980, we attended the Perinatal Intracranial Hemorrhage Conference organized by Jerry Lucey in Washington, D.C. (10) (This conference continued yearly thereafter and evolved into the Hot Topics meeting.) By that time, there had been an ultrasonic boom, and no fewer than 14 presentations were made from 10 different groups in the UK, United States, Canada, and Australia. We showed data on the accuracy of linear-array images (subsequently amplified with numerous illustrations). (11)

In a prospective study of 95 infants born at fewer than 33 weeks of gestation, we had found PVH in 36, hydrocephalus in 2, and loss of brain tissue in 8. The median age of

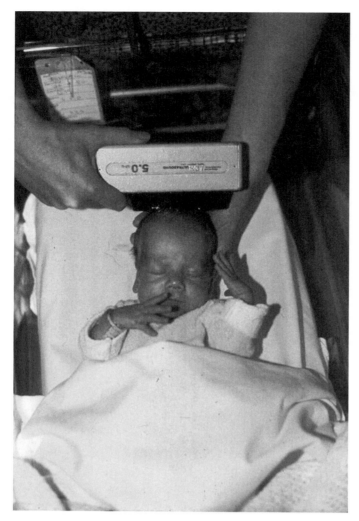

Figure 2. Tony Lipscomb performing the first published fontanelle scan in 1979.

first detection of hemorrhage was the second day, with the maximum extent on the fourth day; very few arose later. The most important predictors of PVH were short gestation and the severity of respiratory illnesses, with pneumothorax being a particularly potent causal antecedent. Very early follow-up showed a correlation between cerebral lesions and a poor outcome. Most other groups in Washington presented data consistent with ours, which were published in full over the next 2 years.

Follow-up of Scanned Infants

We performed sector-scanning in parallel with linear-array from mid-1981 and gradually converted to sector-scanning only, largely carried out by Peter Hope and Pat Hamilton.

For many years, the scanned infants were enrolled for follow-up by Ann Stewart and her colleagues, and numerous publications resulted. For example, in a study of 342 prospectively scanned infants born at fewer than 33 weeks' gestation, it was found that by the time of discharge from the unit, infants could be assigned to groups of either low, intermediate, or high risk of neurodevelopmental impairments detectable at 1 year of age. (12) The largest group comprised 275 infants (80%) with normal scans or uncomplicated PVH (PVH not associated with hemorrhagic parenchymal infarction and not followed by ventricular dilatation with cerebrospinal fluid). These infants were at low risk, with only a 4% probability of a disabling impairment at 1 year. In contrast, a small

group of 26 infants (8%) with posthemorrhagic hydrocephalus or any loss of brain tissue (including PVL and cysts at the site of hemorrhagic infarctions) were at high risk, with a probability of a disabling impairment of 58% (and of any impairment of 88%). Between these two groups lay the 41 infants (12%) with mild ventricular dilatation who were at intermediate risk, with a 27% risk of a disabling impairment. These results were generally confirmed at 4 and 8 years of age, although cognitive impairments (usually minor) were emerging that were not closely related to the ultrasonography findings. (13)

Conclusions

The reason why the UCH group and many others became involved with cranial ultrasonography imaging was to address specific questions about perinatal brain injury, especially in VLBW or very preterm infants. What was the prevalence of potentially brain-damaging lesions, how were they caused, when did they occur, how effective were attempts to prevent and treat them, and what was their long-term significance? Ultrasonography has proved very good at answering these questions for the major lesions that generally lead to a very bad outcome, such as hemorrhagic infarction, hydrocephalus, and loss of brain tissue, including cystic PVL. It is much less effective at identifying hypoxic-ischemic brain injury (including PVL) at a very early stage when intervention might have some hope of success. (14)

Follow-up studies (including ours) have shown that this form of brain injury is a more important cause than PVH of long-term disability in preterm infants, and it is the mechanism of damage to the brain during birth asphyxia in more mature infants. For this reason, new methods of detecting early hypoxic-ischemic injury have been sought. Discussions at UCH in the early 1980s about this problem with Dawood Parker and Dave Delpy (soon joined by Ern Cady and Mark Cope) in the medical physics department and Doug Wilkie and Joan Dawson in physiology led to the introduction of magnetic resonance spectroscopy (MRS) and near-infrared spectroscopy for observing brain oxidative metabolism and hemodynamics

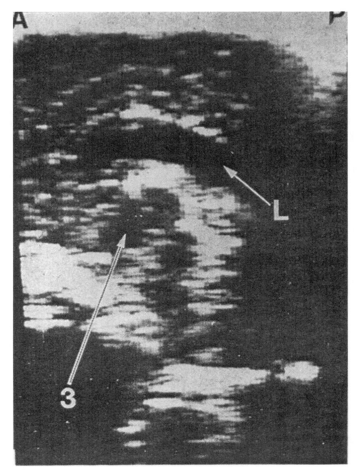

Figure 3. Parasagittal image obtained during the scanning procedure illustrated in Fig 2 (8). A = anterior; P = posterior; L = lateral ventricle; 3 = 3rd ventricle.

(15)(16) Peter Hope, Tony Costello, John Wyatt, and David Edwards were the main clinical protagonists. Magnetic resonance imaging came later to UCH, although David Edwards, who moved to Hammersmith Hospital in 1992, is, with his colleagues there, making

considerable progress in its application to the neonatal, particularly very preterm, brain.

One important aspect of cranial ultrasonography imaging and other objective techniques for investigating the neonatal brain is that the parents of a sick infant can be reasonably reassured if the prognostic indicators are good (eg, normal ultrasonography scan or small PVH), early warning can be given if trouble can be foreseen, and if the outlook is very bad (eg, large bilateral hemorrhagic infarctions, major loss of brain tissue, or severe energy failure diagnosed by MRS), the staff of the unit can discuss rationally with the parents how far intensive care should be pursued. I believe that this approach helps considerably in achieving what must be the major aim of intensive care, namely, to provide the maximum chances of survival for potentially healthy children, but at minimum risk of salvaging hopelessly disabled ones.

Osmund Reynolds, CBE, MD, FRS
Emeritus Professor of Neonatal Paediatrics
University College London
London, United Kingdom

[To read the original article on detection of brain damage in preterm infants via cranial ultrasonography written by Reynolds and colleagues in 1979, which was reprinted with permission from *Lancet*, please go to: http://neoreviews.aappublications.org/cgi/content/full/4/11/e291/DC1]

References

1. Conway M, Durbin GM, Ingram D, et al. Continuous monitoring of arterial oxygen tension using a catheter-tip polarographic electrode in infants. *Pediatrics*. 1976;57:244–250

2. Papile LA, Burstein J, Burstein J, Koffler H. Incidence and evolution of subependymal and intraventricular hemorrhage: a study of infants with birthweights less than 1500 gm. *J Pediatr*. 1978;92:529–534

3. Looking at the unborn: historical aspects of obstetric ultrasound. In: Tansey EM, Christie DA, eds. *Wellcome Witnesses to Twentieth Century Medicine*. Vol 5. London, United Kingdom: Wellcome Trust; 2000:1–77

4. Johnson ML, Mack LA, Rumack CM, Frost M, Rashbaum C. B-mode echoencephalography in the normal and high risk infant. *Am J Radiol*. 1979;133: 375–381

5. Origins of neonatal intensive care in the UK. In: Christie DA, Tansey EM, eds. *Wellcome Witnesses to Twentieth Century Medicine*. Vol 9. London, United Kingdom: Wellcome Trust; 2001:1–75

6. Pape KE, Wigglesworth JS. Haemorrhage, ischaemia and the perinatal brain. *Clinics in Developmental Medicine*. Nos. 69/70. London, United Kingdom: SIMP, Heinemann; 1979

7. Pape KE, Blackwell RJ, Cusick G, et al. Ultrasound detection of brain damage in preterm infants. *Lancet*. 1979;i:1261–1264

8. Lipscomb AP, Blackwell RJ, Reynolds EOR, Thorburn RJ, Cusick G, Pape KE. Ultrasound scanning of brain through anterior fontanelle of newborn infants. *Lancet*. 1979;ii:39

9. Cooke RWI. Diagnosis of periventricular haemorrhage by real time two dimensional ultrasound sector scanning. In: Bath RP, ed. *Fetal and Neonatal Physiological Measurements*. Bath, United Kingdom: Pitman; 1980: 344–355

10. Lipscomb AP, Thorburn RJ, Blackwell RJ, et al. Detection of brain damage in newborn infants by ultrasound and other objective techniques. In: *Perinatal Intracranial Hemorrhage Conference Syllabus*. Columbus, Ohio: Ross Laboratories; 1980:410–446

11. Thorburn RJ, Lipscomb AP, Reynolds EOR, et al. Accuracy of imaging of the brains of newborn infants by linear-array real-time ultrasound. *Early Hum Devel*. 1982;6:31–46

12. Stewart AL, Reynolds EOR, Hope PL, et al. Probability of neurodevelopmental disorders estimated from ultrasound appearance of brain in very preterm infants. *Dev Med Child Neurol*. 1987;29:3–11

13. Reynolds O. Causes and outcome of perinatal brain injury. In: Magnusson D, ed. *The Life-Span Development of Individuals*. Nobel Symposium. Cambridge, United Kingdom: University Press; 1996:52–75

14. Hope PL, Gould SJ, Howard S, Hamilton PA, Costello AM deL, Reynolds EOR. Precision of ultrasound diagnosis of pathologically verified lesions in the brains of very preterm infants. *Dev Med Child Neurol*. 1988; 30:457–471

15. Cady EB, Costello AM de L, Dawson MJ, et al. Non-invasive investigation of cerebral metabolism in newborn infants by phosphorus nuclear magnetic resonance spectroscopy. *Lancet*. 1983;i:1059–1062

16. Wyatt JS, Cope M, Delpy DT, Wray S, Reynolds EOR. Quantitation of cerebral oxygenation and haemodynamics in sick newborn infants by near-infrared spectroscopy. *Lancet*. 1986;ii:1063–1066

Historical Perspectives: Intensive Care and Cranial Ultrasonography at UCH in London: Parts 1 and 2

Alistair G. S. Philip, Osmund Reynolds and Osmund Reynolds

NeoReviews 2003;4;291

DOI: 10.1542/neo.4-11-e291

Transcutaneous Bilirubinometry

*M. Jeffrey Maisels, MB, BCh**

In this 2006 Historical Perspective, Dr Jeffrey Maisels points out that evaluation and quantitation of skin color had been attempted for many years. However, it was not until 1980 that quantitation became more accurately standardized. In that year, Dr Yamanouchi and colleagues in Japan reported on a noninvasive method of estimating serum bilirubin levels.(1) Continuing experience has demonstrated that transcutaneous bilirubinometry continues to have a place in the assessment of newborn infants who have jaundice (2).

Alistair G. S. Philip, MD, FRCPE, FAAP
Editor-in-Chief, NeoReviews

References

1. Yamanouchi I, Yamauchi Y, Igarashi I, Transcutaneous bilirubinometry: preliminary studies of non-invasive transcutaneous bilirubin meter in Okayama National Hospital. *Pediatrics.* 1980;65:195–202
2. Schmidt ET, Wheeler CA, Jackson GL, Engle WD. Evaluation of transcutaneous bilirubinometry in preterm neonates. *J Perinatol.* 2009;29(8):564–569

Introduction

When the bilirubin concentration in the serum increases, bilirubin is deposited in the skin and subcutaneous tissues, (1) producing the (yellow) physical sign of jaundice or icterus. There is a well-established relationship between the total serum bilirubin (TSB) concentration and the intensity of jaundice, and the possibility of quantifying the bilirubin value by assessing skin color is not new. This relationship was documented in 1913 by Ylppö, (2) although he measured the bilirubin concentration in whole blood, not serum. The next major advance was the recognition that bilirubin could be toxic, that its toxicity was related to its concentration, and that it was possible to treat hyperbilirubinemia (and prevent neurologic damage) with exchange transfusion. (3) Pediatricians measured TSB in infants if jaundice appeared early (in the first 24 hours after birth) or appeared excessive for the infant's age. Unfortunately, it is neither possible, nor desirable, to measure the serum bilirubin daily in every infant for the first week after birth. Accordingly, clinicians have used the clinical sign of jaundice as the trigger for deciding when to measure the TSB concentration.

*Department of Pediatrics, William Beaumont Hospital, Royal Oak, Mich.

The Clinical Diagnosis of Hyperbilirubinemia

How Good is the Visual Assessment of Jaundice?

Although there is a clear and semi-quantitative relationship between the yellowness of the skin and the TSB, the variations in color perception by the human eye, differences in neonatal skin pigmentation, and variations in both the intensity and color of the available light affect the ability to estimate the TSB by assessing the degree of jaundice in a newborn. In 1941, Davidson and associates (4) described their experience evaluating the degree of jaundice in 99 infants. They examined each infant in daylight, applying a tongue depressor to the mucous membrane of the lower jaw as well as the skin of the forehead or the chin. Based on the icterus they observed following this procedure, they assigned the infants to one of three categories: no jaundice, moderate jaundice, or marked jaundice. TSB measurements were obtained daily from heel stick samples. The results are shown in Figure 1. Of 99 infants examined, jaundice was noted on at least one occasion in 63 (64%) of the infants. (Hence, the oft-quoted figure that about two thirds of healthy newborns appear jaundiced during the first postnatal week.) The population studied was 90% white, but the number breastfed was not reported.

Although there was a clear relationship between the TSB and the clinical observations of no jaundice, moderate jaundice, or marked jaundice, there was a wide range of TSB values in each category. A few infants whose TSB concentrations were less than 5 mg/dL (85.5 mcmol/L) were categorized as having marked jaundice. More importantly from the clinician's perspective is that in about 5% of the observations, infants who were not jaundiced had TSB levels between 10 and 12 mg/dL (171 and 205 mcmol/L), and in some 10% of nonjaundiced infants, TSB levels were 8 to 10 mg/dL (137 to 171 mcmol/L). Failure to recognize that an infant who has a TSB value of 10 mg/dL (171 mcmol/L) is jaundiced is of no consequence in a 3- or 4-day-old infant, but it is a different matter if that infant is 24 or even 36 hours old, when a value of 10 mg/dL (171 mcmol/L) is above the 95th percentile (6) and calls for further investigation, additional TSB measurements, and close follow up. (7) Wood and associates (8) found that "despite a general alertness for jaundice," infants with TSB values above 12 or even 15 mg/dL (205 to 257 mcmol/L) were not always identified as being jaundiced.

More recent studies confirm these earlier observations (Fig. 2). (9)(10) Moyer and colleagues (10) found that experienced residents, nurse practitioners, and attending physicians provided wide ranges of estimates of TSB concentrations. In addition, agreement between observers was very poor regarding which areas of the body were jaundiced and the estimated TSB. On the other hand, four Israeli neonatologists provided acceptable estimates of TSB concentrations in 283 term newborns. (11)

Cephalocaudal Progression of Jaundice

A potentially useful refinement in the clinical assessment of jaundice is the observation that jaundice appears initially in the face of a newborn and as the TSB increases, becomes apparent on the chest and abdomen and finally, in the extremities (Fig. 3), (12) an observation that has been confirmed using transcutaneous bilirubin (TcB) measurements. (13)(14) Knudsen (14) postulated that the cephalocaudal

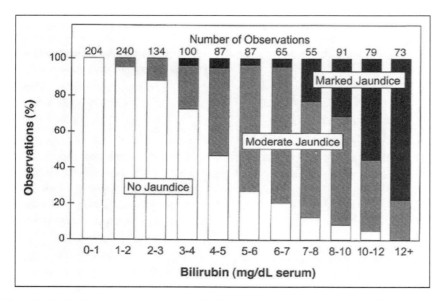

Figure 1. Relationship between total serum bilirubin concentration and the degree of jaundice, with 1,215 observations made on 120 infants during the first postnatal week. Note that some infants were considered to be markedly jaundiced with bilirubin concentrations of less than 3 mg/dL (51 mcmol/L), and some with concentrations of greater than 10 mg/dL (171mcmol/L) were judged to be nonjaundiced. Redrawn from the data of Davidson et al (4) and reproduced from Johnson and Bhutani (5) with permission.

progression of jaundice can be explained by conformational changes of bilirubin albumin complexes. Although the initial binding of bilirubin to albumin is extremely rapid, final conformational changes may not occur for about 8 minutes. Thus, blood leaving the reticuloendothelial system and going to the proximal parts of the body contains bilirubin that is less tightly bound to albumin than that which subsequently reaches the distal parts of the body. Bilirubin that is less tightly bound is more likely to precipitate as bilirubin acid in phospholipid membranes in the skin and subcutaneous tissues, which is why the face appears jaundiced before the abdomen or the legs.

As can be seen from Figure 3, although mean indirect bilirubin levels increase as jaundice progresses from the head to the extremities, the range of bilirubin values in each zone is wide. Bhutani and associates (15) studied 916 infants in six well-baby nurseries. The infants were evaluated by experienced nurses and, if jaundice was present, the zone was noted. At the same time, TcB was measured. The cephalocaudal progression was confirmed, but the rangesof TcB and the overlap were substantial. In zone 1, TcB values ranged from

2.3 to 13.8 mg/dL (39 to 236 mcmol/L) and in zone 2 from 4.3 to 14.2 mg/ dL (74 to 243 mcmol/L).

Comparison With a Color Scale

One method of improving the estimate of TSB values by eye is to compare the infant's skin color with a color scale. In 1960, Gosset (16) described the use of an icterometer (Cascade Healthcare Products, Salem, Ore.) to assess neonatal jaundice. It appears that Dr Gosset painted transverse stripes of five different shades of yellow on a piece of transparent plastic (Fig. 4). The instrument is pressed against the baby's nose, the yellow color of the blanched skin is matched with the appropriate yellow stripe (numbered 1 through 5), and a jaundice score is assigned. If the reading appears to fall between two stripes, a 0.5 score can be assigned (eg, 1.5, 2.5). For each score, the icterometer provides a mean TSB and 2 standard deviations above the mean. As a screening tool, the icterometer has performed as well as far more sophisticated instruments in term (17) and preterm infants, (18) and it has been used effectively in the hospital (19) and by nurses and parents in the home. (20)(21)

Noninvasive Measurements of Bilirubin
Skin Reflectance and Transcutaneous Bilirubinometry

When light is transmitted to the skin, the yellowness of the reflected light can be measured to provide an objective measurement of skin color. Hannemann and coworkers (22)(23) applied these principles to predict TSB levels from skin reflectance. Monochromatic light from a tungsten source was applied to the infant's skin through one branch of a bifurcated fiberoptic bundle while a second branch of the bundle carried the reflected light back to an optical detector. The transduced signals were recorded and processed in a computer. This system was too complex for routine use in the nursery.

The first clinically applicable and easily portable transcutaneous bilirubinometer was introduced by Yamanouchi and associates. (24) Working with the Minolta Camera Company, these investigators developed a handheld instrument that measured the yellow color intensity in the skin. When a photoprobe is pressed against the infant's skin to a pressure of approximately 200 g, a xenon tube produces a strobe light that travels through a fiberoptic filament to the photoprobe (Fig. 5). The bright light penetrates the blanched skin and transilluminates the subcutaneous tissue. The scattered light returns through a second fiberoptic filament and is carried to the spectrophotometric module. Inside the module, the light is divided by a dichroic mirror into two spectra, one of which passes through a blue filter (maximum absorption, 460 nm) and the other through a green filter (maximum absorption, 550 nm). Absorption at these spectra correct for hemoglobin, and the intensity of the yellow color is measured as the difference between the optical densities of blue and green and processed electronically to provide a digital meter reading.

Multiple studies performed with the Minolta jaundice meter have demonstrated a linear relationship between TSB and TcB measurements, (25)(26)(27)(28) and the meter has been used to document the previously described cephalocaudal progression

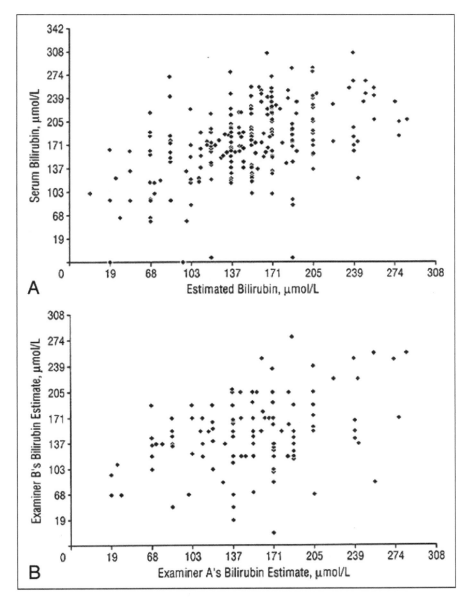

Figure 2. A. Estimates by visual assessment of TSB levels (horizontal axis) compared with laboratory measurements (vertical axis). Experienced residents, nurse practitioners, and attending pediatricians provided the estimates. B. Level of agreement on the visual estimate of TSB levels between observers. Reprinted from *Archives of Pediatrics & Adolescent Medicine*, 118(3):454–458. Copyright (1969) American Medical Association. All rights reserved.

of icterus in the newborn. (13)(14) These studies demonstrated that the jaundice meter could provide an objective measurement of the degree of newborn jaundice and, when used as a screening tool, could identify infants who required a TSB measurement. (25)(26) (27)(28) Routine use of this meter in the nursery reduced costs and the need for TSB measurements. (29)(30) Nonetheless, both the original jaundice meter and the subsequent model had some disadvantages. They did not provide a read-out of the serum

bilirubin concentration; a TcB index was displayed and TSB values were derived from the TcB index on the basis of data obtained in individual hospital laboratories. Further, readings were significantly affected by gestation and skin pigmentation. As a result, these instruments have achieved limited acceptance in hospitals in the United States, although they were widely used in Japan. (27)(31)(32)

Tayaba and associates (9) evaluated the Chromatics Colormate III (Chromatics Color

Sciences International, Inc, New York, NY) in a large population of term and preterm infants. The handheld colorimeter, which contained a xenon flash tube and light sensors connected to a portable computer, measured over a band of wavelengths from 400 to 700 nm, with specific filters used to assess the reflectance of light for specific wavelengths. The algorithm incorporated the underlying color of normal skin, accounting for it in a baseline evaluation. Measurements made on the cheek, back, forehead, and chest showed a close correlation with TSB measurements. (9) The primary disadvantage was the requirement for a baseline measurement of skin color in every infant before the onset of jaundice. This instrument no longer is marketed.

Contemporary Instruments for TcB Measurement

Two handheld devices that use skin reflectance currently are available for the measurement of TcB: the Bili-Chek® (Respironics, Marietta, Ga.) (33)(34) and the Draeger JM-103 (formally the Minolta/Hill-Rom Air-Shields JM-103) (Draeger Medical, Hattboro, Pa.). (35)(36) Although these instruments use different algorithms and measurement techniques, their principles of operation are similar. The BiliChek measures TcB by using the entire spectrum of visible light (380 to 760 nm) reflected by the skin. White light is transmitted into the skin, and reflected light is collected for analysis (Fig. 6). Algorithms have been developed that take into account the effect of hemoglobin, melanin, and dermal thickness, and the absorption of light due to bilirubin in the capillary bed and subcutaneous tissue is isolated by spectral subtraction. The JM-103 has attempted to overcome some of the disadvantages of the earlier model by using two wavelengths and a dual optical path system. (35) The principle of operation includes the formation of two beams, one of which reaches only the shallow areas of the subcutaneous tissue, while the other penetrates the deeper layers. The differences between the optical densities are detected by blue and green photocells. Measurement of bilirubin accumulated primarily in the deeper subcutaneous tissue should decrease the influence of other pigments in the

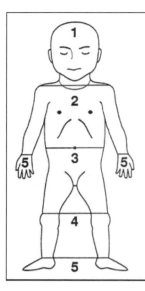

Dermal Zone	Indirect Bilirubin (mg/100 mL)		
	Mean ± SD	Range	Observations
1	5.9 ± 0.3	4.3 – 7.9	13
2	8.9 ± 1.7	5.4 – 12.2	49
3	11.8 ± 1.8	8.1 – 16.5	52
4	15.0 ± 1.7	11.1 – 18.3	45
5		> 15	29

Figure 3. Zones for estimating the cephalocaudal progression of jaundice. The indirect bilirubin values corresponding to each zone are shown in the table. Reprinted from *Archives of Pediatrics & Adolescent Medicine*, 154(4):391–394. Copyright (2000) American Medical Association. All rights reserved.

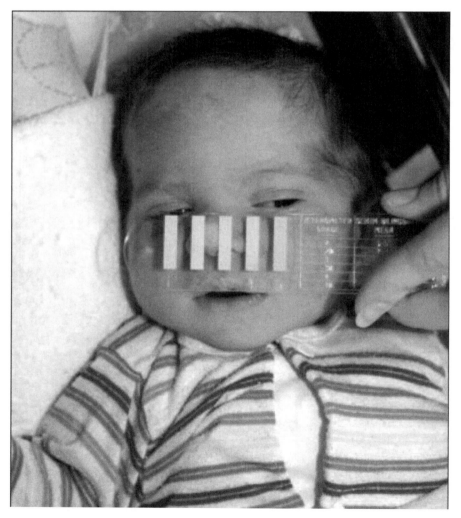

Figure 4. The Gossett icterometer.

skin, such as melanin and hemoglobin. It was hoped that the innovative technologies employed in the BiliChek and the JM-103 would make TcB measurements independent of race, age, gestation, and birth-weight, but these hopes have not been fully realized. Both instruments provide a digital read-out of the actual transcutaneous bilirubin concentration rather than an index that needs to be converted to a TSB value. The BiliChek requires five repeat measurements that are averaged to provide one TcB measurement. The JM-103 provides the option of obtaining one to five measurements that are automatically averaged.

Factors Affecting the Measurement
Effects of Skin Pigmentation and Gestation

Although large studies of both the BiliChek and the JM-103 have shown very good correlations between TcB and TSB measurements, (33)(34)(36)(37) the hope that such measurements would be independent of both race and gestation has not been entirely fulfilled. In the one study that contained a significant number of African-American infants (n = 145), (33) the correlation between BiliChek TcB and high-performance liquid chromatography (HPLC) measurements of the TSB in African-American infants was as good as in Caucasian infants, but TcB measurements by the JM-103 in African-American infants tended to overestimate the TSB measurements. (36) In the other racial groups (East Asian, Middle Eastern, Indian/Pakistani, Hispanic), JM-103 measurements were very similar to the TSB measurements. (36) Nevertheless, both the JM-103 and the BiliChek are less reliable in predicting TSB in more preterm infants, particularly those younger than 30 weeks' gestation. (37)(38)(39)

Site of Sampling

In *77* Japanese infants, JM-103 measurements from the forehead correlated well with TSB measurements and better than measurements obtained with the JM-102. (35) We compared JM-103 measurements from the forehead and sternum in 475 infants and found that the Pearson correlation coefficient (r) was higher for the sternum (0.953) than

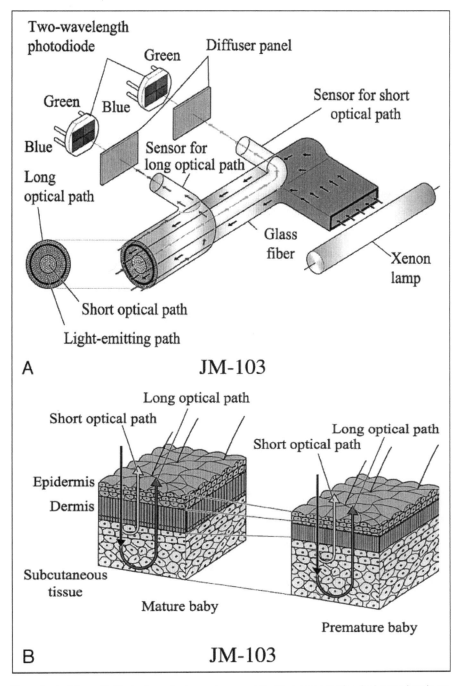

Figure 5. A. Schematic illustration of a transcutaneous bilirubinometer. B. The dual optical path system. Reproduced with permission from Draeger Medical.

Poland and associates (41) found that brow readings were 20% lower than TSB values, but chest readings were only 5% lower. They suggested that exposure to ambient light might result in lower TcB readings. On the other hand, Ebbesen and colleagues, (37) in their study of Danish infants, found that Bili-Chek measurements from the forehead in a neonatal intensive care unit population predicted the TSB better than measurements from the sternum; in the well baby population, measurements at both sites were equally reliable. They also found, as did Engle, (40) that the BiliChek tended to underestimate the TSB, a discrepancy that increased when the TSB was 10 mg/dL (171 mcmol/L) or greater.

Laboratory Measurements and TcB

TcB is a measurement of bilirubin in the skin, not the serum. Currently, we use the TSB value for making decisions about when to initiate investigations, what type of surveillance is necessary, and when to initiate treatment. (7) Some investigators have compared TcB measurements with HPLC measurements of serum bilirubin; (33)(34) others have compared the TcB measurement with standard laboratory measurements of TSB. The variability of TSB measurements within and between different laboratories is well documented, (42) so that comparisons with TcB measurements vary in different institutions. In addition to these variations, we occasionally have laboratory errors. Indeed, we have had occasions in our nursery where the measured TSB diverged widely from the TcB. When the laboratory test was repeated, the initial measurement was shown to be in error.

HPLC measurements sometimes are considered the putative "gold standard" for measuring serum bilirubin, and in one study, (34) BiliChek TcB measurements correlated more closely than did standard laboratory TSB measurements with HPLC TSB measurements. On the other hand, no data document the variability of HPLC measurements within or between different laboratories; the assumption that this is the gold standard against which TcB measurements should be compared remains to be proven.

the forehead (0.914). (36) Because the forehead is exposed to ambient light, both in the nursery and following discharge (while the sternum almost always is covered), measurements from the sternum might be a better choice.

Studies with the BiliChek have used both forehead (33)(34) and sternum as sampling sites. (37) Engle and associates (40) studied a Hispanic population and found that BiliChek measurements from the forehead tended to underestimate TSB, particularly when the TSB exceeded 10 mg/dL (171 mcmol/L). However, in a small study of 31 infants comparing outpatient BiliChek measurements from the brow and the sternum,

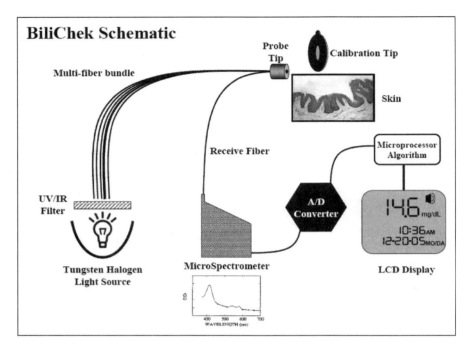

BiliChek Schematic

Multi-fiber bundle

Probe Tip

Calibration Tip

Skin

Receive Fiber

Microprocessor Algorithm

UV/IR Filter

A/D Converter

14.6 mg/dL

10:36 AM
12-20-05 MO/DA

Tungsten Halogen Light Source

MicroSpectrometer

LCD Display

Figure 6. Schematic diagram of the BiliChek TcB meter. Reproduced with permission from Philips Children's Medical Ventures.

Phototherapy

Because phototherapy bleaches the skin, both visual assessments of jaundice and TcB measurements in infants undergoing phototherapy are not reliable but probably can be taken about 18 to 24 hours after cessation of phototherapy. (39)(43)

Who is Doing the Measurement?

Virtually all of the published studies performed with the BiliChek and the JM-103 have been performed under the relatively rigorous conditions of clinical investigation, with TcB measurements obtained by research nurses or technicians. Such studies almost certainly provide more accurate and precise results than those obtained with "real world" measurements by many different nurses or physicians in different environments and in the course of a normal day's work.

Impact of TcB on Blood Sampling and Costs

We and others have shown a significant reduction in TSB measurements in our nurseries when TcB measurements were used as a screening tool. (29)(44) Currently, every infant in our nursery is screened with a JM-103 TcB measurement during the midnight

shift. This has resulted in a decrease in the number of infants who have at least one TSB measurement during their nursery stay from 27.6% to 9%, which represents a 67% reduction in TSB measurements. Ebbesen and associates (37) estimated that TcB measurements in their nursery would save 80% of the infants from blood sampling.

How Should We Use TcB Measurements?

At present, TcB measurements should be used as a screening tool. They can help to answer the questions "Should I worry about this infant?" and "Should I obtain a TSB on this infant?" (45) Our primary goals are to avoid an unnecessary heel stick and to avoid missing a high TSB level (ie, a false-negative TcB measurement). To achieve these goals, we can set a value for a TcB measurement (based on the infant's age in hours and other risk factors) above which a TSB level always should be obtained.

In Ebbesen's nursery, (37) if the TcB value is 70% of the TSB level recommended for the use of phototherapy, a TSB measurement is obtained. In our nursery, the nurses automatically obtain a TSB if the TcB is above the 75th percentile. (6) Although we readily

accept the likelihood that we will obtain several unnecessary TSB measurements, we do not want to miss a TSB level that will change our management. In our study with the JM-103, (35) the chance of a TcB measurement underestimating the TSB level by 3 mg/dL (51 mcmol/L) or more was only 0.6%, so choosing the 75th percentile as a cut point seemed reasonable. Bhutani and colleagues (33) found that as long as the TcB was less than the 75th percentile, 0 of 349 infants had a TSB above the 95th percentile (a negative predictive value of 100%).

An alternative approach is: "If the real TSB value is TcB + 3 mg/dL (51 mcmol/L), is there a reasonable chance that this will change my management?" If the answer is yes, a TSB should be measured, which allows the clinician to take into account other risk factors, including the gestation. With this approach, no infant who has significant hyperbilirubinemia should be missed, and many infants and their families will be spared the trauma, cost, and inconvenience of having a laboratory measurement of serum bilirubin. In an outpatient study of a primarily Hispanic population, no infant who had a JM-103 level of 13 mg/dL (222 mg/dL) or less had a TSB of greater than 17 mg/dL (291 mcmol/ L), (46) and 50% of TSB determinations were avoided.

Conclusion

Although TcB measurements provide a good estimate of the TSB level, they are not a substitute for TSB values, and they never should be considered in isolation. Further, critical decisions should not be made from a single TcB measurement. Any measurement has the potential for error, and if the clinical assessment of jaundice differs from the TcB reading, a TSB should be measured.

Measurements of TcB in the nursery, the office, or other outpatient settings, including the home, provide a noninvasive, instantaneous estimate of the TSB. This has been of enormous value in our nursery as well as our outpatient follow-up clinic and should prove equally valuable in an office practice. TcB measurements can help to avoid the potential errors associated with clinical estimation of bilirubin levels.

Unfortunately, because of cost concerns, very few pediatric offices are currently equipped with an instrument for measuring the TcB. The CPT code for measuring TcB is 88400. A private pediatric group affiliated with our hospital found that about 50% of 250 TcB measurements performed in the office were reimbursed by third party payers at an average of about $6 per test (S. Clune MD, personal communication).

Before we had pulse oximetry, we assessed the oxygen saturation of a newborn or a child who had asthma by eye, and we were often wrong. Today, it is difficult to imagine managing such children without the benefits of pulse oximetry. It is likely that TcB measurements soon will be considered similarly indispensable in the care of the jaundiced newborn.

References

1. Rubaltelli FF, Carli M. The effect of light on cutaneous bilirubin. *Biol Neonate.* 1971;18:457–472

2. Ylppö A. Icterus neonatorum (incl. I. n. gravis) und Gallenfarbstoffsekretion beim Foetus and Neugeboren. *Z Kinderheilkd.* 1913;9:208

3. Hsia DYY, Allen FH, Gellis SS, Diamond LK. Erythroblastosis fetalis. VIII. Studies of serum bilirubin in relation to kernicterus. *N Engl J Med.* 1952;247:668–671

4. Davidson LT, Merritt KK, Weech AA. Hyperbilirubinemia in the newborn. *Am J Dis Child.* 1941;61:958–980

5. Johnson L, Bhutani VK. Guidelines for management of the jaundiced term and near-term infant. *Clin Perinatol.* 1998;25:555–574

6. Bhutani VK, Johnson L, Sivieri EM. Predictive ability of a predischarge hour-specific serum bilirubin for subsequent significant hyperbilirubinemia in healthy-term and near-term newborns. *Pediatrics.* 1999;103:6–14

7. Maisels MJ, Baltz RD, Bhutani V, et al. Management of hyperbilirubinemia in the newborn infant 35 or more weeks of gestation. *Pediatrics.* 2004;114:297–316

8. Wood B, Culley P, Roginski C, Powell J, Waterhouse J. Factors affecting neonatal jaundice. *Arch Dis Child.* 1979;54:111–115

9. Tayaba R, Gribetz D, Gribetz I, Holzman IR. Noninvasive estimation of serum bilirubin. *Pediatrics.* 1998;102:e28. Available at: http://pediatrics.aappublications.org/cgi/content/full/102/3/e28

10. Moyer VA, Ahn C, Sneed S. Accuracy of clinical judgment in neonatal jaundice. *Arch Pediatr Adolesc Med.* 2000;154:391–394

11. Riskin A, Kuglman A, Abend-Weinger M, Green M, Hemo M, Bader D. In the eye of the beholder: how accurate is clinical estimation of jaundice in newborns? *Acta Paediatr.* 2003;92:574–576

12. Kramer LI. Advancement of dermal icterus in the jaundiced newborn. *Am J Dis Child.* 1969;118:454–458

13. Hegyi T, Hiatt M, Gertner I, et al. Transcutaneous bilirubinometry: the cephalocaudal progression of dermal icterus. *Am J Dis Child.* 1981;135:547

14. Knudsen A. The cephalocaudal progression of jaundice in newborns in relation to the transfer of bilirubin from plasma to skin. *Early Hum Dev.* 1990;22:23–28

15. Bhutani VK, Meloy LD, Poland RL, et al. Correlation of clinical assessment of jaundice, transcutaneous and total serum bilirubin levels in healthy term and near-term infants. *Pediatr Res.* 2004;55:591A

16. Gossett IH. A Perspex icterometer for neonates. *Lancet.* 1960;1:87–88

17. Schumacher RE, Thornbery J, Gutcher GR. Transcutaneous bilirubinometry: a comparison of old and new methods. *Pediatrics.* 1985;76:10–14

18. Merritt KA, Coulter DM. Application of the Gosset icterometer to screen for clinically significant hyperbilirubinemia in premature infants. *J Perinatol.* 1994;14:58–65

19. Madlon-Kay DJ. Recognition of the presence and severity of newborn jaundice by parents, nurses, physicians, and icterometer. *Pediatrics.* 1997;100:e3. Available at: http://pediatrics.aappublications.org/cgi/content/full/100/3/e3

20. Madlon-Kay DJ. Maternal assessment of neonatal jaundice after hospital discharge. *J Fam Prac.* 2002;51:445–448

21. Madlon-Kay DJ. Home health nurse clinical assessment of neonatal jaundice. *Arch Pediatr Adolesc Med.* 2001;155:583–586

22. Hannemann RE, DeWitt DP, Hanley EJ, Schreiner RL, Bonderman P. Determination of serum bilirubin by skin reflectance: effect of pigmentation. *Pediatr Res.* 1979;13:1326–1329

23. Hannemann RE, DeWitt DP, Wiechel JF. Neonatal serum bilirubin from skin reflectance. *Pediatr Res.* 1978;12:207–210

24. Yamanouchi I, Yamauchi Y, Igarashi I. Transcutaneous bilirubinometry: preliminary studies of noninvasive transcutaneous bilirubin meter in the Okayama National Hospital. *Pediatrics.* 1980;65:195

25. Maisels MJ, Conrad S. Transcutaneous bilirubin measurements in full-term infants. *Pediatrics.* 1982;70:464–467

26. Hegyi T, Hiatt IM, Indyk L. Transcutaneous bilirubinometry. I. Correlations in term infants. *J Pediatr.* 1981;98:454–457

27. Yamauchi Y, Yamanouchi I. Transcutaneous bilirubinometry. Evaluation of accuracy and reliability in a large population. *Acta Paediatr Scand.* 1988;77:791–795

28. Schumacher RE. Non-invasive measurements of bilirubin in the newborn. *Clin Perinatol.* 1990;17:417–435

29. Maisels MJ, Kring E. Trancutaneous bilirubinometry decreases the need for serum bilirubin measurements and saves money. *Pediatrics.* 1997;99:599–601

30. Briscoe L, Clark S, Yoxall C. Can transcutaneous bilirubinometry reduce the need for blood tests in jaundiced full term babies? *Arch Dis Child Fetal Neonatol Ed.* 2002;86:F190–F192

31. Yamauchi Y, Yamanouchi I. Transcutaneous bilirubinometry in normal Japanese infants. *Acta Paediatr Jpn.* 1989;31:65–72

32. Yamauchi Y, Yamanouchi I. Transcutaneous bilirubinometry: effect of postnatal age. *Acta Paediatr Jap.* 1991;33:663–667

33. Bhutani V, Gourley GR, Adler S, Kreamer B, Dalman C, Johnson LH. Noninvasive measurement of total serum bilirubin in a multiracial predischarge newborn population to assess the risk of severe hyperbilirubinemia. *Pediatrics.* 2000;106:e17. Available at: http://pediatrics.aappublications.org/cgi/content/full/106/2/e17

34. Rubaltelli FF, Gourley G.R., Loskamp N, et al. Transcutaneous bilirubin measurement: a multicenter evaluation of a new device. *Pediatrics.* 2001;107:1264–1271

35. Yasuda S, Itoh S, Isobe K, et al. New transcutaneous jaundice device with two optical paths. *J Perinat Med*. 2003;31:81–88

36. Maisels MJ, Ostrea EJ, Jr, Touch S, et al. Evaluation of a new transcutaneous bilirubinometer. *Pediatrics*. 2004;113:1628–1635

37. Ebbesen F, Rasmussen LM, Wimberley PD. A new transcutaneous bilirubinometer, BiliChek, used in the neonatal intensive care unit and the maternity ward. *Acta Paediatr*. 2002;91:203–211

38. Maisels MJ, Kring EA. Accuracy of transcutaneous bilirubin (TcB) measurements in preterm infants. *Pediatr Res*. 2004;55:458A

39. Knupfer M, Pulzer F, Braun L, Heilmann A, Robel-Tillig E, Vogtmann C. Transcutaneous bilirubinometry in pre-term infants. *Acta Paediatr*. 2001;90:899–903

40. Engle WD, Jackson GL, Sendelbach D, Manning D, Frawley W. Assessment of a transcutaneous device in the evaluation of neonatal hyperbilirubinemia in a primarily Hispanic population. *Pediatrics*. 2002;110:61–67

41. Poland RL, Hartenberger C, McHenry H, Hsi A. Comparison of skin sites for estimating serum total bilirubin in in-patients and out-patients: chest is superior to brow. *J Perinatol*. 2004;24:541–543

42. Vreman HJ, Verter J, Oh W, et al. Interlaboratory variability of bilirubin measurements. *Clin Chem*. 1996;42:869–873

43. Tan KL, Dong F. Transcutaneous bilirubinometry during and after phototherapy. *Acta Paediatr*. 2003;92:327–331

44. Dai J, Krahn J, Parry DM. Clinical impact of transcutaneous bilirubinometry as an adjunctive screen for hyperbilirubinemia. *Clin Biol*. 1996;29:581–586

45. Schumacher R. Transcutaneous bilirubinometry and diagnostic tests: "the right job for the tool." *Pediatrics*. 2002;110:407–408

46. Engle WD, Jackson GC, Stehel EK, Sendelbach DM, Manning M.D. Evaluation of a transcutaneous jaundice meter following hospital discharge in term and near-term neonates. *J Perinatol*. 2005;25:486–490

Historical Perspectives: Transcutaneous Bilirubinometry

M. Jeffrey Maisels

NeoReviews 2006;7;e217-e225

DOI: 10.1542/neo.7-5-e217

The Early Development of Neonatal Magnetic Resonance Imaging

Malcolm I. Levene, MD, FRCPCH*

The ability to evaluate the neonatal brain changed enormously in the late 1970s, first with computed tomography (CT) scanning and then with cephalic ultrasonography. Instead of guessing whether or not an infant might have an intracranial hemorrhage, based on a falling hematocrit and deteriorating clinical status, it was now possible to obtain images that could define the size and location of hemorrhage or to virtually exclude it.

Soon afterwards, nuclear magnetic resonance imaging (MRI) in children was reported by Dr Malcolm Levene and colleagues at the Hammersmith Hospital in London (1). Several of the children were neonates. Despite the difficulties inherent in performing these studies (with the need to transport the infants to the magnet and give sedation, rather than being able to do it at the bedside), it was clear that information could be obtained that was not available with CT or ultrasound imaging. This information included abnormal myelination, periventricular edema, and asphyxial injury. This is described in detail in this 2006 Historical Perspective by Professor Levene.

At about this time too, magnetic resonance spectroscopy (MRS) in neonates was being developed at University College Hospital, London (2). While MRS is less readily available, MRI has become the preferred method of evaluating the brain for prognostic purposes (3) and also for evaluating other organ systems in both the fetus and newborn (4).

Alistair G. S. Philip, MD, FRCPE, FAAP
Editor-in-Chief, NeoReviews

References

1. Levene MI, Whitelaw A, Dubowitz V, et al. Nuclear magnetic resonance imaging of the brain in children. *Br Med J.* 1982;285:774–776
2. Delpy DT, Gordon RE, Hope PL, et al. Non-invasive investigation of cerebral ischemia by phosphorus nuclear magnetic resonance. *Pediatrics.* 1982;70:310–313
3. Mirmiran M, Barnes PD, Keller K, et al. Neonatal brain magnetic resonance imaging before discharge is better than serial cranial ultrasound in predicting cerebral palsy in very low birth weight preterm infants. *Pediatrics.* 2000;114:992–998
4. Barth RA, Rubasova E. Fetal magnetic resonance imaging: anomalies of the neck, chest and abdomen. *NeoReviews.* 2007;8:e313–e335

Introduction

Imaging of the central nervous system is the most important advance in clinical neurology in the 20th century, providing for the first time a "window on the brain." Initially, the view was somewhat opaque, but successive generations of scanning techniques and modifications to technology resulted by the end of the century in images of remarkable anatomic-like clarity. Although such advances have provided access to the brains of patients in all age groups, the study of the neonatal brain has particularly benefited

clinicians at a time when survival of very immature infants was increasing dramatically and concern was developing about the causes of neurodevelopmental disability in the surviving child.

The brain of the immature infant initially was imaged using computed tomography (CT) scanning by Papile and colleagues (1) from Albuquerque in 1978, and in the following year, Karen Pape, (2) a Canadian working in London, described the diagnosis of brain damage in preterm babies scanned with real-time ultrasonography. These and subsequent articles showed that intraventricular hemorrhage occurred commonly in preterm infants, most of the babies who had these

lesions survived, and a surprisingly high proportion showed few abnormal clinical signs at the time of the hemorrhage. In 1983, we at the Hammersmith Hospital in London used real-time ultrasonography to diagnose hemorrhagic periventricular leukomalacia with the evolution to cystic degeneration in surviving sick preterm infants. (3)

Although these two techniques led to a massive new interest in causation and prevention of brain pathology in preterm infants, both suffered from a number of disadvantages. CT exposed the babies to potentially high levels of X-irradiation and, therefore, could be performed only infrequently. In addition, the baby had to be transported from the intensive care environment to the scanner, which might be situated a considerable distance away. Ultrasonography had the great advantage of portability, and even the sickest babies could be scanned in their intensive care incubators, but some brain regions were invisible to the ultrasound beam due to problems with contact and absorption of sound by the ossifying skull. Resolution of pathology in the white matter was a particular problem with ultrasound techniques and, to a lesser extent, continues to prove problematic, even with modern equipment.

In the early 1980s, nuclear magnetic resonance (NMR) or magnetic resonance (MR), as the technique now is called, was shown to be valuable in clinical practice and subsequently revolutionized the approach to demonstrating both structure and function of the brain and other organs to the benefit of almost every medical speciality. Development of this technique represents the multidisciplinary efforts of physicists, radiologists, clinicians, and technicians.

The development of NMR to analyze the composition of chemical compounds was accomplished independently in 1946 by Felix Bloch at Stanford University and Edward Purcell at Harvard University, who were jointly awarded the Nobel prize for physics in

*Professor of Pediatrics and Child Health, University of Leeds, Leeds, England.

1952. Raymond Damadian, a medical doctor working in New York in 1971, showed that NMR could be used to characterize normal from abnormal tissue, (4) and in 1973, Paul Lauterbur published the first description of image construction using NMR, which he described as "zeugmatography."(5) Further advances in two-dimensional scanning were made possible by using computer algorithms developed by Godfrey N. Hounsfield (another Nobel laureate) for constructing CT images. Due to the nonionizing nature of MR compared with CT, the former rapidly took over from the latter as a preferred imaging modality.

The widespread application of MR in clinical practice required the commercial development of wide-bore magnets that produced a uniform magnetic field into which the patient could be placed. In the United Kingdom, three independent groups working in London, Nottingham (England), and Aberdeen (Scotland) developed prototype machines for clinical imaging. These included Young working at Picker Ltd (a subsidiary of GEC) in conjunction with radiologists at Hammersmith Hospital; Steiner, Bydder, Mansfield, and Moore in Nottingham; and Mallard and Hutchinson in Aberdeen.

MR Neonatal Brain Imaging

A prototype machine was installed at Hammersmith Hospital in the early 1980s, and permission was obtained from the Ethics Committee to scan pediatric and infant patients in 1981. In September 1982, Levene and colleagues (6) were the first to describe the appearance of the brain in babies subjected to MR and showed that this relatively new modality gave important insight into brain development and pathology that could not be obtained with other imaging devices available at that time.

The original machine was housed in a small room within the radiology department of Hammersmith Hospital. It comprised a 0.15-T cryomagnet with a receiver coil around the baby's head (Fig. 1). The children usually were sedated with chloral hydrate (75 mg/kg) or occasionally scanned when they were asleep after a feeding. Because of the strong magnetic field, monitoring the babies using any device containing metal was impossible,

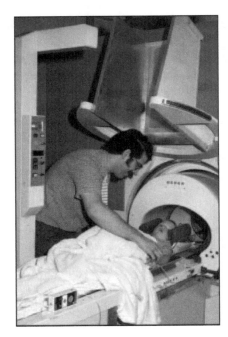

Figure 1. The author placing a child in the prototype magnet at Hammersmith Hospital in 1981.

but patient safety during the scan was paramount to avoid a catastrophe that would severely limit the use of MR in infants for years to come. Initially, attempts at assessing patient well-being during image acquisition were relatively crude. For the first patients studied, the neonatologist lay in the core of the magnet at the other end to the baby with a finger on the infant's pulse during the examination. This was not totally successful and very uncomfortable for the clinician. A second method for monitoring the babies used an esophageal stethoscope, which involved placing a plastic tube into the child's esophagus, with the other end attached to earpieces similar to those provided to passengers on long airline journeys. The neonatologist listened to the neonatal heart through the stethoscope during the examination. In older children, a surface respiratory monitor was used. This small, flat, air-filled plastic capsule was strapped to the baby's abdomen and attached by a very long plastic extension tube out of the magnet-containing room to a monitor that provided an audible signal on every breath. An alarm was sounded if no signal was detected after 20 seconds. These methods worked very well, and no baby ever came to any harm during the course of the early studies at Hammersmith Hospital.

Because we had little idea what information these brain images would provide, a variety of babies and young children who had different forms of pathology were investigated. These included infants who had ultrasonographically detected ventricular dilatation, probable rubella embryopathy, neuromuscular disorders, inborn errors of metabolism, congenital brain anomalies, and hypoxic-ischemic encephalopathy as well as infants who had been born very preterm. Good images of brain structure were obtained both in the normal brain and in babies who had structural abnormalities, including ventricular dilatation, porencephaly, and partial agenesis of the corpus callosum.

The imaging sequences chosen were repeated free induction decay for proton density, inversion recovery, and spin echo. The significant differences in water content within the immature brain compared with adult patients who had been scanned up to that time required adjustment of sequences and acquisition times to obtain satisfactory images. Up to 10 slices were performed in each child, with at least one of each type of sequence in each study.

Although myelination was known to be particularly sensitive in adult studies to inversion-recovery (IR) sequences, showing long T1 regions in these areas, we were surprised at how little myelination was apparent on IR sequences in the immature brain. We then attempted to develop standard myelination appearances in four normal children (usually belonging to staff members) at term birth and at 6 months, 20 months, and 5 years of age. Little or no myelination was present in the periventricular white matter in a term infant, but was present in the posterior internal capsule and thalamooccipital radiation. In a healthy 20-month-old infant, myelination signal was present within the white matter of the periventricular region of both cerebral hemispheres, and the signal became much more extensive by 5 years of age (Fig. 2). Such appearances of the rapid myelination in the immature brain never had been demonstrated in vivo before.

Structural abnormalities well seen on MR included ventricular dilatation, porencephalic cysts, and congenital malformations such as

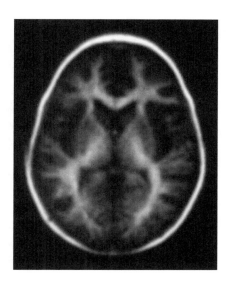

Figure 2. A normal scan from the prototype magnet of a 5-year-old volunteer made in 1982.

partial agenesis of the corpus callosum. In the first report, delay in myelination was observed in two babies, both of whom had significant developmental delay. One baby presented a particular startling abnormal appearance, with long T1 and short T2 areas in the periventricular white matter. This baby had congenital muscular dystrophy and probably represented a rare dysmyelinating (Fukuyama) form of this condition.

A subsequent report from the Hammersmith group in 1983 (7) described a larger cohort of infants and children who had more varied pathology. Eight healthy children and 52 children who had a wide variety of conditions were scanned and confirmed the value of this technique in providing accurate and new information of clinical relevance, such as the appearances of cerebral artery infarction. Five babies were scanned after acute hypoxic-ischemic insult, three of whom were term infants. The scans showed a new appearance of long T1 in the periventricular regions on IR scans that was considerably more extensive than that seen in healthy term babies. Long T2 was seen in the same areas using spin echo sequences, which also were more prominent than in healthy term babies. These appearances were believed to be possibly due to cerebral edema, but this still remains uncertain. These results first were presented orally to a pediatric audience at the Second Special Ross Laboratories Conference on Perinatal Intracranial Hemorrhage in Washington, DC, in 1983.

The Hammersmith Hospital group continued to develop the imaging equipment, improving the image resolution by using smaller diameter RF coils and newer image reconstruction software. In 1987, they described studies on 177 patients, of whom 10 were healthy volunteers and many of whom were neonates. (8)

MR Spectroscopy

As discussed previously, NMR was used initially in the 1940s for tissue characterization prior to its development for clinical imaging. MR spectroscopy later was used as an in vivo clinical tool and first described for study of the neonatal brain in 1983. (9) This work was pioneered at University College Hospital, London, under the direction of Reynolds and Wilkie, with the collaboration of the department of medical physics and bioengineering at Oxford Research Systems, using a small-bore 1.9-T magnet of only 20 cm diameter housed in the basement of the hospital. This limited the application to only the neonatal head because the baby's body was too large to enter the core of the magnet.

This group used phosphorus NMR spectroscopy to measure noninvasively the intracellular concentrations of all the phosphorus metabolites free in solution, including those in intracellular energy metabolism. They studied seven infants who had severe intrapartum asphyxia or brain abnormalities detected by cranial ultrasonography. The three asphyxiated babies all showed low phosphocreatine/inorganic phosphorus (PCr/Pi) ratios, with an increase in the subsequent few weeks. Further work by this group showed that the cerebral energetics changed with time following a severe hypoxic-ischemic insult, with a honeymoon period during the first day, followed by a progressive abnormal PCr/Pi ratio after 18 to 24 hours. Infants who had the greatest fall in cerebral phosphorus energetics had the poorest prognoses. (10)

In the United States, the first babies were studied with a 25-cm diameter 1.9-T MR spectroscopy unit placed at the hospital of the University of Pennsylvania, Philadelphia. (11) Investigators described 15 preterm infants who had hypoxic-ischemic insult at birth and were studied between 1 and 88 days after birth, showing similar findings to the London group.

A further development with MR spectroscopy was the introduction of proton spectroscopy used to examine the neonatal brain, which was pioneered by the diagnostic radiology/ neonatal group at Hammersmith Hospital. (12) They showed separation between N-acetylaspartate (NAA) molecules, choline-containing compounds (Cho), and creatinine plus phosphocreatinine (Cr). The NAA/ Cho ratio remained lowest in infants who had the most severe neurologic abnormality. In a follow-up study of 11 infants born at term following severe hypoxic-ischemic injury, the NAA/Cho and NAA/Cr ratios best reflected clinical outcome. (13)

The acquisition of data for both MR spectroscopy and imaging in neonates using one magnet was first described by Boesch and Martin in 1988, (14) who used a more powerful 2.35-T system housed at the University Children's Hospital, Zurich, Switzerland. Their first report described the findings from 105 babies and children (more than 20 neonates) who were studied on 142 occasions. The larger-bore diameter of the magnet (35 cm) allowed study of children up to the age of 9 years. This state-of-the-art facility combined the potential for MR brain imaging with acquisition of spectroscopic data from proton and phosphorus images.

During the 1980s, the application of MR imaging and spectroscopy to neonatal and pediatric patients became much more widespread. Reports were published in the literature of MR studies involving the evaluation of disease in children's hearts using both imaging (15) and spectroscopy, (16) spinal dysraphism, (17) abdominal masses, (18) hips, (19) thorax, (20) pediatric gynecologic disorders, (21) tumors, (22) and liver disorders. (23) Today, MR is used ubiquitously to study almost every organ in the body, and many thousands of neonates are screened annually using these techniques.

Fetal Imaging

The first description of fetal MR imaging was from the pioneering group in Aberdeen, Scotland in 1983. (24) They described imaging six 12 to 20 weeks' gestation fetuses immediately prior to termination of pregnancy, and in 1984, they described imaging a more mature fetus in the third trimester. (25) Although imaging was possible, the lack of differentiation between some fetal tissues and the slow acquisition time made fetal movement during imaging a major problem. Another early fetal imaging group from Nottingham, England, found that movement artefact was less of a problem when mature fetuses were required to remain still during the 2-minute scan time due to their relative physical restriction and paucity of movement. (26) The first report from the United States was by McCarthy and associates, (27) who described the scans of nine fetuses of 34 to 36 weeks' gestation, reporting that heart and lungs were particularly well delineated, but the brain was relatively featureless due to the lack of grey-white matter differentiation.

These early articles showed that MR could be applied to the fetus, but because ultrasonography was such a safe, convenient, and accurate method of examining the fetus, few applications of MR for the fetus were reported until ultrafast imaging sequences such as fast spin echo and other techniques were developed. Today, MR has a useful role in assessing the fetus when abnormalities are suggested with ultrasonography.

Conclusion

The development of MR has provided clinicians with a unique and invaluable tool to study the human in health and disease. The basic scientists who developed this technique have been awarded three Nobel prizes for their work, which underscores the unique contribution that MR has made to medicine. The original use of MR in the neonate and infant was opportunistically based on prototype magnets placed in a small number of centers and the collaboration of radiologists and neonatologists. In contrast, clinical MR spectroscopy was developed specifically with the baby's head in mind, and the early magnets were limited to smallbore devices that allowed placement of only small babies inside.

In the 1990s and later, further great developments have been made in the application of MR to pediatric and neonatal brain disorders. Many applications currently are only in experimental settings and include diffusion-weighted imaging, cerebral perfusion and blood flow, functional MR assessment of cerebral oxygen metabolism, tractography, and estimates of differential brain growth. We will continue to see further developments using this technique, which should have direct application to the neonatal brain to understand normal development, pathology, and function.

References

1. Papile LA, Burstein J, Burstein R, Koffler H. Incidence and evolution of subependymal and intraventricular hemorrhage: a study of infants with birthweights less than 1,500 gm. *J Pediatr.* 1978;92:529–534

2. Pape KE, Blackwell RJ, Cusick G, et al. Ultrasound detection of brain damage in preterm infants. *Lancet.* 1979;i:1261–1264

3. Levene MI, Wigglesworth JS, Dubowitz V. Hemorrhagic periventricular leukomalacia: a real-time ultrasound study. *Pediatrics.* 1983;71:794–797

4. Damadian R. Tumor detection by nuclear magnetic resonance. *Science.* 1971;171:1151–1153

5. Lauterbur PC. Image formation by induced local interactions: examples of employing nuclear magnetic resonance. *Nature.* 1973;242:190–191

6. Levene MI, Whitelaw A, Dubowitz V, et al. Nuclear magnetic resonance imaging of the brain in children. *Br Med J.* 1982;285:774–776

7. Johnson MA, Pennock JM, Bydder GM, et al. Clinical NMR imaging of the brain in children: normal and neurologic disease. *Am J Neuroradiol.* 1983;4:1013–1026

8. Johnson MA, Pennock JM, Bydder GM, Dubowitz LMS, Thomas DJ, Young IR. Serial MR imaging in neonatal cerebral injury. *Am J Neuroradiol.* 1987;8:83–92

9. Cady EB, Dawson MJ, Hope PL, et al. Non-invasive investigation of cerebral metabolism in newborn infants by phosphorus nuclear magnetic resonance spectroscopy. *Lancet.* 1983;i:1059–1062

10. Hope PL, Costello AM, Cady EB. Cerebral energy metabolism studied with phosphorus NMR spectroscopy in normal and birth-asphyxiated infants. *Lancet.* 1984;ii:366–370

11. Leonard JC, Younkin DP, Chance B, et al. Nuclear magnetic resonance: an overview of its spectroscopic and imaging applications in pediatric patients. *J Pediatr.* 1985;106:757

12. Peden CJ, Cowan FM, Bryant DJ, et al. Proton MR spectroscopy of the brain in infants. *J Comp Asst Tomography.* 1990;14:886–894

13. Peden CJ, Rutherford M, Sargentoni J, Cox IJ, Bryant DJ, Dubowitz LM. Proton spectroscopy of the neonatal brain following hypoxic-ischaemic injury. *Dev Med Child Neurol.* 1993;35:502–510

14. Boesch C, Martin E. Combined application of MR imaging and spectroscopy in neonates and children: installation and operation of a 2.35-T system in a clinical setting. *Radiology.* 1988;168:481–488

15. Goldman MR, Pohost GM. Nuclear magnetic resonance imaging. The potential for cardiac evaluation of the pediatric patient. *Cardiol Clin.* 1983;1:521–525

16. Whitman GJ, Chance B, Bode H, et al. Diagnosis and therapeutic evaluation of a pediatric case of cardiomyopathy using phosphorus-31 nuclear magnetic resonance spectroscopy. *J Am Coll Cardiol.* 1985;5:745–749

17. Kuharik MA, Edwards MK, Grossman CB. Magnetic resonance evaluation of pediatric spinal dysraphism. *Paed Neurosci.* 1985;12:213–218

18. Merten DF, Kirks DR. Diagnostic imaging of pediatric abdominal masses. *Pediatr Clin North Am.* 1985;32:1397–1425

19. Toby EB, Koman LA, Bechtold RE. Magnetic resonance imaging of pediatric hip disease. *J Pediatr Orthop.* 1985;5:665–671

20. Laurin S, Williams JL, Fitzsimmons JR. Magnetic resonance imaging of the pediatric thorax: initial experience. *Eur J Radiol.* 1986;6:36–41

21. Sanfilippo JS, Booth RJ, Fellows RA. Ultrasonography in the pediatric gyn patient. *Pediatr Ann.* 1986;15:607–613

22. Ringertz H, Ehman RL, McNamara MT, Gooding CA, Brasch RC. Magnetic resonance imaging in pediatric haematology/oncology. Part II. Illustrative cases and assessment of technique. *Crit Rev Onc-Hematol.* 1986;6:7–18

23. Weinreb JC, Cohen JM, Armstrong E, Smith T. Imaging the pediatric liver: MRI and CT. *Am J Roentgen.* 1986;147:785–790

24. Smith FW, Adam AH, Phillips WDP. NMR imaging in pregnancy. *Lancet.* 1983;i:61–62

25. Smith FW, MacLennan F, Abramovich DR, MacGilivray I, Hutchinson JM. NMR imaging in human pregnancy: a preliminary study. *Mag Res Imag.* 1984;2:57–64

26. Johnson IR, Symonds EM, Kean DM, et al. Imaging the pregnant human uterus with nuclear magnetic resonance. *Am J Obstet Gynecol.* 1984;148: 1136–1139

27. McCarthy S, Stark DD, Higgins CB. Demonstration of the fetal cardiovascular system by MR imaging. *J Comp Asst Tomogr.* 1984;8:1168–1169

Historical Perspectives: The Early Development of Neonatal Magnetic Resonance Imaging

Malcolm I. Levene

NeoReviews 2006;7;e329-e333

DOI: 10.1542/neo.7-7-e329

Extracorporeal Membrane Oxygenation (ECMO)

Despite the fact that his group had previously performed many animal experiments and reported success with a series of 45 human newborns in 1982, the 1985 report by Dr Bartlett and colleagues in human neonates, to which he refers in this 2005 Historical Perspectives column, generated considerable skepticism. This was because they had used an unusual statistical analysis called "Play the winner" for their randomized trial.

Their report was followed by another study of ECMO by O'Rourke et al in 1989, which was also criticized for its statistical method, but the results were striking. Despite the criticisms, many people were persuaded that ECMO was a useful therapeutic modality, because it had been highly successful in situations associated with very high mortality rates. In the United States, many ECMO centers were established and the neonatologists involved had lost equipoise, making it impossible to mount a randomized controlled trial.

In the United Kingdom, skepticism persisted and an ECMO trial was organized. It came as no great surprise to neonatologists in the United States, who had established ECMO centers, when the results of the British trial showed convincingly that ECMO could save lives. This study was published in 1995.

At the present time, ECMO is used less frequently than it was 20 years ago. This is because the primary reason for using ECMO is persistent pulmonary hypertension of the newborn (PPHN). More recently, inhaled nitric oxide therapy and newer approaches to assisted ventilation, as well as other pharmacologic treatments, have been successful in relieving severe hypoxemia in many cases of PPHN (1).

Alistair G. S. Philip, MD, FRCPE, FAAP
Editor-in-Chief, NeoReviews

References

[See also Dr Bartlett's reference list]
1. Steinhorn RH, Farrow KN. Pulmonary hypertension in the neonate. *NeoReviews.* 2007;8:e14–e21

Introduction

In 1984 and 1985, we conducted a prospective randomized trial of extracorporeal life support (ECLS) versus conventional treatment in neonatal respiratory failure that was reported in *Pediatrics* in 1985. (1) Two decades, later ECLS is standard treatment for neonatal respiratory failure that is unresponsive to other methods of management. The editors of *NeoReviews* have invited this commentary on the development and clinical implementation of ECLS in neonatal respiratory failure.

The Heart-Lung Machine

The heart-lung machine was invented by John Gibbon and initially used clinically in 1954 to replace heart and lung function long enough to allow operations on the heart. The entire field of cardiac surgery resulted from this invention. However, the heart-lung machine itself caused blood damage and multiple organ failure when used for more than 1 hour. The major cause of blood damage was direct exposure of the blood to oxygen gas. In the 1960s, some laboratories and medical device companies developed gas exchange devices in which a silicone rubber membrane was interposed between the blood and the oxygen. This modification (and others) allowed the use of a heart-lung machine for days or weeks.

Evolution to ECMO

In 1971, prolonged extracorporeal circulation was used successfully to treat a young man who had acute respiratory distress syndrome (ARDS) after trauma. (2) In the next few years, several other cases were reported using prolonged extracorporeal support to treat cardiac failure and respiratory failure from a variety of causes. Because the membrane type of artificial lung was the unique part of the device, the entire technology of prolonged ECLS came to be known as extracorporeal membrane oxygenation (ECMO). Of course, the technology involves much more than oxygenation, but that acronym has remained.

In 1975, the National Institutes of Health (NIH) sponsored a prospective, randomized, multicenter trial of ECMO for ARDS in adult patients. (3) Only 10% of both ECMO and control groups survived, effectively stopping research on ECMO for adult respiratory failure for the next 15 years.

Improving Membrane Oxygenators

Our work on prolonged extracorporeal circulation began in 1965 with efforts to improve the efficiency of membrane oxygenators. The primary motivation was the very high mortality following surgery for complex congenital heart diseases. Low cardiac output, oliguria, acidosis, respiratory failure, and death occurred in 50% of children after complex cardiac surgery. Encouraged by Dr Robert Gross and supervised by Dr Francis Moore, Phil Drinker (an engineer from the Massachusetts Institute of Technology) and I designed, built, and tested membrane oxygenators in the laboratories of the Peter Bent Brigham Hospital and Harvard Medical School.

We developed techniques to improve the efficiency of membrane oxygenators, (4) but more importantly, we began to study the technology and physiology of prolonged extracorporeal circulation. In 1970, Dr Allan Gazzaniga and I (two residents recently graduated from the Brigham program) joined the small surgical faculty at the new medical school at the University of California - Irvine. Dr John Connolly was the chairman of the department, and he recruited surgeons with training and certification in general, thoracic, vascular, and pediatric surgery. Al and I were responsible for the day-to-day surgical care at the Orange County Medical Center (later the UCI Medical Center). Dr Connolly provided laboratory space, and we undertook the serious study of prolonged extra-corporeal circulation, using sheep as the experimental model. (5) Our research, initially supported by the NIH in 1971, continues today.

Clinical Trials

We instituted clinical trials with the ECMO apparatus that we were using in the laboratory. Our first successful case was in a 2-year old patient who had cardiopulmonary failure following a Mustard operation for transposition in 1972. In 1975, we used ECMO for support of a newborn who had meconium aspiration and persistent fetal circulation. This child survived, and other successful newborn respiratory failure cases soon followed. (6) The use of ECLS for neonatal respiratory failure had been attempted by John White (7) and by Bill Dorson (8) in the past. Both used the umbilical vessels and had major problems with bleeding and device failure. Building on their experience and our own laboratory experiments, we used the jugular and carotid arteries for vascular access and titrated anticoagulation to very low levels.

The American Society for Artificial Internal Organs (ASAIO) is the primary venue for physicians, engineers, researchers, and practitioners who are studying the development and use of artificial organs. We reported our first clinical cases of ECMO for cardiopulmonary support in infancy at the meeting of ASAIO in April 1976. (6) Of the 13 infants treated, 9 were neonates who had respiratory failure, and 3 of these survived. By the next year, we had used ECMO for 16 infants who had neonatal respiratory failure, 9 of whom improved and 6 of whom ultimately survived. This series was presented at the meeting of the American Association for Thoracic Surgery and published in the *Journal of Thoracic and Cardiovascular Surgery*. (9) Although the artificial organs researchers and the thoracic surgeons received these reports with cautious optimism, the community of pediatrics and neonatologists was very skeptical. Robin Jefferies, a surgical resident, presented our results at the Society for Pediatric Research in 1977 and was met with skepticism and criticism.

As our clinical experience grew, pediatric and cardiac surgeons visited Irvine to learn the technique and review the patients. Neonatal ECMO programs were established at the Medical College of Virginia by Tom Krummel (10) and at the University of Pittsburgh by Bob Hardesty and Bart Griffith. (11)

In 1980, I moved from UCI to the University of Michigan, bringing the laboratory and research projects on extracorporeal circulation. In 1982, we reported 45 cases of neonatal respiratory failure with 55% survival. (12) Other centers reported similar results. A few young neonatologists who were frustrated by the high mortality associated with conventional treatment for neonatal respiratory failure came to Ann Arbor to learn the technology and established the first ECMO programs. These neonatologists were accused publicly of "academic suicide" by one of the deans of neonatology, but they persisted on behalf of their patients. Many of these neonatologists have become prominent in academic neonatology and pediatrics. They included Larry Cook, Bill Kanto, Devn Cornish, Billie Short, Deiter Roloff, Bob Schumacher, Tom Green, Martin Keszler, Pearl O'Rourke, Ernesto Gangiatano, and others.

By 1984, we had improved the technology to the point that the survival rate was 90% for most cases of neonatal respiratory failure and 70% for hypoplasia associated with diaphragmatic hernia. We knew the technique well enough to propose a controlled, randomized trial. We immediately encountered the logistical and ethical problems of conducting a randomized trial of a complex life support technique in which the end point is death. The NIH adult trial had addressed this issue by creating a category of "de jure" death, that is, patients in the control group defined as "will surely die" who could be crossed over to ECMO support. The criteria were arbitrary, which was one of many flaws in the NIH adult trial. Therefore, we determined that death would be the end point, but we knew we could select patients who had a 90% risk of dying with conventional treatment, and we knew that 90% of the ECMO patients would survive.

To attempt to minimize the ethical problem, we used a statistical method that had been described in the statistical literature but never used for a clinical trial. Dr Richard Cornell, chairman of Biostatistics at the University of Michigan, was our statistical collaborator. We used a method described by Wei and Durham (13) in which the first patient is truly randomized, and subsequent patients are randomized, but the treatment assignment is based on the outcome of all of the previous patients in the trial. If there is no difference between the two treatment arms, patients accrue at the same rate in both arms. If there is a major difference between the two methods of treatment, patients accrue more rapidly in the more successful arm. This type of adaptive design was well suited for our study. The study design was called "randomized play the winner" by the original authors.

We conducted two simultaneous studies, one in term infants and one in preterm infants. Three patients were entered into the preterm study, and two died of intracranial bleeding, which prompted cessation of the preterm study. In contrast, among the term infants, the first ECMO infant survived, and the next patient was a conventional treatment patient who died. The next ECMO patient survived, so the odds of being assigned to ECMO grew with each successive case. By the time 12 patients had been entered into the term neonatal trial, Dr Cornell called to report that we had reached statistical significance with a P value of .00000001. There were 11 patients in the treatment group, who all survived, and one patient in the control group, who died.

The report of this study was submitted to two journals, which declined to publish it because of the unusual statistical method. It was accepted by *Pediatrics*. Several conversations with the editor, Jerry Lucey, preceded acceptance for publication. This was to be the first publication of successful neonatal ECMO technology in the pediatric literature. Most neonatologists still considered ECMO a radical, unproven, and unnecessary technology. After all, the NIH adult ECMO trial had proven that the technique was unsuccessful. The suggestion of a prospective, randomized trial proving that ECMO was better than conventional care for neonatal respiratory failure was worrisome to most neonatologists, including the reviewers for *Pediatrics*. The treatment of neonatal respiratory failure at the time emphasized hyperventilation with induced respiratory alkalosis to decrease pulmonary vascular resistance. This often entailed the use of high ventilator pressure. Jen Wung, neonatologist at Columbia Presbyterian Hospital, had been using low-pressure ventilation for neonatal respiratory failure and had prepared a report of his phase I experience. (14) *Pediatrics* published our randomized trial adjacent to Dr Wung's paper, along with several invited commentaries, all of which criticized the ECMO report. I responded to these criticisms with a letter to the editor that never was published.

The most articulate of the critics from the Boston Children's Hospital sniffed that "a proper study has yet to be done." (15) Pearl O'Rourke of that institution conducted a second randomized trial, using a different type of adaptive design, and demonstrated that survival was much better in the ECMO-treated patients. (16) Meanwhile, many neonatal centers learned and implemented the technology. By 1990, every major children's

hospital had an ECMO team or a plan for triaging ECMO patients. In 1990, the NIH convened a workshop on diffusion of high-tech medicine from bench to clinic, using neonatal ECMO as the prototype example. (17)

Conclusion

Stimulated by the neonatal experience, ECMO is used today for cardiac and pulmonary failure in all age groups. The availability of ECMO as a rescue treatment facilitated the study of inhaled nitric oxide, high-frequency oscillation, and other methods of treatment. Today, many infants who would have received ECMO in 1995 improve with simpler methods. However, using ECMO as "rescue" after other treatments fail results in unnecessary death and chronic lung and neurologic disease. (18) Early use of ECMO (at 50% mortality risk) improves outcome without increasing cost. (19) As technology improves, ECLS will be used much earlier in all patients, including

newborns. (20) One major import of our article was to stimulate discussion of the problems and methodology of randomized trials of life support systems. The United Kingdom neonatal ECMO trial resulted from this discussion. (21) The methodology of that study defines a nearly ideal design for randomized trials of life support in which the end point is death.

Robert H. Bartlett, MD
Department of Surgery
University of Michigan
Ann Arbor, Mich.

[To read the original article on ECMO written by Barlett and associates and published in *Pediatrics* in 1985, please go to: http://neoreviews.aappublications.org/cgi/content/full/6/6/e251/DC1 or http://pediatrics.aappublications.org/cgi/content/abstract/76/4/479]

References

1. Bartlett RH, Roloff DW, Cornell RG, Andrews AF, Dillon PW, Zwischenberger JB. Extracorporeal circulation in neonatal respiratory failure: a prospective randomized study. *Pediatrics*. 1985;76:479–487

2. Hill JD, O'Brien TG, Murray JJ, et al. Extracorporeal oxygenation for acute post-traumatic respiratory failure (shock-lung syndrome): use of the Bramson membrane lung. *N Engl J Med*. 1972;286:629–634

3. Zapol WM, Snider MT, Hill JD, et al. Extracorporeal membrane oxygenation in severe acute respiratory failure: a randomized prospective study. *JAMA*. 1979;242:2193–2196

4. Bartlett RH, Isherwood J, Moss RA, Olszewski WL, Polet H, Drinker PA. A toroidal flow membrane oxygenator: four day partial bypass in dogs. *Surg Forum*. 1969;20:152–153

5. Bartlett RH, Fong SW, Burns NE, Gazzaniga AB. Prolonged partial venoarterial bypass: physiologic, biochemical and hematologic responses. *Ann Surg*. 1974;180:850–856

6. Bartlett RH, Gazzaniga AB, Jefferies R, Huxtable RF, Haiduc N, Fong SW. Extracorporeal membrane oxygenation (ECMO) cardiopulmonary support in infancy. *Trans Am Soc Artif Intern Organ*. 1976;22:80–88

7. White JJ, Andrews HG, Risemberg H, et al. Prolonged respiratory support in newborn infants with a membrane oxygenator. *Surgery*. 1971;70:288–296

8. Dorson WJ, Baker E, Cohen ML, et al. A perfusion system for infants. *ASAIO Trans*. 1969;15:155

9. Bartlett RH, Gazzaniga AB, Huxtable RF, Schippers HC, O'Connor MJ, Jefferies MR. Extracorporeal circulation (ECMO) in neonatal respiratory failure. *J Thorac Cardiovasc Surg*. 1977;74:826–833

10. Kirkpatrick BV, Krummel TM, MuellerDG, et al. Use of extracorporeal membrane oxygenation for respiratory failure in term infants. *Pediatrics*. 1983;72:872–876

11. Hardesty RL, Griffith BP, Debski RF, et al. Extracorporeal membrane oxygenation: successful treatment of persistent fetal circulation following repair of congenital diaphragmatic hernia. *J Thorac Cardiovasc Surg*. 1981; 81:556–563

12. Bartlett RH, Andrews AF, Toomasian JM, Haiduc NJ, Gazzaniga AB. Extracorporeal membrane oxygenation (ECMO) for newborn respiratory failure: 45 cases. *Surgery*. 1982;92:425–433

13. Wei LJ, Durham S. The randomized play-the-winner rule in medical trials. *J Am Stat Assoc*. 1978;73:840–843

14. Wung JT, James LS, Kilchevsky E, et al. Management of infants with severe respiratory failure and persistence of the fetal circulation without hyperventilation. *Pediatrics*. 1985;76:488–494

15. Ware JH, Epstein MF. Extracorporeal circulation in respiratory failure. [Commentaries]. *Pediatrics*. 1985;76:849–851

16. O'Rourke PP, Krone R, Vacanti J, et al. Extracorporeal membrane oxygenation and conventional medical therapy in neonates with persistent pulmonary hypertension of the newborn: a prospective randomized study. *Pediatrics*. 1989;84:957–963

17. Wright L, ed. *Report of the Workshop on Diffusion of ECMO Technology*. Bethesda, Md: National Institutes of Health; 1993: NIH Pub. #93–3399

18. Campbell BT, Braun TM, Schumacher RE, Bartlett RH, Hirschl RB. Impact of ECMO on neonatal mortality in Michigan (1980–1999). *J Pediatr Surg*. 2003;38:290–295

19. Schumacher RE, Roloff DW, Chapman R, Snedecor S, Bartlett RH. Extracorporeal membrane oxygenation in term newborns: a prospective cost-benefit analysis. *ASAIO J.* 1993;39:873–879

20. Bartlett RH. Extracorporeal circulation in 2050: a speculation. *Perfusion.* 2003;18:207–209

21. UK collaborative randomized trial of neonatal extracorporeal membrane oxygenation. UK Collaborative ECMO Trial Group. *Lancet.* 1996;348:75–82

Historical Perspectives: Extracorporeal Membrane Oxygenation (ECMO)

Robert H. Bartlett

NeoReviews 2005;6;e251-e254

DOI: 10.1542/neo.6-6-e251

History of Pulse Oximetry in Neonatal Medicine

*William W. Hay, Jr, MD**

In this 2005 Historical Perspective, my coeditor at *NeoReviews*, Dr Bill Hay, traces the development of the application of pulse oximetry to the neonate. While it is clear that he played an important role in the careful assessment of this new technology, the date of its introduction for neonatal use is less clear. Anesthesiologists may have used it before neonatologists (1). The technology expanded very rapidly in neonatal intensive care units, and as Dr Hay states, oxygen saturation is now the "fifth vital sign," together with heart rate, respiration rate, temperature, and blood pressure. Nevertheless, we continue to debate the appropriate norms (range) for oxygen saturation in preterm infants, especially in the delivery room and in the first weeks after birth (2).

Alistair G. S. Philip, MD, FRCPE, FAAP
Editor-in-Chief, NeoReviews

References

1. Sendak MJ, Harris AP, Rogers MC et al. Pulse oximetry in newborn infants in the delivery room. *Anesthesiology.* 1985;63:739–740
2. Finer N, Leone T. Oxygen saturation monitoring for the preterm infant: the evidence basis for current practices. *Pediatr Res.* 2009;65:375–380

Introduction

Although pulse oximetry in neonatal medicine was introduced fewer than 25 years ago, today it is the principal form of oxygen monitoring around the world in nearly all clinical situations that require measurement of oxygen in neonates. It has become, in fact, the fifth vital sign in neonatal medicine. For the near future, it holds center stage as the primary form of oxygen monitoring for a large international commitment to determine, after more than 50 years of mistakes, mistrials, and misunderstandings, the appropriate level of oxygen supply and blood oxygenation in preterm infants. Hopefully, these studies and the unique advantages of pulse oximetry will help to eliminate, or at least diminish, the adverse effects of too much oxygen, such as retinopathy of prematurity (ROP), without increasing the incidence of complications of hypoxia, such as patent ductus arteriosus (PDA) and pulmonary hypertension. The purpose of this review is to look back at how oximetry began, how "pulse" oximetry was developed, and how this new technology has revolutionized oxygen monitoring in neonatal medicine.

Early Developments

Oximetry, or the use of light to measure the amount of oxygen carried in the blood, began in about 1874, when Karl von Vierordt attempted to measure blood saturation in the human hand. Quantitative oximetry began with Krogh in Copenhagen just after World War I in 1918. In the 1930s, Millikan and Wood developed the two-wavelength ear oximeter that later was modified in 1935 by Matthes into the first oxygen saturation meter using red and green filters (personal communication, W. Clifford, 2004). Squire developed an instrument for measuring the quantity of blood and its degree of oxygenation in the web of the hand in 1940, and Goldie developed a device for continuous indication of oxygen saturation in circulating blood in adults in 1942. (1)(2)(3)(4) In 1949, Wood and Geraci (5) added a pressure capsule to try to obtain absolute oxygen saturation values and developed a photoelectric determination of arterial saturation. In 1964, Shaw assembled the first absolute-reading ear oximeter using eight wavelengths of light, which was commercialized by Hewlett

Packard manufacturing (personal communication, W. Clifford, 2004).

Pulse oximetry began in 1972, when Takuo Aoyagi at Nihon Kohden in Japan invented conventional pulse oximetry using the ratio of red-to-infrared light absorption of pulsating components at the measuring site. The idea of pulse oximetry developed when Aoyagi attempted to measure cardiac output using the dye dilution method with the addition of Wood's oximeter principle to make the measurements less invasive. In Wood's method, the earlobe was compressed to make it ischemic, and the transmitted light was measured. Pressure then was released, and after blood flow returned, the transmitted light was measured again. The first value was regarded as incident light, the second as transmitted light, and the ratio of the two yielded the optical density of blood, which can be correlated with the relationship of Sao_2 by a predetermined nomogram. The addition of two wavelengths of light, 805 nm and 900 nm, allowed discrimination between hemoglobin and the injected dye. Importantly, the 900-nm light was found to be sensitive to oxygen, and its response proved to be opposite in direction to the effect of oxygen in the red wavelengths. Specifically, desaturation of oxygen from blood increased infrared light transmission of blood but decreased red light transmission, thus providing the now universal application of red and infrared as the two wavelengths of light in all pulse oximeters to discriminate changes in the amount of oxygen bound to hemoglobin.

While extending these pilot studies in animals, Aoyagi noticed that arterial pulsations overlapped the dye curve, and he realized that the amplitude of the pulsation carried important color information that was unique to the arterial component of the blood. Because the pulsation showed the color of arterial blood, the effect of venous blood on the color could be excluded (and, thus, the probe could be placed across any tissue that had arterial pulsations, such as a finger, not just the ear lobe), and there was no need to

*Director, Neonatal Clinical Research Center, Department of Pediatrics, University of Colorado School of Medicine and The Children's Hospital, Denver, Colo.

compress and then release the pressure over the tissue, making the application of the probe noninvasive. Aoyagi developed the method into a single instrument at Hokkaido University and, in 1974, presented his work at the Conference of the Japan Society of MEBE in Osaka. (6) The instrument was developed reproducibly by Nihon Kohden, which submitted a patent application in Japan and produced and sold the world's first pulse oximeter, the OLV 5100. Nihon Kohden did not apply for international patents, and Aoyagi left this line of work in 1975. The first medical paper on this pulse oximeter was published in 1975. (7)

Minolta, the Japanese camera maker, extended commercialization of a pulse oximeter in 1977. The OXIMET added the novel approach of making measurements through a pair of optical fibers (hence, future developments of the cable connecting the probe to the instrument). Miyasaka used both the Minolta OXIMET and the Nihon Kohden OLV5100 for research studies, but also was the first to point out that the device could be used as a clinical monitor. Trials were conducted in Japan (8)(9) and in the United States at Stanford University in the Department of Anesthesiology by William New, Jr, (10) who along with engineer Jack Lloyd, subsequently founded Nellcor Inc. The new pulse oximetry instruments and the unique methodology caught the attention of several other entrepreneurs, who embarked on highly competitive development of clinical pulse oximeters and evaluation of their application in a variety of clinical situations. Specifically, conventional pulse oximetry was commercialized in the United States by BIOX/Ohmeda (Scott Wilber and Mike Hickey) in 1981. BIOX and Nellcor (*New*, *Ll*oyd, *Cor*man) almost simultaneously added LEDs and pulsatile signal measurements in 1983 that were correlated with predetermined Sao_2 values to produce an algorithm that determined Spo_2 from the ratio of red-to-infrared light transmission across tissues. (10)

Personal Story Regarding BIOX/Ohmeda

Mike Hickey of BT, Inc, (Biox Technology, Inc) brought a prototype Biox instrument to

me, a very junior neonatologist, in about 1982 at the suggestion of Dr Ernest Cotton, Head of Pediatric Critical Care and Pulmonology in the Department of Pediatrics at the University of Colorado School of Medicine in Denver. I asked our newly established Neonatal Clinical Research Center research nurses (who represented our National Institutes of Health-funded Pediatric General Clinical Research Center) to assist me in trying the instrument on a variety of infants in the neonatal intensive care unit (NICU) and the well baby nursery. Mike Hickey used the data we collected to enhance his instrument's algorithm. (11)(12) Not long after that, Mike sold BT, Inc, to Ohmeda for about $26 million dollars. In contrast, I received a free pulse oximeter from Ohmeda for use in my laboratory and NICU and a free trip to Zurich, Switzerland, to present the results of our pulse oximetry trials in preterm and term infants in the NICU at an early meeting of people interested in oxygen monitoring, organized by Albert and Renate Huch.

Early Studies of Accuracy and Reliability

With the new Ohmeda instruments, an enterprising University of Colorado student sat at the bedside of stable and unstable infants in the NICU and collected the first detailed set of data correlating pulse rate with heart rate and Spo_2 with Pao_2 and $TCPo_2$. (13) Unique to this set of data was the strict adherence to measurement of Spo_2 only when the pulse rate exactly equaled the heart rate and when these rates and the Spo_2 value were unchanging for at least 10 seconds. (14)(15) Very few subsequent studies provided this strict approach to correlating pulse rate and heart rate, perhaps contributing to unexpected sources of error, differences between Sao_2 and Spo_2, and other variability.

New Applications of Pulse Oximetry in Neonatal Medicine

Hay and associates (15)(16) compared Spo_2 with simultaneously measured Sao_2 and Pao_2 (using blood from arterial catheters) and $TCPo_2$ values. Spo_2 mimicked Sao_2 over the physiologic range from 80% to 100% with sufficient accuracy that hemoglobin-oxygen

affinity curves could be determined. These studies showed that Spo_2 values between 90% and 96% would, at least 95% of the time, prevent simultaneous Pao_2 values from drifting below 50 torr or above 100 torr, thus defining for the first time a reasonably safe range of Spo_2 values to prevent adverse effects of hypoxemia (opening of the ductus arteriosus, constriction of pulmonary vasculature) and hyperoxia (generally accepted then as Po_2 values more than 100 torr), such as ROP. Spo_2 also could be used to confirm that simultaneous $TCPo_2$ values were inaccurate, usually due to leak of air under the probe or to abnormal peripheral blood flow to the skin at the site of the probe.

Additional studies confirmed that infants who had chronic lung disease or bronchopulmonary dysplasia could be studied just as well with pulse saturation as healthy infants or acutely ill infants, contrary to results from currently used transcutaneous Po_2 instruments. (17)(18) Further studies provided reassurance that interfering substances and conditions (eg, dark skin color, dyes, dyshemoglobins, fetal hemoglobin, bilirubin, and other pigments) did not interfere with pulse oximetry readings, and ambient light could be blocked with opaque drapes. (19)(20)(21)(22) These and other technical advances helped secure pulse oximetry as both safe and effective in nearly all conditions.

Determination of Normal Spo_2 Values, Sea Level and Altitude

Thilo and colleagues (23) showed that Spo_2 values were slightly lower in Denver, Colorado (5,280 ft elevation) compared with sea level values. The investigators did not report hemoglobin concentrations in the infants, which tend to be slightly higher at altitude than at sea level, but not enough to account for the lower Spo_2 at the modestly increased altitude in Denver, thus indicating that the lower Spo_2 values in babies in Denver were due to the lower atmospheric Po_2 and the resulting lower Pao_2.

Nursing and Medical Procedures

Additional studies were conducted in term and preterm infants in a variety of clinical situations, all showing the considerable versatility of pulse oximetry. (16) House and associates

(24) showed that SpO_2 increased minute-by-minute following delivery, reaching normal values often well after 10 to 15 minutes following birth, evidence of the increase in pulmonary blood flow, ventilation, and ventilation-perfusion matching as well as closing of the ductus arteriosus. Sendak and colleagues (25) and Kopotic and Lindner (26) also showed that infants born by cesarean section could be distinguished from those born vaginally by having lower postnatal SpO_2 values for many minutes after birth, indicative of delayed opening of alveoli, clearing of lung fluid, and effective ventilation and ventilation-perfusion in infants delivered by elective cesarean section.

Detection of Hyperoxemia and Hypoxemia and Determination of PaO_2 at Various SpO_2 Values

Brockway and Hay (27) considered that for pulse oximetry to replace most, if not all, invasive or percutaneous PO_2 measurements, clinicians must have confidence that the SpO_2 value displayed by the pulse oximeter reliably predicts PaO_2. To prove this, they studied infants who were being weaned off oxygen as respiratory distress improved and who had arterial catheters in place to monitor blood PaO_2. They fixed SpO_2 at selected values (90%, 92%, 94%, 96%, and 98%) for periods up to 1 minute in duration, and when the pulse and heart rate also were stable during these periods, they obtained an arterial blood gas sample. SpO_2 clearly predicted PaO_2 accurately, but with increasing variability at higher values where, expectedly, the oxyhemoglobin affinity relationship was flatter and PaO_2 values could vary considerably with progressively smaller changes in saturation.

The Fifth Vital Sign

Within the short span of only about 15 years, pulse oximetry developed universal application, not just in the operating room, but in every adult, pediatric, and neonatal intensive care unit, as well as in the emergency department, doctors' offices, and on transport units. No one receiving oxygen or who had unstable conventional vital signs was allowed not to have pulse oximetry

monitoring. This new technology clearly had become the fifth vital sign. (28)

Newer Developments of Pulse Oximetry
Motion Artifact

The major difficulty with pulse oximetry is that it requires motion—the arterial pulse—to detect arterial oxygenation. Thus, any other motion adds signal to the nonarterial components of the tissue through which the two wavelengths of light are transmitted, producing motion artifact contributions to the arterial pulse signals. The situation worsens under low blood flow conditions, when the motion-induced pulse artifact becomes increasingly large relative to the weakening arterial pulse signal. To limit motion artifact as much as possible and make the instruments more versatile by being more accurate in low flow conditions, Diab and Kiani in 1989 at Masimo Corporation, an offshoot of Ohmeda, invented Signal Extraction Pulse Oximetry using adaptive filters and unique software calculations to separate the arterial signal from noise, allowing oximeters to monitor patients accurately during motion and low perfusion. (29) In 1998, Masimo SET was marketed internationally, and in 2002, Hay and colleagues (30) provided some of the first testing of successful measurements during motion in preterm infants in the NICU.

Assessment of Bradycardias and Apneas

Poets and colleagues (31)(32)(33) and Hay and colleagues, (30) among other investigators, have addressed how pulse oximetry can be used to monitor perplexing clinical conditions in the preterm infant. One of the most vexing is the relationship between bradycardias, apneas, and hypoxemia in preterm infants. Improved pulse detection with reduction of motion artifact has allowed simultaneous recording of pulse rate and SpO_2 along with heart rate and respiratory rate. This has been made even easier with new monitors that have all vital sign recordings in one instrument and the capacity to store data for later evaluation as well as simultaneous visual observation. Few systematic studies have been conducted yet, but anecdotally, it appears that

apneas, bradycardias, and desaturation events frequently are not temporally linked, indicating a mixture of physiologic, pathologic, and technical contributions to this heretofore well-recognized triad.

Perfusion Index

Pulse oximetry also has been used as an indicator, if not a measure, of peripheral blood flow, according to the perfusion index mode, or the measurement of the strength of the photo-plethysmographic signal at the sensor site, (34) which measures the change in the optical path length of light from the sensor as it passes through pulsating tissue. Path length change is the result of arterial bed expansion as blood flows through it. This mode recognizes that pulse amplitude can be quantified by the pulse oximeter probe and used as an indicator of the volume of blood pulsating through the tissue under the probe. It has been used most effectively as a precatheterization assessment for peripheral arterial line placement and assessment of distal circulation in patients who have long-term arterial lines. Hand surgeons also have used the perfusion index as a vascular study at the bedside for evaluation of collateral circulation to the hand.

Potential for Automated Oxygen Delivery Using Pulse Oximetry

Although not produced or marketed commercially, there is some potential for using very accurate and reliable pulse oximetry instrumentation for automatic adjustment of oxygen flow and oxygen concentration in incubators and oxygen hoods to prevent prolonged periods of desaturations or hyperoxia when attendants are too busy to adjust them manually. (35) At present, the risks of this use of pulse oximetry have outweighed potential advantages, but it is an intriguing development that might place pulse oximetry into a more regulatory role than simply as an alarm and recording device.

Level of Blood Oxygenation for Preterm Infants

Based on the successful application of pulse oximetry and the development of relatively motion artifact-free pulse oximetry technology, a variety of new studies are now underway around the world to try to determine, after more than 50 years of not knowing, what level of blood oxygenation is appropriate and what levels are harmful in preterm infants over both short- and long-term periods. (36) The NICHD-NEI STOP-ROP study in the United States (37)(38) and the BOOST study in Australia were the first to use pulse oximetry to test whether hyperoxia would therapeutically prevent or ameliorate the severity of ROP once prethreshold conditions had been reached in a baby's eyes, assuming that the hyperoxia would constrict the rapidly proliferating retinal vasculature and limit progression of the ROP to retinal detachment. Results were disappointing, with no clear evidence that the proposed outcome was improved and even some indication that the chronic hyperoxia led to other respiratory complications. Still, these studies did show that pulse oximetry was sufficiently accurate to maintain infants at different blood oxygen saturation values for both short and long periods. The successful pulse oximetry approach now is being used to guide studies of how low oxygen saturation should be to reduce the incidence of hyperoxic injuries such as ROP without increasing the incidence of hypoxia-related growth failure, PDA, and pulmonary vascular resistance with pulmonary hypertension. Perhaps one of the most important applications of neonatal pulse oximetry might be determination of the right dose of oxygen, resolving one of the longest standing dilemmas in neonatal medicine.

Remaining Problems
Accuracy at Low Blood Oxygen Saturation Levels: The Real-life Situation

Gerstman and associates (39) recently published data from a variety of clinical neonatal situations and using several different commercial pulse oximeters. They found increasingly high Spo_2 values at progressively lower Sao_2 values, a phenomenon that has been seen before in some studies, but not in most. Nonetheless, it raises the question of what contributes to accuracy of pulse oximetry and blood oxygen saturation measurements. No deviation between Spo_2 and Sao_2, even to values as low as 60%, were seen in the study by Hay and associates in 1989, (13) in which heart rate and pulse rate were strictly correlated before sampling blood and recording the Spo_2. Also, the Gerstman study (39) showed considerable variation among instruments, leading to the speculation that different software and hardware applications for the different instruments may be partly responsible for the Spo_2-Sao_2 discrepancy noted at lower blood oxygenation values. For example, instruments that eliminated motion artifact more effectively were less prone to the discrepancy. These investigators also speculated that laboratory calibration did not account for different tissue volumes and unique characteristics of sick infants in the NICU. Regardless of the accuracy of these results and the potential mechanisms for any such discrepancy, if real, this study is important for alerting caregivers who apply pulse oximetry and the industry that reliability and accuracy must continue to be monitored and perfected.

Industry Standardization

Currently, the United States Food and Drug Administration (FDA) is in the process of improving their evaluation processes for pulse oximeters. (40) For example, for neonatal accuracy claims, the FDA considered the requirement that every new pulse oximeter and sensor be compared in neonates using arterial blood samples measured on co-oximetry over the range from 70% to 100% in at least 10 patients, with at least 200 samples evenly spread over the range. This has been the industry standard for adult use of pulse oximetry, but it seems logistically undoable, potentially dangerous, and most likely unethical in neonates. Other approaches have involved comparison of published data that have noted adult laboratory accuracy variation of 2%, but as much as 3.3% in hospitalized patients. Similar results, both in controlled study situations and in hospitalized neonates, have shown about the same percentage accuracy variation as reported with the adult studies.

Conclusions

Pulse oximetry is here to stay. It has become more than the fifth vital sign. It is the principal first measurement applied to newborns and to patients needing oxygen monitoring in nearly every other clinical setting. Perhaps most exciting and important today, pulse oximetry is at the heart of new research into the role of oxygen in producing toxicity in newborns and regarding how oxygen therapy should be managed to avoid both hyperoxic and hypoxic complications. It is hard to believe that this exciting technology is barely 25 years old! (41)

Acknowledgments

Supported in part by grant MO1-RR00069, General Clinical Research Centers Program, NCRR, NIH (WWH, Associate Director).

References

1. Astrup PB, Severinghaus JW. *The History of Blood Gases, Acids and Bases.* London, England: Butterworth; 1986

2. Severinghaus JW, Honda Y. Pulse oximetry. *Int Anesthesiol Clin.* 1987;25: 205–215

3. Squire JR. Instrument for measuring quantity of blood and its degree of oxygenation in web of the hand. *Clin Sci.* 1940;4:331–339

4. Goldie EAG. Device for continuous indication of oxygen saturation of circulating blood in man. *J Sci Instrum.* 1942;19:23

5. Wood E, Geraci JE. Photoelectric determination of arterial oxygen saturation in man. *J Lab Clin Med.* 1949;34:387–401

6. Aoyagi T, Kishi M, Yamaguchi K, Watanabe S. Improvement of an earpiece oximeter [in Japanese]. *Abstracts of the 13th Annual Meeting of the Japan Society of MEBE.* 1974:90–91

7. Nakajima S, Hirai Y, Takase H, et al. Performances of new pulse wave earpiece oximeter. *Respir Circ.* 1975;23:41–45

8. Nakajima S, Ikeda K, Nishioka H, et al. Clinical application of a new (fingertip type) pulse wave oximeter. *Jpn J Surg.* 1979;41:57–61

9. Yoshiya I, Shimada Y, Tanaka K. Spectrophotometric monitoring of arterial oxygen saturation in the fingertip. *Med Biol Eng Comput.* 1980;18:27–32

10. Yelderman M, New W Jr. Evaluation of pulse oximeter. *Anesthesiol.* 1983;59:349–352

11. Hay WW Jr. *Application of Pulse Oximetry in Neonatal Medicine: Technical Report, Ohmeda.* Boulder, Colo: BOC Group, Inc; 1986

12. Hay WW Jr. Physiology of oxygenation and its relation to pulse oximetry in neonates. *J Perintol.* 1987;7:309–319

13. Hay WW Jr, Brockway J, Eyzaguirre M. Neonatal pulse oximetry: accuracy and reliability. *Pediatrics.* 1989;83:717–722

14. Monaco F, Feaster WW, McQuitty JC, et al. Continuous noninvasive oxygen saturation monitoring in sick newborns. *Respir Care.* 1983;28:1362

15. Hay WW Jr. The uses, benefits and limitations of pulse oximetry in neonatal medicine: consensus on key issues. *J Perinatol.* 1987;7:347–349

16. Hay WW, Brockway J, Eyzaquirre M. Application of the Ohmeda Biox 3700 pulse oximeter to neonatal oxygen monitoring. *Adv Exp Med Biol.* 1987;220:165–170

17. Solimano AJ, Smyth JA, Mann TK, et al. Pulse oximetry: advantages in infants with bronchopulmonary dysplasia. *Pediatrics.* 1986;78:844–849

18. Lafeber HN, Fetter WPF, Wirl AR, et al. Pulse oximetry and transcutaneous oxygen tension in hypoxemic neonates and infants with bronchopulmonary dysplasia. *Adv Exp Med Biol.* 1987;220:181–186

19. Mok J, Pintar M, Bensen L, et al. Evaluation of noninvasive measurements of oxygenation in stable infants. *Crit Care Med.* 1986;14:960–963

20. Ralston AC, Webb RK, Runciman WB. Potential errors in pulse oximetry III: effects of interference, dyes, dyshaemoglobins and other pigments. *Anaesthesia.* 1991;46:291–295

21. Veyckemans F, Baele P, Guillaume JE, Willems E, Robert A, Clerbaux T. Hyperbilirubinemia does not interfere with hemoglobin saturation measured by pulse oximetry. *Anesthesiology.* 1989;70:118–122

22. Pologe JA, Raley DM. Effects of fetal hemoglobin on pulse oximetry. *J Perinatol.* 1987;7:320–322

23. Thilo EH, Park-Moore B, Berman ER, Carson BS. Oxygen saturation by pulse oximetry in healthy infants at an altitude of 1610 m (5280 ft.). What is normal? *Am J Dis Child.* 1991;145:1137–1140

24. House JT, Schultetus RR, Gravenstein N. Continuous neonatal evaluation in the delivery room by pulse oximetry. *J Clin Monit.* 1987;3:96–100

25. Sendak MJ, Harris AP, Rogers MC, et al. Pulse oximetry in newborn infants in the delivery room. *Anesthesiology.* 1985;63:739–740

26. Kopotic RJ, Lindner W. Assessing high-risk infants in the delivery room with pulse oximetry. *Anesth Analg.* 2002;94:S31–S35

27. Brockway J, Hay WW Jr. Prediction of arterial partial pressure of oxygen with pulse oxygen saturation measurements. *J Pediatr.* 1998;133:63–66

28. Neff TA. Routine oximetry: a fifth vital sign? *Chest.* 1998;94:227

29. Goldman JM, Petterson MT, Kopotic RJ, Barker SJ. Masimo signal extraction pulse oximetry. *J Clin Mon.* 2000;16:475–483

30. Hay WW, Rodden DJ, Collins SM, Melara DL, Hale KA, Fashaw LM. Reliability of conventional and new pulse oximetry in neonatal patients. *J Perinatol.* 2002;22:360–366

31. Poets CF, Urschitz MS, Bohnhorst B. Pulse oximetry in the neonatal intensive care unit (NICU): detection of hyperoxemia and false alarm rates. *Anesth Analg.* 2002;94:S41–S43

32. Poets CF, Stebbens VA, Samuels MP, Southall DP. The relationship between bra-dycardia, apnea, and hypoxemia in preterm infants. *Pediatr Res.* 1993;34:144–147

33. Bohnhorst B, Peter CS, Poets CF. Pulse oximeters' reliability in detecting hypoxemia and bradycardia: comparison between a conventional and two new generation oximeters. *Crit Care Med.* 2000;28:1565–1568

34. De Felice C, Latini G, Vacca P, Kopotic RJ. The pulse oximeter perfusion index as a predictor for high illness severity in neonates. *Eur J Pediatr.* 2002;161:561–562

35. Urschitz MS, Von Einem V, Seyfang A, Poets CF. Use of pulse oximetry in automated O_2 delivery to ventilated infants. *Anesth Analg.* 2002;94;S37-S40

36. Silverman WA. A cautionary tale about supplemental oxygen: the albatross of neonatal medicine. *Pediatrics.* 2004;113:394–396

37. STOP-ROP. The STOP-ROP Multi-center Study Group. Supplemental therapeutic oxygen for prethreshold retinopathy of prematurity (STOP-ROP), a randomized, controlled trial. *Pediatrics.* 2000;105:295–310

38. Cole CH, Wright KW, TarnowMordi W, Phelps DL, Pulse Oximetry Saturation Trial for Prevention of Retinopathy of Prematurity Planning Study Group. Resolving our uncertainty about oxygen therapy. *Pediatrics.* 2003;112:1415–1419

39. Gerstmann D, Berg R, Haskell R, et al. Operational evaluation of pulse oximetry in NICU patients with arterial access. *J Perinatol.* 2003;23:378–383

40. Batchelder P, Clifford D, Goldman JM. Pulse oximetry: real world performance. Presented at the *24th International Symposium on Intensive Care and Emergency.* 2004

41. Hay WW. Pulse oximetry: as good as it gets? *J Perinatol.* 2000;20:181–183

Historical Perspectives: History of Pulse Oximetry in Neonatal Medicine

William W. Hay, Jr

NeoReviews 2005;6;e533-e538
DOI: 10.1542/neo.6-12-e533

History of Surgery for Congenital Diseases of the Heart

Abraham M. Rudolph, MD*

The accompanying 2005 article, written by Dr Abraham Rudolph, is based on the Thomas E Cone Jr, MD, Lecture on Perinatal Medicine, delivered at the meeting of the Perinatal Section of the AAP at the National Conference and Exhibition in Boston in October 2003.

Alistair G. S. Philip, MD, FRCPE, FAAP
Editor-in-Chief, NeoReviews

Introduction

The frequency of congenital diseases of the heart is generally quoted as about 8 per 1,000 live births. However, this estimate was based on autopsy or clinical assessments prior to the era of cardiac ultrasonography. It is now appreciated that many infants are born with ventricular septal defects that close soon after birth, that the aortic valve is bicuspid in 1% to 2% of individuals, and that a small "silent" patent ductus arteriosus may be detected by ultrasonography in as many as 0.3% to 0.5% of infants. Persistent patency of the ductus arteriosus in a large proportion of preterm infants also has been recognized. Thus, the frequency of congenital cardiac lesions may be as high as 4% to 5%.

In Sir James Mackenzie's book *Diseases of the Heart* in 1913, the chapter on Congenital Affections of the Heart occupied one page; in the section on Treatment, he stated, "If the heart maintains the circulation well, no treatment is required. In more serious cases, beyond attending to the child's comfort and nourishment, special treatment of the heart is of little benefit..." Now, about 90 years later, the majority of those lesions that do not improve spontaneously can be corrected or palliated.

Lord Ritchie-Calder stated that, "In science, there are those that make it happen, and those that make it possible." This discussion reviews some remarkable achievements and the individuals who made them possible or were responsible for their execution.

*Emeritus Professor of Pediatrics and Senior Staff, Cardiovascular Research Institute, University of California, San Francisco, Calif.

Classification

Case reports of several congenital cardiac lesions had been reported earlier, such as ventricular septal defect (maladie de Roger) and tetralogy of Fallot, but in the late 19th and early 20th century, Maude Abbott (Fig. 1), through intensive study of pathologic specimens, described the various types of congenital defects of the heart and developed a classification.

She was born in 1869 and named Maude Elizabeth Seymour Babin. During her infancy, her father abandoned the family, and her mother died of tuberculosis. She was formally adopted by her 62–year-old maternal grandmother, named Abbott, and reared in St. Andrews East in Quebec province. She won a scholarship to attend McGill University in Montreal, or rather, the Donalda Department for Women, a branch of McGill. She became attached to McGill University and applied to the Medical School, but was denied admission because women were not accepted. She made public petitions to have women admitted, but even though the Abbott family had helped to establish McGill University, the Medical School persevered. She was admitted to the Faculty of Medicine at Bishop's College in Quebec as the only woman in the class.

After graduating, Dr Abbott set up a private practice, but also worked as a curator at the McGill Medical Museum. To learn how to classify the specimens, she visited several medical museums in the United States. While in Baltimore at Johns Hopkins Hospital, she encountered Sir William Osler, who became very impressed with her abilities. He persuaded her to concentrate her efforts on classification of congenital cardiac disorders.

She returned to McGill and was appointed Curator of the Medical Museum. William Osler was so impressed with her work on congenital heart disease that he invited her to contribute a chapter on the topic to his book, *Systems of Modern Medicine*, which was published in 1908. In 1910, she was awarded an honorary MD degree by McGill, but not until 1925 was she appointed to an Assistant Professorship. During her tenure as Curator of the Museum, she reviewed the records of 1,000 cases of congenital lesions of the heart. Based on this material, she developed a new classification, which was published in the *Atlas of Congenital Cardiac Disease* by the American Heart Association.

Clinical Diagnosis

In her descriptions of congenital cardiac anomalies, Maude Abbott provided only limited information about the clinical manifestations of the various lesions. It remained for Helen Taussig to define the signs and symptoms of the different cardiac lesions. Furthermore, she provided detailed descriptions of radiologic and fluoroscopic features as well as electrocardiographic changes.

Although Taussig was born in Cambridge, Mass., in 1898, almost 30 years after Maude Abbott, she had similar experiences of discrimination against women by the academic and medical community. After attending Radcliffe College for 2 years and subsequently completing the BA degree at the University of California, Berkeley, she applied to Harvard Medical School, but was denied admission because she was a woman. Having decided that the next best thing was to enter public health, she applied to the Harvard School of Public Health. She was told by the Dean that she could be admitted to the courses, but only with the stipulation that

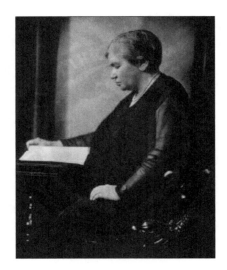

Figure 1. Maude Abbott. Courtesy of the National Library of Medicine.

she could not earn a degree because these were not conferred on women. She records that she asked the Dean, "Who is going to be such a fool as to spend four years studying and not get a degree?" to which the Dean responded "No one, I hope." She replied "Dr Rosen, I will not be the first to disappoint you." She then studied anatomy under the guidance of the Dean and Professor of Anatomy at Boston University. He was so impressed with her abilities that, after 2 years, he persuaded her to apply for medical training at Johns Hopkins University. Here women were being accepted because Elizabeth Garrett, who made a major donation to establish the Medical School, had stipulated that women be admitted on an equal basis as men. After completing the MD degree, she applied for a medical internship, which was denied because the Department of Medicine did not accept women. Therefore, she trained in Pediatrics. In 1930, Edward Park, the Chairman of the Pediatrics Department, appointed her as head of the pediatric cardiac clinic and urged her to apply fluoroscopy and electrocardiography to the study of heart disease in children. Over the next 15 years, she provided detailed descriptions of the clinical features and radiographic and electrocardiographic manifestations of the various congenital cardiac lesions. These were described in the classic *Congenital Malformations of the Heart* published by the Commonwealth Fund in 1947.

Cardiac Catheterization

It was not until the development of cardiac catheterization techniques that more precise diagnosis and detailed information about altered hemodynamics of the various lesions became available. In 1929, while a trainee in surgery at the hospital in Eberswalde, a small town near Berlin, Werner Forssmann (Fig. 2) worried that the insertion of a long needle through the chest wall into the heart to treat emergencies could result in serious complications. He embarked on an attempt to inject drugs directly into the heart without using a transthoracic needle. With local anesthesia of his left antecubital fossa, he isolated a vein and inserted a lubricated radio-opaque ureteric catheter into the vein and advanced it 65 cm, a distance he estimated would place the tip in the heart chambers. With the catheter in place, he walked to the stairs, went down to the radiography department, and took a radiograph to confirm the catheter position with the tip in the right atrium. He repeated this procedure on himself six more times. It is surprising that the technique was not immediately used for cardiac diagnosis.

Forssmann continued his surgical training in Berlin and discussed the procedure with the Professor of Surgery, the eminent Ferdinand Sauerbrach, who responded, "You might lecture in a circus about your tricks, but never in a respectable German university." When he persisted with the discussion, he was told to get out and leave the department immediately. He returned to the small hospital in Eberswalde to relative obscurity and practiced urology. It was as much as 12 years later that Cournand and Richards again performed cardiac catheterization. Their interest in the procedure was not for diagnostic purposes, but rather for obtaining a mixed venous blood sample to use in analysis of perfusion-ventilation relationships in the lung. In 1956, the Nobel Prize in Medicine and Physiology was awarded to Andre Cournand, Werner Forssmann, and Dickinson Richards "for their discoveries concerning heart catheterization and pathological changes in the circulatory system." Soon after they described the procedure, it was applied to the diagnosis of

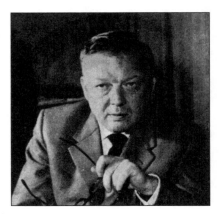

Figure 2. Werner Forssmann. Courtesy of the National Library of Medicine.

congenital cardiac lesions by Lewis Dexter and Rudolph Bing. However, in 1950, Keith and Munn wrote that "cardiac catheterization is especially valuable for older children, but is difficult or impractical in infants." The techniques were developed for infants over the next 10 years by Adams and Lind, Rowe and James, and Rudolph and Cayler.

Angiocardiography

The ability to visualize the vascular system by radiography was demonstrated by Haschek and Lindenthal in 1896 by injecting mercuric sulfide into the arterial system of an amputated hand. In 1931, Forssmann attempted to perform selective angiograms by injecting the contrast medium uroselectan, which was then used for pyelography, through the catheter he had advanced into the heart. A radiograph was taken during the injection. Unfortunately, this was not too successful because the contrast agent was injected by hand pressure through small catheters and, thus, too slowly to provide adequate visualization of the vascular system. Subsequently, by increasing the rate of delivery of contrast, Agustin Castellanos in Cuba was able to define the interior of the heart and great vessels as well as flow patterns and to apply the technique to the diagnosis of congenital cardiac lesions. The primary disadvantage of the initial procedure was that still radiographs were taken in rapid succession to define the course of the injected contrast medium; elaborate and very expensive radiograph film changer systems were developed to obtain six or more pictures per second. This drawback was resolved by the introduction of cineradiography in the late 1950s and early 1960s. The use of selective cineangiography for diagnosis of congenital cardiac anomalies was promoted by Mason Sones at the Cleveland Clinic.

Development of Techniques for Vascular Surgery

The first concerted efforts to develop surgical techniques for repairing blood vessels were initiated in Lyon, France, toward the end of the 19th century. Mathieu Jaboulay reported in 1898 on a method for suturing arteries by using "vertical mattress sutures," U-shaped sutures that everted the vessel edges, thereby avoiding projection of the suture line into the lumen. These procedures were performed on carotid arteries of donkeys.

Alexis Carrel (Fig. 3) was born in 1873 in a village near Lyon. When he was a medical student, the President of France, Sadi Carnot, suffered a tear in the portal vein from an assassin's attack. He died from hemorrhage because the surgeons did not have the technique or skills to suture blood vessels. Carrel decided that it would be his life's mission to design procedures for repairing blood vessels.

He frequently assisted Jaboulay in his work on vessel suture, and Jaboulay suggested that results could be improved if smaller needles and finer thread could be used. Carrel asked his mother where he could purchase these.

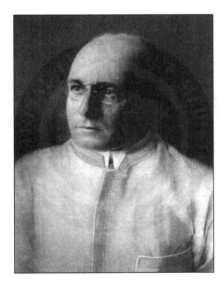

Figure 3. Alexis Carrell. Courtesy of the National Library of Medicine.

She referred him to her embroideress, Mme Leroudier, who not only advised him where he could obtain fine needles and thread, but also, Carrel acknowledged, instructed him in the fine art of sewing. Working in Professor Soulier's laboratory, he developed the "triangulation method" for suturing blood vessels. This consisted of placing three equidistant sutures around the circumference of the vessel edges; by pulling on two of these, suturing was facilitated by providing a straight edge.

Carrel earned an excellent reputation in Lyon, but was disliked by many because he did not recognize their contributions to his work or to his education. It was not surprising, therefore, that when the opportunity presented, he was told he would never be successful in examinations or in obtaining positions in the hospital. This arose in relation to an incident on a visit to Lourdes. It was customary for a physician to accompany groups traveling to Lourdes for the cures by the magical waters. In 1903, as a favor to a friend, Carrel agreed to join the pilgrimage. On the trip was a young woman, Marie Bailly, who was extremely ill with a diagnosis of tuberculous peritonitis, and there was concern that she would not survive the trip. However, after the holy water had been sprinkled on her abdomen, she rapidly improved and eventually made a complete recovery. Carrel, whose mother was very religious and who himself was very religious, was most impressed and recorded the entire incident in great detail. He was reluctant to publicize his observations, but with pressure from the church, he appeared with Marie Bailly to make a statement to the newspapers. The faculty in Lyon thought he was extremely gullible and that his behavior was both medically unethical and in poor taste. As a result, he became *persona non grata* and, realizing he would not be offered a position in Lyon, he moved to Paris. His reputation followed him there, so he became disillusioned with medicine and decided to embark on ranching in the Canadian West.

In 1904, Carrel left for Montreal, where he accidentally encountered a surgeon who had been very impressed with his publications from Lyon and subsequently arranged for him to deliver a lecture. As a result, he was

invited to work in surgical laboratories in Chicago. However, he first traveled to Western Canada and California and became disenchanted with the idea of ranching. Therefore, he worked in an experimental laboratory with Charles Guthrie in Chicago and was extremely productive. In 1906, he was invited by Simon Flexner to the staff of the Rockefeller Institute, where he continued his researches on vascular suture and applied it to transplantation of organs in animals. In 1912, he was awarded the Nobel Prize "in recognition of his work on vascular suture and the transplantation of blood vessels and organs."

It is difficult to explain why Carrel's laboratory work on vascular surgery and its recognition by the award of the Nobel Prize did not stimulate an immediate interest in applying his techniques in humans. Possibly the advent of World War I and the Depression accounted for the lack of interest. It was not until the late 1930s that interest in cardiovascular surgery was rekindled.

Surgery for Congenital Cardiac Lesions

Robert Gross (Fig. 4) is considered the "father of surgery for congenital heart disease" because he performed the "first successful ligation of a ductus arteriosus." While a resident in surgery at the Children's

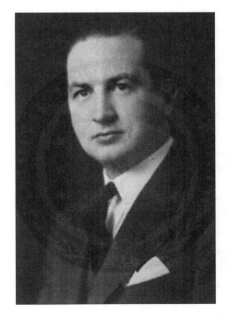

Figure 4. Robert Gross. Courtesy of the National Library of Medicine.

Hospital, Boston, with the help of a pediatrician, John Hubbard, he planned a surgical approach to the ductus. He proposed the procedure to the chief of surgery, William Ladd, who expressed his strong opposition and told him not to do it. On August 16, 1938, while the chief was on vacation, with the concurrence of Thomas Lanman, Gross successfully ligated the ductus in a 7-year-old girl. On his return, Ladd was furious and fired Gross from the residency, but because the procedure received widespread acclaim, he subsequently relented. Eighteen months prior to this procedure, John Strieder, at the Massachusetts Memorial Hospital in Boston, had ligated a ductus arteriosus, but the patient died after 4 days from an infection. What is not generally known is that Emil Karl Frey had successfully ligated a ductus arteriosus earlier in 1938 in Germany.

The successful ligation of the ductus provided the impetus to attempt to correct other congenital heart lesions. Charles Hufnagel, working with Gross in the laboratory, designed a method for reanastomosing the ends of a severed aorta in dogs, with the objective of repairing coarctation of the aorta. Clarence Crafoord from Stockholm, Sweden, visited the laboratory in Boston and observed the procedure. On October 19, 1944, he successfully resected a coarctation in a 12-year-old boy. Gross operated on a 5-year-old boy with aortic coarctation on June 28, 1945, but the child died at the end of the procedure. He successfully resected a coarctation in a 12-year-old girl a week later.

Soon after the first aortic coarctation repair had been performed, the first systemic arterial-to-pulmonary arterial shunt was performed on November 29, 1944, at Johns Hopkins Hospital. Helen Taussig had come to recognize that children who had cyanosis due to pulmonary stenosis with decreased pulmonary blood flow and a right-to left shunt survived longer and were less symptomatic if the ductus arteriosus remained patent. She hypothesized that cyanotic children who had reduced pulmonary blood flow could be improved if some way could be developed to provide additional blood flow. She visited Gross in Boston and discussed with him the possibility of producing a

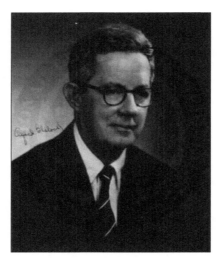

Figure 5. Alfred Blalock. Courtesy of the National Library of Medicine.

ductus arteriosus surgically. He told her he was interested in closing ductuses, not creating them, and suggested she return to Baltimore. Alfred Blalock (Fig. 5) had recently arrived from Vanderbilt University to assume the Chairmanship of Surgery at Johns Hopkins. Taussig overheard a discussion between him and Edward Park, the Chairman of Pediatrics, in which Park suggested that it might be possible to bypass a coarctation of the aorta by connecting the left subclavian artery to the descending aorta. She asked Blalock if it was perhaps possible to connect the left subclavian artery to the left pulmonary artery. By coincidence, this procedure had already been accomplished in Blalock's laboratory in dogs.

As a member of the surgical faculty at Vanderbilt University in Nashville, Tennessee, Blalock had instituted an active laboratory research program. As he became increasingly active in clinical surgery, much of the experimental surgery was performed by his assistant, Dr William Longmire, and a technician, Vivien Thomas. Vivien Thomas, a young African-American man, left college during his first year for financial reasons. He became an aid in Blalock's laboratory, but because he demonstrated outstanding skills with surgical technique, he soon became a technician. Blalock was interested in developing a model of pulmonary arterial hypertension and proposed anastomosing the left subclavian artery to the left pulmonary artery. Longmire and Thomas perfected the surgical

technique for this procedure. They designed a special clamp for partial occlusion of the pulmonary artery so the anastomosis could be accomplished without significant bleeding. This clamp was named the "Blalock Clamp." When Blalock left Nashville for Baltimore in 1941, he invited Thomas to supervise the surgical research laboratory at Johns Hopkins, which he did for 35 years.

Helen Taussig persuaded Blalock to create a subclavian-to-pulmonary artery anastomosis in a child with tetralogy of Fallot. With some trepidation, Blalock agreed and on Nov. 29, 1944, performed the first Blalock-Taussig shunt in a 15-month-old girl. Blalock insisted that Thomas stay close to him during the operation to advise him and guide him through the procedure. The shunt was achieved, but the child had a very stormy passage. Subsequent procedures were more successful; with the third patient, when the clamps were removed, the anesthetist, remarked, "She is now a lovely color." Blalock's contribution to relieving cyanosis in infants and children who had many congenital cardiac anomalies was acclaimed worldwide. Taussig and Thomas, however, received little immediate recognition. On one occasion, Taussig remarked, "Over the years I've gotten recognition for what I did, but I didn't at the time. It hurt for a while. It hurt when Dr Blalock was elected to the National Academy of Arts and Sciences and I didn't even get promoted from an assistant to associate professor." She did, however, receive recognition years later, and among other awards, she received the Presidential Medal of Freedom in 1964. Thirty years after the first operation, Vivien Thomas was appointed Instructor of Surgery and awarded an honorary Doctor of Law degree by Johns Hopkins University.

Intracardiac Surgery

All the surgical procedures for congenital cardiac lesions discussed previously involved surgery on blood vessels and did not address approaches to correction of lesions in the heart itself. In early efforts to approach cardiac chambers by clamping vessels entering the heart, it was quickly recognized that such clamping could be done for only a short period without causing severe cerebral and cardiac damage or death. In 1950, Bigelow showed that dogs that had been cooled to 20°C could survive 15 minutes of total circulatory arrest and suggested that hypothermia with arrest could be used to perform intracardiac surgery. In 1953, Lewis and Taufic repaired an atrial septal defect in a 5-year-old girl during circulatory arrest after surface cooling. Also, Horiuchi repaired ventricular septal defects in 18 infants younger than 1 year of age during total circulatory arrest after surface cooling to 25°C. However, there was great concern about the duration of circulatory arrest and the possibility of damage to the brain.

Robert Gross and Elton Watkins developed the atrial well technique for closing atrial septal defects. They designed a rubber well with an opening in the bottom, the edges of which were sutured to the atrial wall, which was incised. Because right atrial pressure is low, blood was contained within the well. The atrial septal defect was approached blindly and sutured directly or patched by feel. In the first patient, the tricuspid valve was inadvertently sutured, and the child died. Subsequently, the procedure was applied successfully, but soon was abandoned after it became possible to visualize the cardiac chambers directly.

In 1955, Lillehei reported the closure of ventricular septal defects in eight children, five of whom were younger than 1 year of age, by use of "controlled cross-circulation." An adult was used as the "oxygenator." Venous blood was pumped from the child's venae cava to the femoral vein in the adult and from the adult femoral artery returned to the child. Flow rates that were used were very low, based on the so-called "azygos flow principle." Six of the eight children survived. This approach was developed at the time that cardiopulmonary bypass was being introduced and soon was supplanted.

Cardiopulmonary Bypass

In 1930, John Gibbon (Fig. 6), while working as a research fellow with Edward Churchill at the Massachusetts General Hospital, was involved in the care of a young woman who had a pulmonary embolus. The possibility of removing the embolus by opening the

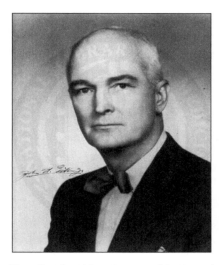

Figure 6. John Gibbon. Courtesty of the National Library of Medicine.

pulmonary artery was proposed, but it had been shown that if the main pulmonary artery was clamped for more than 6 minutes, dire consequences or death ensued. As the woman's condition deteriorated, the decision was made to operate. The pulmonary artery was occluded and the clot removed through an incision distal to the clamp. However, by the time the artery was sutured and the clamp removed, 7 minutes had elapsed, and the patient died. This incident stimulated Gibbon to try to develop a method for approaching the interior of the heart and great vessels for a longer period. He envisioned a machine that could bypass the heart and lungs and assume the functions of oxygenating blood and maintaining the circulation. He moved to Philadelphia with his wife, who had been a technician in Churchill's laboratory, and together they worked on designing such a machine. By 1935, they had constructed a pump-oxygenator that maintained a cat's circulation and respiration for 3 hours 50 minutes. The cat is a small animal compared with humans, and they were confronted with the problem of designing equipment that was large enough to be used in humans. By 1939, they were able to support a dog on cardiopulmonary bypass, but the machine was so large it could not fit into an elevator. Further developments were curtailed by his service in World War II.

After his return from service, Gibbon assumed the position of Professor of Surgery at Jefferson Medical College and resumed his work on developing the bypass machine. He was approached by a medical student who told him that IBM might have an interest in the machine. Gibbon approached Thomas Watson, Chairman of the Board at IBM. He agreed to help in the development and provided financial assistance as well as the service of machinists. In May 1953, after 23 years of apparatus design, Gibbon successfully closed an atrial septal defect in an 18-year-old girl, Cecilia Bavolek, using cardiopulmonary bypass. It should be noted that, in March 1952, Gibbon attempted to close an atrial septal defect in a 15-month-old baby, who died. The clinical diagnosis had been incorrect; the child had a patent ductus arteriosus. After the successful surgery in 1953, the next two attempts resulted in death of the patients. Gibbon imposed a 1-year moratorium. John Kirklin at the Mayo Clinic modified the apparatus designed by Gibbon and successfully operated on a large series of patients with a variety of intracardiac defects in the ensuing years.

The development of cardiopulmonary bypass made it possible to design surgical approaches to either correct or palliate almost all congenital cardiac abnormalities. In addition to closing atrial and ventricular septal defects and relieving pulmonary and aortic stenosis, imaginative approaches to treating complex lesions were introduced. In 1959, Senning described a procedure for redirecting flows in the atrial chambers to treat aortopulmonary transposition. In 1976, Jatene described an operation to reconnect the aorta and pulmonary artery (the arterial switch procedure) in infants who had transposition. In 1967, Rastelli used a valved aortic homograft from the right ventricle to the pulmonary artery to bridge an atretic right ventricular outflow tract.

Many other surgical approaches have been designed, and new procedures certainly will be introduced in the future. The success in managing congenital diseases of the heart has been truly remarkable, and it is important to recognize those who have contributed to these achievements.

Julius Comroe points out that the surgeon did not make one giant step to reach the pinnacle, but climbed up the back of the mountain using the knowledge and assistance of many others.

Acknowledgments

In preparing this manuscript, I have found two resources particularly helpful. I would like to express my appreciation to:

Exploring the Heart by Julius H. Comroe, Jr, published in 1983 (W.W. Norton, New York, NY) and *The Two Lions of Lyons* by Angelo M. May and Alice G. May, published in 1992 (Kabel Publishers, Rockville, Md.).

Historical Perspectives: History of Surgery for Congenital Diseases of the Heart
Abraham M. Rudolph
NeoReviews 2005;6;e447-e453
DOI: 10.1542/neo.6-10-e447

Contents by Category

Index